RAPID PREPARATION
for the
USMLE
Step 1

J&S

J&S PUBLISHING COMPANY, INC.

THE PRINCETON REVIEW

AUTHORS

The George Washington University School of Medicine, Washington, DC

Kurt E. Johnson, PhD, Professor of Anatomy and Cell Biology

Frank J. Slaby, PhD, Associate Professor of Anatomy and Cell Biology

Ronald C. Bohn, PhD, Associate Professor of Anatomy and Cell Biology

Ajit Kumar, PhD, Professor of Biochemistry and Molecular Biology

Gerald V. Stokes, PhD, Associate Professor of Microbiology and Immunology

Frank N. Miller, MD, Emeritus Professor of Pathology

Julia B. Frank, MD, Associate Professor of Psychiatry and Behavioral Science

Nadia Krupnokova, MD, Assistant Professor of Psychiatry and Behavioral Science

Medical College of Virginia, Richmond, Virginia

Emma R. Jakoi, PhD, Associate Professor of Physiology and Neurology

Pennsylvania State University College of Medicine, Hershey Pennsylvania

Melvin L. Billingsly, Professor of Pharmacology

Uniformed Services University of the Health Sciences, Bethesda, Maryland

Mark R. Adelman, PhD, Associate Professor of Anatomy and Cell Biology

Louisiana State University School of Medicine, New Orleans, Louisiana

Raymond F. Gasser, PhD, Professor of Anatomy

With an introduction by Patrick Burnett, MD-PhD candidate, The Johns Hopkins School of Medicine, and Master Trainer and teacher, The Princeton Review

First edition

All of the items found in this book are drawn from the series of books, *Review for the New National Boards*, which have been previously published by J&S Publishing Company Inc., Alexandria, Virginia.

ISBN 1-888308-02-8

Library of Congress catalog card number 97070680

Editorial: Kurt E. Johnson, PhD, David P. Kelley, Evan R. Schnittman
Production: Lisa Ruyter and Susan Keats
Designer: John Bergdahl and Meher Khambata

Printed in the United States of America

9 8 7 6 5 4 3 2 1

How to Use this Book

The simple method behind the J&S Publishing Company's success has been to provide medical students and graduates with extensive review exercises to complete in a short period of time before the boards. The J&S Publishing Company publishes books for all of the basic sciences, with over 500 questions in each.

Extensive practice with problem-solving techniques has long been the hallmark of The Princeton Review in its courses, books, and software. Each of the live, preparatory courses for the USMLE Step 1 offered by The Princeton Review devotes many hours of instruction to completing assessment exams, classroom drills, homework, and clinical case studies, and to reviewing all those problems with instructors who have aced the boards with high scores.

Both J&S Publishing and The Princeton Review believe that the best preparation for the USMLE Step 1 includes

- reviewing and integrating the clinically-relevant topics in basic science, and
- teaching students to apply that knowledge and resolve problems, just like those on Step 1

Because our mission and methods for USMLE Step 1 preparation are similar, our two companies decided to work together to publish a single volume covering all of the basic sciences.

We conceived of and designed this book to accomplish both of the above goals by exposing you to the types of items found on the test while providing detailed tutorials with all of the answers. Each tutorial includes a full explanation of the answers and incorrect options, so that you don't need to consult another book to clarify the points made by the correct answer choice.

Each of the basic sciences is reviewed in a separate chapter, covering only the highest-yield topics on the boards. We recommend that you complete the items in each chapter in a single sitting over a specified period of time, and then immediately review the tutorials for each set, found in the back of each subject chapter. Completing an entire chapter at once will help you understand the big picture for each subject on the boards. Completing the entire book within a short time span will help you integrate across the subjects, which is important for the boards.

If you need more information about the USMLE Step 1, call The Princeton Review at 1-800-2REVIEW. The Princeton Review offers free seminars to get acquainted with the marathon of medical licensing and live courses to successfully prepare for the medical boards in over 20 cities in the United States.

To purchase the full complement of the J&S series, *Review for the New National Boards*, please call 1-703-823-9833, or visit your medical school bookstore.

We wish you the best success in sitting for your board exams.

Kurt E. Johnson, PhD

Professor of Anatomy and Cell Biology
The George Washington University Medical Center
Washington D.C.
and
President and Publisher
J&S Publishing Company, Inc.
Alexandria, Virginia

David P. Kelley

Director of Medical Licensing Programs
The Princeton Review
New York, NY

ACKNOWLEDGMENTS

The Princeton Review staff, J&S Publishing Company Inc., and the authors of this book would like to thank the following people for their invaluable contributions in preparing this first edition and the questions within it.

Michael Holliday, Jeremy Topin, Lisa Ruyter, John Bergdahl, Jose Freire, Chris Thomas, Greta Englert, Patricia Acero, Evelyn Sanchez, Mabel Villanueva, Robert McCormack, Carmine Raspaolo and Len Small.

Table of Contents

INTRODUCTION

"Where should I start?", you might be thinking. The USMLE Step 1 seems like the standardized test to end all standardized tests. You may have been taking them forever, from the PSAT to the MCAT, if you were educated in the United States. While this particular standardized test requires more test-taking stamina that any other test you have probably taken, many academic and commercial institutions are very interested in your success. As recently as 1989, the options for boards prep were extremely limited, and aspiring physicians sitting for the boards were completely left to their own devices to find their collective way through studying for and passing the NBME, the FMGEMS, and the FLEX. All that has changed because many options are available to you now. You do not have to do this all by yourself.

I do not intend to replace or even duplicate the abundant Step 1 general information found in the revered *First Aid for the USMLE Step 1*, with which you are likely already familiar. In this introduction, I only want to acquaint you with my own experience in studying and teaching for the Step 1.

Step-by-step
There are as many ways to prepare for USMLE Step 1 as there are people taking the exam each year. I have found that all of the approaches share some common elements. Efficient preparation takes discipline, organization and self-confidence. Here are some pointers from students and graduates who have fared well against this 2-day, 12-hour, 720-question devil.

Know the enemy
Register to sit for the exam as early as you can so that you can get the booklet which outlines the Step 1 and gives you a 3-hour practice test with 180 items. The sample items section is an invaluable tool to see how the questions are written. Aside from that, the booklet describes the exam structure, item style, subjects and topics tested within each subject. A number of boards preparation enterprises, often including your own medical school, provide seminars to describe the Step 1 in depth if you want more information.

Talk to students or graduates who have already passed Step 1, in particular, to people who have taken the last two or three administrations. Ask them how they allocated their time and what they saw on their boards. But keep in mind that topics tested can vary noticeably from one administration to another, and that about 60-80 of the questions found throughout all four booklets are unscored, experimental items. You must attain a sense of the scope and the common denominators across multiple administrations. Do not make the mistake of talking only to people who sat for the SAME administration of the Step 1.

Your medical school faculty may also be a good source of information. They are generally as invested in your success as you are, so they may know what topics in their field are most likely to be tested.

Start now
Do not put this off. It is better to start too early than too late. It always takes more time than one thinks to read, comprehend, and review even the most basic topics. Most importantly, realize that each student is different and in the end you must make a decision about how much time you will devote to preparing for this exam. Do not let this decision be made for you by waiting too long to get started.

Schedule your time
You need to determine what your strengths and weaknesses are. Decide how much time you are going to devote to each area and schedule every moment of your study time. Once you have made your schedule, stick to it.

Get lean
Find good review materials. In teaching both USMLE Step 1 and MCAT courses for The Princeton Review, I have learned to cut to the chase. You have to believe in the materials you are working with and realize that you only have so much time to prepare. Too many medical students and graduates latch on to every textbook or review book in the basic sciences in order to prepare for the exam. That is a dangerous and risky proposition given the abundance of material out there. Remember—you will only have 720 questions to show what you know. Whichever materials you select, make sure the subject reviews are clearly written, explicitly identify Step 1 topics and how they will be tested, and contain abundant visual material.

A picture is worth a thousand words
If you can draw out or map a concept or principle, then you are in good shape. Taking the time after reading several pages of material or discussing a complex pathway to condense your understanding into a table, flow chart, graph or concept map will boost your confidence and fix your comprehension. Many books and course materials do this for you, but as an exercise, doing it yourself cannot be beaten.

Practice makes perfect
The first day of the test is not a good time to find out that it takes you 2 minutes just to even understand what a test item is really asking. You have a minute per item, on average, on the actual Step 1. Unless you make yourself complete timed sections of USMLE Step 1 practice items, you will have no idea if you can keep pace and apply your knowledge on the testing days.

Schedule time to tackle practice questions at regular intervals during your studying. Study from questions written in the current, integrated style, which focuses on clinical application of knowledge just like the real exam. Make sure those questions also have detailed explanations for the answers, so you not only confirm why the answer is right, but understand why the other options are wrong.

Eliminate distraction
During your scheduled study time, it is crucial that you become engrossed in the task at hand, preparing for the boards. While the best environment for studying will be different from person to person, the key is to focus. Choose a place where you will not be interrupted.

Study with friends
Studying with friends who are also preparing for the boards can be helpful because you can help answer each other's questions. Teaching others will affirm your knowledge and increase your confidence. However, schedule a specific time to meet with them, keeping that time separate from your regular, personal study time.

Take care of yourself
While you should stick to a heavy and structured study routine, it's essential that you stay healthy. Schedule time for exercise and fun and establish a consistent sleeping pattern. A daily dose of exercise, complemented by regular sleep will keep you from burning out and becoming a nervous wreck. You need that break every day or the effects of cumulative stress will impair your chances of getting your best boards score. Extra tip: about 2-3 weeks in advance, start setting your alarm for the time of morning when you will need to arise to take the actual test on those two mornings. This will help set your "internal clock." Eat properly. Your nutrition leading up to the exam is important. There is only one thing worse than going into the exam tired, and that is going in sick. Exercise, sleep and proper nutrition will ward off fatigue and strain.

The home stretch
In the final 48-72 hours before the test, make sure you specifically schedule short-but-frequent blocks of time for reviewing memory-intensive material such as often-cited drugs, equations, and biochemical pathways. While much of the Step 1 tests application of knowledge, you cannot avoid a certain amount of memorization. This is the time to brush up on those hard-to-remember items.

These guidelines I have described have helped me and many other medical students succeed in achieving great USMLE Step 1 scores. Part of my success owes to the thorough review I received from completing the subject-based review books published by J&S. When I was asked to help prepare a "best of..." edition, I was more than happy to help spread the word. While teaching for The Princeton Review, I have fine-tuned the above strategies to help US medical school students and international graduates get great scores. I am confident that this book will help you achieve the same success.

Study hard, and good luck!

Sincerely,

Patrick Burnett

Baltimore, MD

Patrick is a USMLE Step 1 Teacher and Master Trainer for The Princeton Review as well as an MD-PhD student at The Johns Hopkins School of Medicine.

DIRECTIONS

Each of the following nine chapters contains approximately 100 items that have been written and designed strategically to walk you through problems in the highest-yield topics on the USMLE Step 1. Completing each chapter in a single sitting for the indicated periods of time will build your stamina for the long sections on the actual testing days, sharpen your test-taking skills, and train you to keep a decent pace on the actual test. Do not stop after each item or set of items to see if you answered correctly. Do not consult other textbooks while answering the items. Tackle all of the items until you are instructed to stop, just like on any standardized test.

After you've answered all the items, the book reviews the content. The answers to all of these review problems may be found at the end of the chapter, along with an extensive tutorial annotation for each item or set of items. Again, we encourage you to answer all of the questions before moving on to the answers and tutorial. The tutorials have been specifically written to anticipate the most frequent mistakes made in selecting answer choices. If you haven't already selected an answer before reading the tutorial, your reading of the tutorial won't be as valuable.

CHAPTER 1

Gross Anatomy and Neuroanatomy

DIRECTIONS (Items 1-53): For each of the numbered items that proceed, you must select the single best answer from among the lettered options listed.

Some of the numbered items will pose a question or incomplete sentence that is followed by a list of 4-5 lettered options. In all cases, select the ONE lettered option that best answers the question or completes the sentence given.

Some of the numbered items are preceded by 5-24 lettered options. In these sets, the lettered options will be preceded by a single instruction asking you to match one of the lettered options to each numbered item most closely associated with it. In all matching sets, you may use any of the lettered options once, more than once or not at all, but you should still only select ONE lettered option per numbered item.

If you wish to simulate actual USMLE testing conditions, you should aim to complete all the items in this chapter in 55 minutes.

Do NOT look at the answers and tutorials until you have completed all of the items in this chapter.

Good luck!

Item 1

1. A 28-year-old woman suffers an injury to the left arm during an automobile accident. Radiographs of the left arm show an oblique fracture through the mid-shaft of the humerus. Which nerve is most likely to be injured by the mid-shaft fracture of the humerus?

   (A) axillary nerve
   (B) median nerve
   (C) musculocutaneous nerve
   (D) radial nerve
   (E) ulnar nerve

Items 2-3

A loop of ileum becomes entrapped in the right inguinal canal of a 10-year-old boy who has had a patent processus vaginalis here.

2. If pain fibers in the entrapped ileal loop produce visceral pain, in which abdominal region will the patient most likely feel the visceral pain?

   (A) epigastric region
   (B) umbilical region
   (C) hypogastric region
   (D) right inguinal region
   (E) right lumbar region

3. Sensory fibers from the jejunum, ileum and cecum enter the spinal cord at spinal cord segment levels

   (A) C3, C4 and C5
   (B) T5, T6, T7, T8 and T9
   (C) T8, T9, T10, T11 and T12
   (D) T10, T11, T12, L1 and L2
   (E) L1, L2, S2, S3 and S4

Item 4

4. A 38-year-old woman with septic thrombosis of the cavernous sinus complains of double vision whenever she looks downward. The two images are farthest apart when she looks downward and to the left. The physical exam shows that the patient can move her right eyeball directly to the left. However, when the cornea of her right eyeball faces directly medially, the patient is unable to move her right eyeball so that the cornea also looks downward. Which muscle of her right eye is not acting effectively?

   (A) superior rectus
   (B) inferior rectus
   (C) lateral rectus
   (D) inferior oblique
   (E) superior oblique

Items 5-6

A 42-year-old man enters the emergency department (ED) complaining of dyspnea and severe chest pain. The physical findings suggest pericardial tamponade. An electrocardiagram (ECG) showing total electrical alternans and an echocardiogram showing pericardial effusion confirm the diagnosis.

5. Which jugular vein is commonly the best barometer of the patient's central venous pressure?

   (A) right anterior jugular vein
   (B) right external jugular vein
   (C) right internal jugular vein
   (D) left external jugular vein
   (E) left internal jugular vein

6. If the head, neck and trunk of the patient are elevated 30-45 degrees from the horizontal, what is the normal vertical distance above the level of the sternal angle where pulsatile activity will be observed in the jugular veins?

   (A) 0-1 cm
   (B) 2-3 cm
   (C) 4-5 cm
   (D) 6-7 cm
   (E) 8-9 cm

Items 7-8

7. Where along the course of the large intestine do colic branches of the superior mesenteric artery anastomose with colic branches of the inferior mesenteric artery?

   (A) near the border between the cecum and ascending colon
   (B) near the hepatic flexure
   (C) near the splenic flexure
   (D) near the border between the descending colon and sigmoid colon
   (E) near the border between the sigmoid colon and rectum

8. The vagus nerves provide preganglionic parasympathetic innervation to the large intestine as far distally as the region

   (A) near the border between the cecum and ascending colon
   (B) near the hepatic flexure
   (C) near the splenic flexure
   (D) near the border between the descending colon and sigmoid colon
   (E) near the border between the sigmoid colon and rectum

Item 9

9. A 49-year-old woman reports upper abdominal pain of 5 days duration. The history and physical exam reveal pain typical of biliary colic, intermittent fevers with chills, yellowish sclera and oral mucosa, a tender gallbladder, and an enlarged and tender liver. Ultrasound examination of the patient's biliary tract shows gallstones in the lumen of the gallbladder, dilated intrahepatic biliary ducts and a gallstone lodged in the lower part of the common bile duct. The history, physical exam and radiological findings suggest ascending cholangitis (ascending sepsis of the extrahepatic and intrahepatic biliary ducts and the gall-bladder). Which set of spinal nerves innervates the patient's skin in the center of the right upper quadrant of the anterolateral abdominal wall?

   (A) T4, T5 and T6 on the right side
   (B) T7, T8 and T9 on the right side
   (C) T10, T11 and T12 on the right side
   (D) L1 and L2 on the right side
   (E) L3 and L4 on the right side

Items 10-12

A 32-year-old woman suffers an injury to the left arm during an automobile accident. Radiographs of the left arm show a displaced fracture of the medial epicondyle of the humerus.

10. Which nerve is most likely injured in this patient?

   (A) axillary nerve
   (B) median nerve
   (C) musculocutaneous nerve
   (D) radial nerve
   (E) ulnar nerve

11. Assuming that this nerve is injured, which of the following deficits is LEAST LIKELY to be present in this patient?

   (A) weakness in holding a piece of paper between the ring and little fingers against resistance
   (B) weakness in holding a piece of paper between the middle and ring fingers against resistance
   (C) weakness in holding a piece of paper between the index and middle fingers against resistance
   (D) weakness in flexing the distal phalanx of the little finger against resistance
   (E) weakness in flexing the distal phalanx of the thumb against resistance

12. Which muscle can adduct the ring finger?

   (A) 2nd palmar interosseous
   (B) 3rd palmar interosseous
   (C) 1st dorsal interosseous
   (D) 2nd dorsal interosseous
   (E) 3rd dorsal interosseous

Item 13

13. A chief abductor of the thigh is

   (A) piriformis
   (B) gracilis
   (C) quadratus femoris
   (D) gluteus medius
   (E) gluteus maximus

Items 14-15

The parents of a 6-year-old boy report that their son has started walking with a limp. The pediatrician learns that the boy has been in good health for the past few months. His sublingual temperature is 98.5° F. The patient states that he walks with a limp because of right hip pain that started a week ago. The hip pain is aggravated by weightbearing and relieved by rest. Trendelenburg's sign is observed when the boy is asked to stand on the right lower limb only. Radiographs of the hip joints show periarticular soft tissue swelling about the right hip joint. A bone scan reveals diminished activity in the anterolateral aspect of the right capital femoral epiphysis.

14. The patient's pain may be referred to any of the following regions EXCEPT the

    (A) groin
    (B) anterior aspect of the thigh
    (C) medial aspect of the thigh
    (D) medial aspect of the knee
    (E) leg

15. The arteries that are the chief source of blood supply to the patient's capital femoral epiphysis are

    (A) arteries in the ligament to the head of the femur
    (B) medullary arteries of the metaphysis
    (C) arteries derived from the medial and lateral circumflex femoral arteries
    (D) arteries derived from the superior gluteal artery
    (E) arteries derived from the inferior gluteal artery

Item 16

16. A 51-year-old woman complains of recent, progressive clumsiness in sewing and writing with her right hand and reports numbness and tingling in her right hand upon awakening in the morning from sleep. She says that shaking the right hand relieves the numbness and tingling. Examination reveals slight atrophy of the muscle mass underlying the thenar eminence of the right hand and difficulty in drawing the thumb of the right hand across the palm in order to touch the base of the little finger with the tip of the thumb. Light percussion on the lateral (radial) side of the palmaris longus tendon produces a tingling sensation in the right hand whose distribution is similar to that experienced by the patient upon awakening in the morning. Which nerve is impaired in the patient's right upper limb?

    (A) anterior interosseous branch of the median nerve
    (B) median nerve
    (C) ulnar nerve
    (D) deep branch of the ulnar nerve
    (E) superficial branch of the ulnar nerve

Items 17-18

A 24-year-old man is thrown out of a pick-up truck during an accident and sustains an injury to the left upper limb. Examination in the ED does not reveal any cuts, fractures, or dislocations in the left upper limb. However, a number of motor and sensory deficits are found which suggest that the patient has sustained a traction injury to one or more parts of the brachial plexus.

17. The biceps brachii stretch reflex involves sensory and motor nerve fibers in primarily spinal nerves

    (A) C5 and C6
    (B) C6 and C7
    (C) C7 and C8
    (D) C8 and T1
    (E) T1 and T2

18. The triceps brachii stretch reflex involves sensory and motor nerve fibers in primarily spinal nerves

    (A) C5 and C6
    (B) C6 and C7
    (C) C7 and C8
    (D) C8 and T1
    (E) T1 and T2

Item 19

19. An 8-year-old girl's right hand is clawed by a cat. Examination of the child 1 day later reveals evidence of lymphatic dissemination of a hand infection. Which group of axillary lymph nodes is clustered about the region where the cephalic vein pierces deep fascia to extend toward its union with the axillary vein?

    (A) anterior group of axillary nodes
    (B) posterior group of axillary nodes
    (C) lateral group of axillary nodes
    (D) central group of axillary nodes
    (E) deltopectoral (infraclavicular) group of axillary nodes

Items 20-22

In the following items, match each structure with an image of one of its borders in **Figure 1.1**, a PA radiograph of the chest.

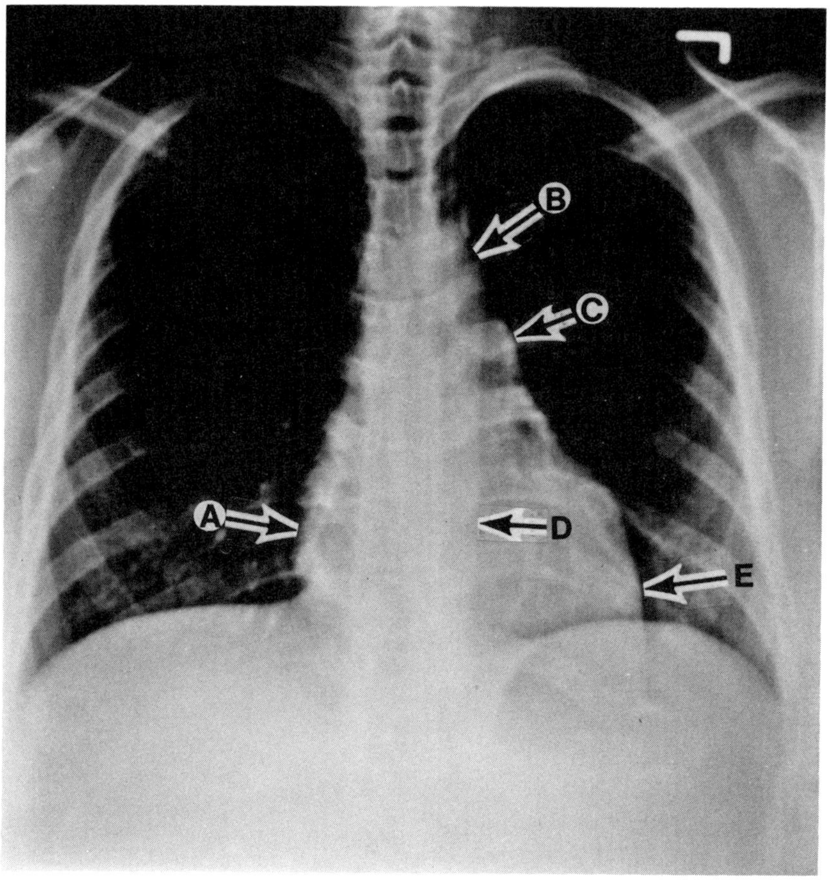

Figure 1.1

20. Aortic arch (aortic knob)

21. Pulmonary trunk

22. Left ventricle

Items 23-25

The three computerized tomography (CT) scans pictured in **Figure 1.2** below are adjacent 10 mm-thick thoracic scans. In the following items, match each structure with its image in the labeled CT scan.

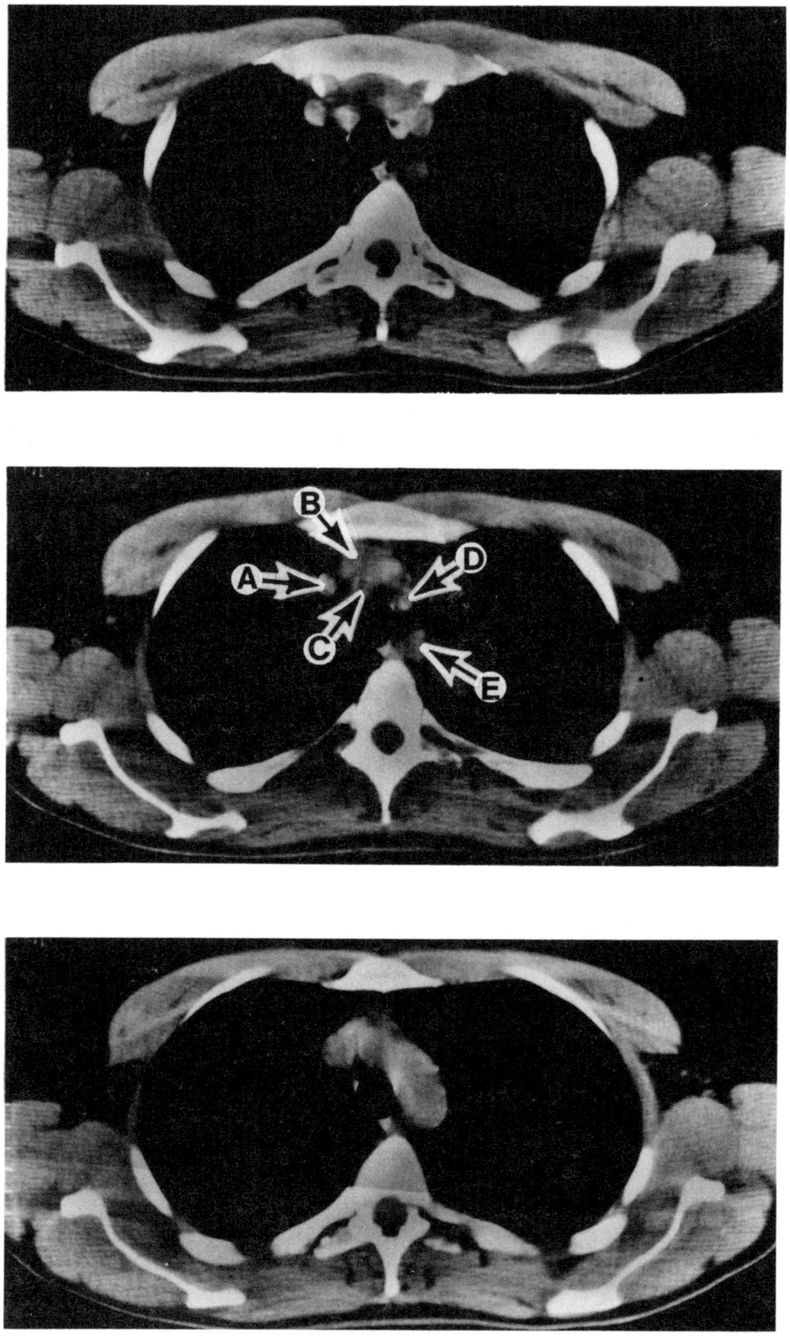

Figure 1.2

23. Right brachiocephalic vein

24. Brachiocephalic trunk

25. Left common carotid artery

Items 26-32

A helpful way to understand the anatomy of the abdomen and pelvis is to visualize in the order shown the placement of the following five groups of organs:

[1] the retroperitoneal viscera of the abdomen

[2] the secondarily retroperitoneal viscera of the abdomen

[3] the intraperitoneal segments of the small and large intestines in the mid and lower abdomen

[4] the liver and gallbladder and the intraperitoneal viscera in the upper abdomen, and

[5] the pelvic viscera

26. All of the following viscera are retroperitoneal EXCEPT

(A) abdominal aorta
(B) spleen
(C) right kidney
(D) left adrenal gland
(E) inferior vena cava

27. All of the following viscera are secondarily retroperitoneal EXCEPT

(A) ascending colon
(B) head of the pancreas
(C) body of the pancreas
(D) tail of the pancreas
(E) descending colon

28. All of the following segments of the small and large intestines are intraperitoneal EXCEPT

(A) 2nd, 3rd and 4th parts of the duodenum
(B) jejunum
(C) ileum
(D) transverse colon
(E) sigmoid colon

29. All of the following regions of the abdominal and pelvic cavities are located in the greater sac EXCEPT

(A) region anterior to the mesentery of the small intestine
(B) left lateral paracolic gutter
(C) hepatorenal recess (Morrison's pouch)
(D) region posterior to the stomach
(E) rectouterine pouch (pouch of Douglas)

30. All of the following statements regarding the epiploic foramen are correct EXCEPT

(A) The epiploic foramen is a passageway between the greater and lesser sacs of the peritoneal cavity.
(B) A part of the caudate lobe of the liver borders the foramen superiorly.
(C) The proximal half of the 1st part of the duodenum borders the foramen inferiorly.
(D) The portal vein borders the foramen posteriorly.
(E) The free right margin of the lesser omentum borders the foramen anteriorly.

31. All of the following peritoneal ligaments border a part of the lesser sac EXCEPT

(A) lesser omentum
(B) lienorenal ligament
(C) gastrophrenic ligament
(D) gastrocolic ligament
(E) falciform ligament

32. All of the following statements concerning peritoneal relationships in the female pelvis are correct EXCEPT

(A) The fundus of the uterus is covered with peritoneum.
(B) In the midline region, the peritoneum which covers the anterior surface of the middle third of the rectum is continuous anteriorly with the peritoneum that covers the uppermost posterior surface of the vagina.
(C) In the midline region, the peritoneum which covers the anterior surface of the uterus is continuous anteriorly with the peritoneum that covers the uppermost anterior surface of the vagina.
(D) The superior surface of the urinary bladder is covered with peritoneum.
(E) The ovary is attached by the mesovarium to the posterior peritoneal layer of the broad ligament of the uterus.

Items 33-35

The two CT scans pictured below in **Figure 1.3** are adjacent 10 mm-thick abdominal sections. Segments of the upper gastrointestinal tract are partially filled with contrast material. In the following items, match each structure with its image in the labeled CT scan.

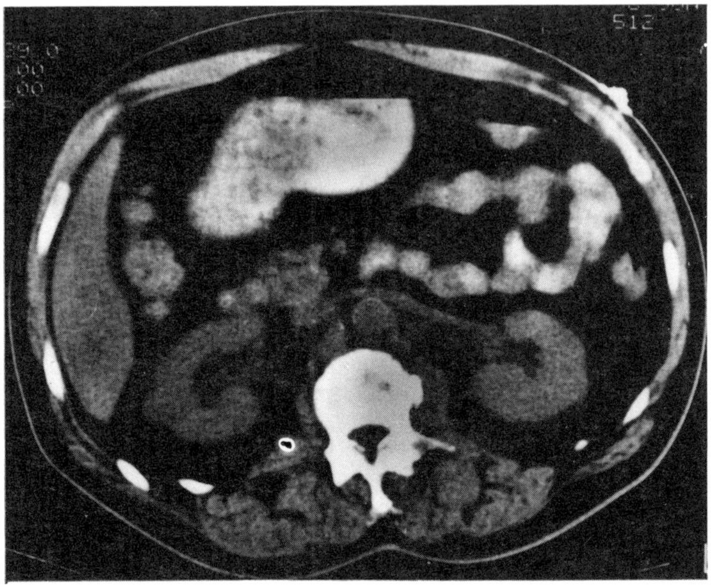

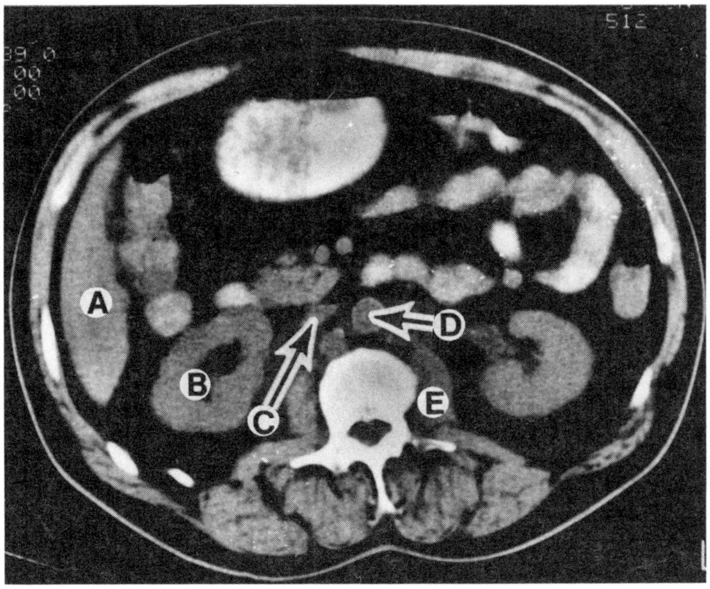

Figure 1.3

33. Inferior vena cava

34. Liver

35. Abdominal aorta

Items 36-38

The two CT scans pictured below in **Figure 1.4** are adjacent 10 mm-thick scans of an individual's head. Contrast material was administered intravenously prior to the scans. Match each item with its image in the labeled CT scan.

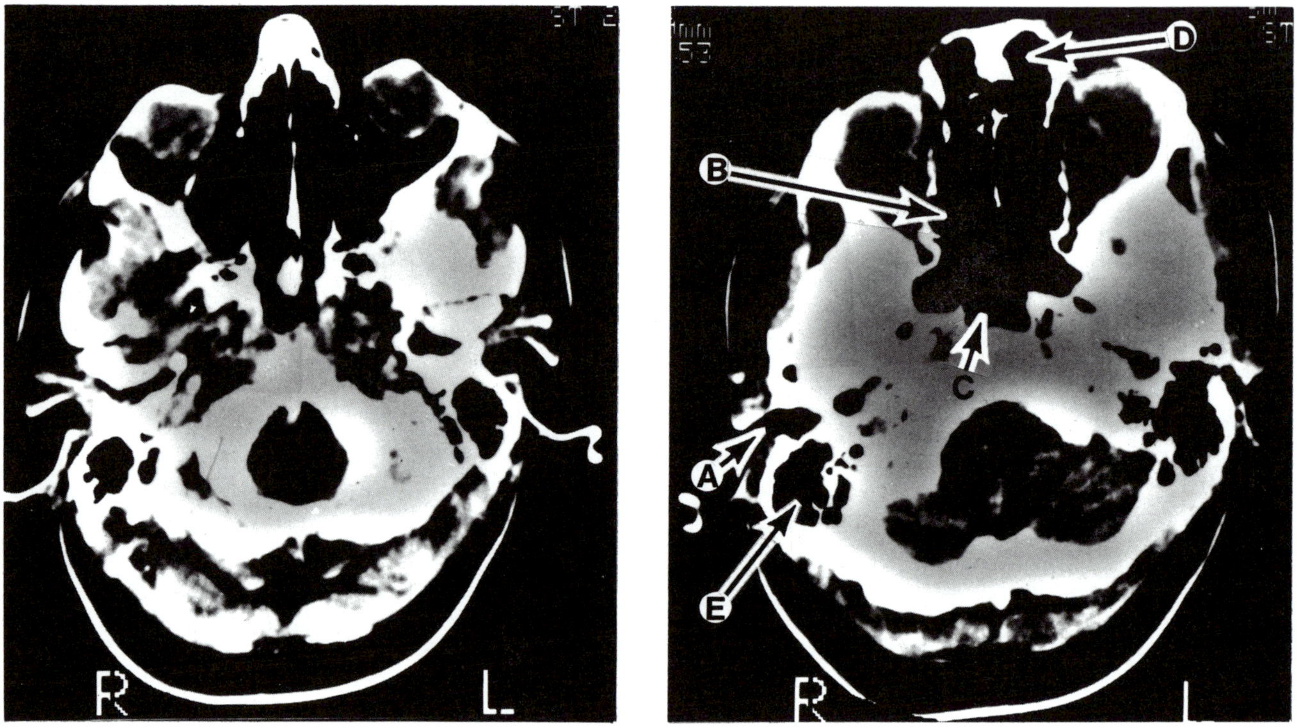

Figure 1.4

36. Mastoid air cells

37. Sphenoid sinuses

38. External auditory meatus

Items 39-42

A 33-year-old woman complains of double vision and a drooping of her upper eyelids. She states that, initially, the visual problems and drooping were transient, but they are now constant. When she speaks, it is noted that her voice is nasal and weak, and with prolonged talking, her voice fatigues to the point of unintelligibility. She states that her throat becomes tired when she eats a large meal. Her face shows little movement and when she attempts to smile, her expression resembles a snarl more than a smile. As she speaks, she holds a hand under her jaw. Blood tests reveal the patient has a abnormally high serum titer of antibodies to human acetylcholine receptors.

39. The diagnosis for this patient is most likely

    (A) Raynaud's disease
    (B) Parkinson's disease
    (C) Weber's syndrome
    (D) myasthenia gravis
    (E) Reye's syndrome

40. The symptoms shown by this patient are the consequence of a

    (A) loss of acetylcholine receptors at the neuromuscular junction
    (B) lesion within the caudate nucleus
    (C) lesion within the red nucleus and substantia nigra
    (D) loss of skeletal muscle fibers
    (E) loss of ventral horn motor neurons

41. Innervation of the skeletal muscle that raises the upper eyelid is by cranial nerve

    (A) III
    (B) VII
    (C) V
    (D) IV
    (E) VI

42. The clinician orders a CT scan of the mediastinum for this patient because

    (A) there may be an aneurysm of the aortic arch
    (B) the patient may have left ventricular hypertrophy
    (C) the thymus gland may have some pathogenetic role in this patient's disease process
    (D) there may be an esophageal stenosis or atresia
    (E) there may be a congenital heart defect

Items 43-48

Figure 1.5, below, is an MRI scan of a midsagittal slice through the head. For each number item below, select the letter which points to the proper site.

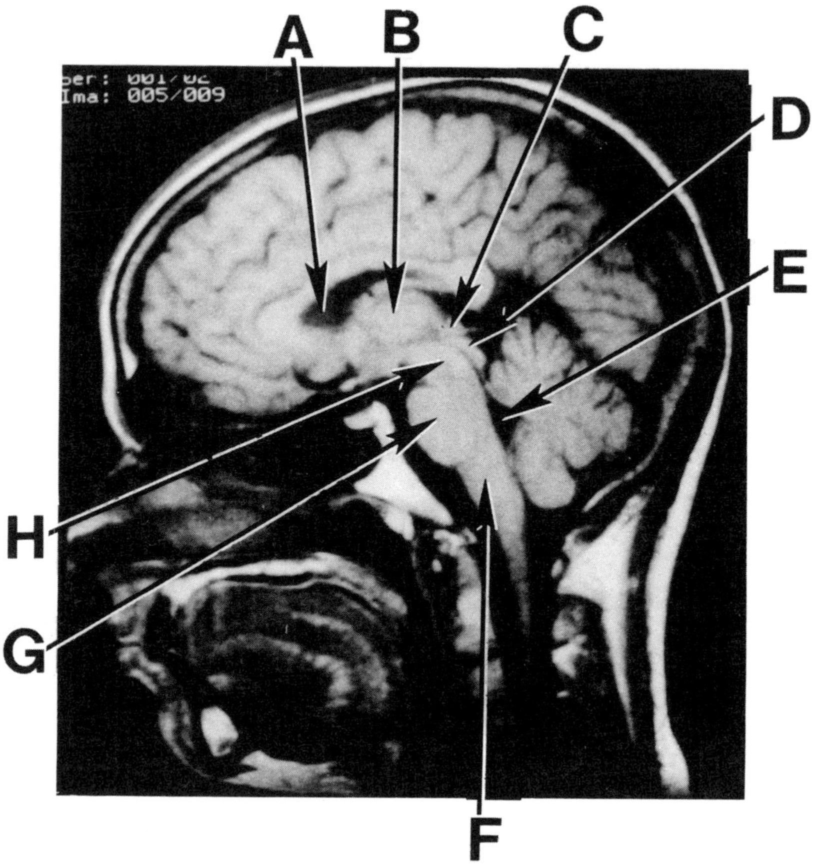

Figure 1.5

43. Region of the brain known as the corpora quadrigemina whose function is to control visual and auditory reflexes.

44. Portion of the ventricular system where cerebrospinal (CSF) exits into the subarachnoid space via the foramen of Magendie and foramina of Luschka.

45. Site of tumor of the pineal gland which could compress aqueduct of Sylvius.

46. Region of the brain that is described as the major sensory relay nucleus of the brain.

47. Region of brain where a vascular accident could compromise the red nucleus and substantia nigra.

48. Region of the brain that contains the principle sensory nucleus of and gives origin to the fibers of the trigeminal nerve.

Items 49-53

Figure 1.6 below represents a cross-section through the brainstem.

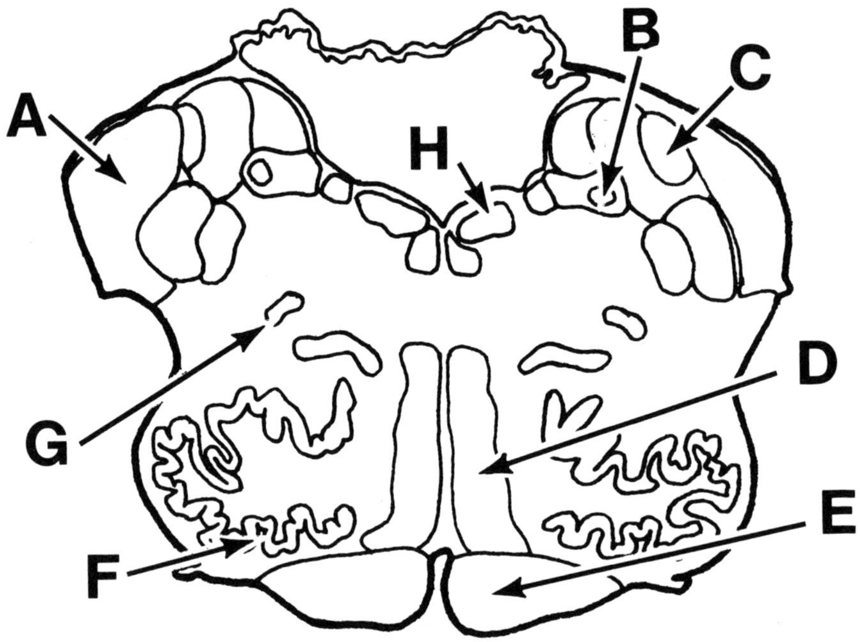

Figure 1.6

49. The cross-section represents what portion of the brainstem?

(A) rostral pons
(B) midbrain
(C) rostral medulla
(D) caudal medulla
(E) caudal pons

50. Which labeled structure carries proprioceptive information from the limbs?

(A) A
(B) B
(C) C
(D) D
(E) E

51. The origin of most of the axons found in structure E is the

(A) cerebellum
(B) motor and premotor cortex
(C) spinal cord
(D) caudate nucleus
(E) red nucleus

52. Which structure provides motor innervation to the muscles of the soft palate and pharynx?

(A) D
(B) E
(C) F
(D) G
(E) H

53. The portion of the ventricular system found at this level of the brainstem is the

(A) open portion of the 4th ventricle
(B) cerebral aqueduct
(C) 3rd ventricle
(D) central canal
(E) lateral ventricle

STOP.

YOU HAVE COMPLETED THIS SECTION.

Notes

Gross Anatomy and Neuroanatomy

Answers and Tutorials

Answer and Tutorial on Item 1

The answer is **D.** The **radial nerve** (RN) arises from the posterior cord (PC) of the brachial plexus (**Figure 1.7**). As the radial nerve extends through the mid-region of the arm (alongside the profunda brachii, a branch of the brachial artery), both the radial nerve and profunda brachii lie against the spiral groove of the shaft of the humerus. The close relation of the radial nerve to the mid-shaft of the **humerus** renders the radial nerve especially susceptible to injury from fractures of the mid-shaft of the humerus. Injury to the radial nerve along its course beside the spiral groove of the humerus may cause partial denervation of triceps and partial or complete denervation of any of the forearm muscles innervated by either the radial nerve (brachioradialis and extensor carpi radialis longus) or the deep branch of the radial nerve (supinator, extensor carpi radialis brevis, extensor carpi ulnaris, abductor pollicis longus, extensor pollicis brevis, extensor pollicis longus, extensor digitorum, extensor indicis and extensor digiti minimi). Weakness in extending, abducting and adducting the hand at the wrist against resistance may occur because of partial loss of action of the chief extensors of the hand (extensor carpi radialis longus, extensor carpi radialis brevis and extensor carpi ulnaris), two of the chief abductors of the hand (extensor carpi radialis longus and extensor carpi radialis brevis) and one of the chief adductors of the hand (extensor carpi ulnaris). Weakness in supinating the forearm against resistance may occur because of partial loss of action of one of the two supinators of the forearm (supinator). Weakness in flexing the hand against resistance will not occur because none of the flexors of the hand are innervated by either the radial nerve or its deep branch. Brachioradialis can flex the forearm and stabilize it in the mid-prone position. It does not exert any action across the wrist joint.

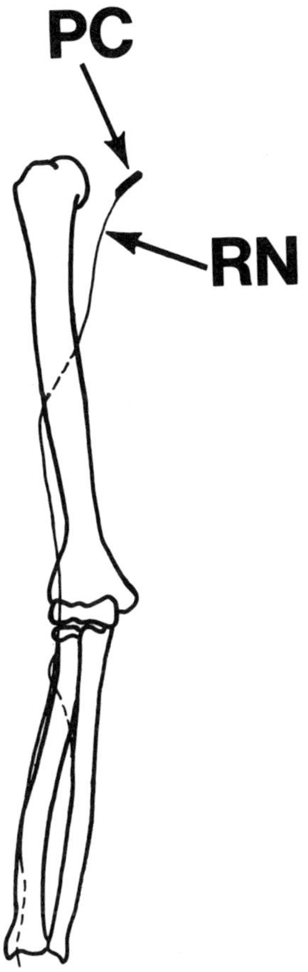

Figure 1.7

Answers and Tutorial on Items 2-3

The answers are: **2-B; 3-C. Abdominal visceral pain** is dull and sickening pain. It is poorly localized to one or more of the midline abdominal regions (epigastric, umbilical or hypogastric). Visceral pain is produced by the stimulation of visceral pain fibers. Visceral pain fibers are sensitive to acute stretching and anoxia. Disease or injury of the abdominal viscera supplied by the superior mesenteric artery produces visceral pain that is most commonly localized to the umbilical region. The greater, lesser and least splanchnic nerves provide almost all the preganglionic sympathetic innervation for the viscera supplied by the superior mesenteric artery. The sensory fibers that innervate the viscera supplied by the superior mesenteric artery enter the spinal cord at those spinal cord segments that provide preganglionic sympathetic innervation for the viscera (specifically, the sensory fibers enter at the T8-T12 levels).

An **indirect inguinal hernia** is a hernia whose contents protrude into the inguinal canal through the deep inguinal ring (DIR) (**Figure 1.8**). The neck of the sac of an indirect inguinal hernia thus always lies lateral to the inferior epigastric artery (IEA). An indirect inguinal hernia almost always occurs in an individual with a patent processus vaginalis. A **direct inguinal hernia** is a hernia whose contents protrude into the inguinal canal through a distention of its posterior wall. The neck of the sac of a direct inguinal hernia always lies medial to the origin of the inferior epigastric artery and within the inguinal, or **Hesselbach's, triangle**. The inguinal triangle is the area within the inguinal region bounded by the inferior epigastric artery (IEA) laterally, the lateral edge of rectus abdominis (RA) medially, and the inguinal ligament (IL) inferiorly (**Figure 1.8**). A **femoral hernia** is a hernia whose contents protrude through the femoral ring (FR) into the femoral canal (Fig. 1.8). The neck of the sac of a femoral hernia always lies immediately lateral and inferior to the pubic tubercle (PT). The lower free borders of internal oblique and transversus abdominis form the roof of the inguinal canal.

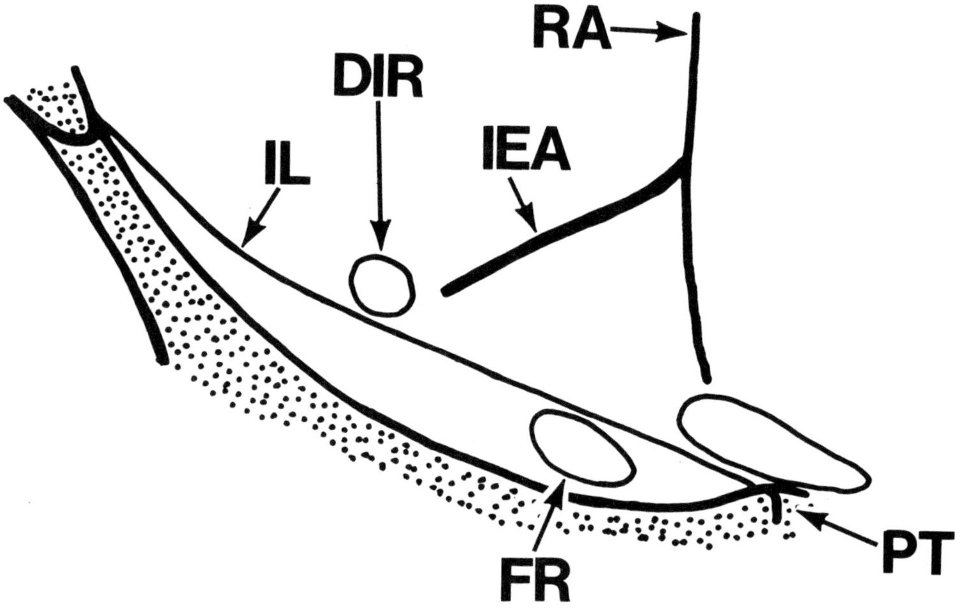

Figure 1.8

Answer and Tutorial on Item 4

The answer is **4-E.** The **cavernous sinus** lies medial to the temporal lobe of the cerebral hemisphere. **Septic thrombosis** of the cavernous sinus may inflame and injure the nerves that extend through the interior of the sinus or its lateral wall. The lateral wall of the cavernous sinus transmits segments of the oculomotor nerve, the ophthalmic and maxillary divisions of the trigeminal nerve and the trochlear nerve. The interior of the cavernous sinus is traversed by segments of the abducent nerve and the internal carotid artery (and accompanying postganglionic sympathetic fibers, some of which innervate dilator pupillae).

The **medial and lateral rectus muscles** move the eyeball from its primary position to orientations in which the cornea faces, respectively, directly medially and laterally. The activities of the medial and lateral rectus muscles are tested during a physical exam by asking the patient to look in directions that directly match the actions of these muscles. For example, to test the activity of the medial rectus, the patient is asked to try to look at the nose. In this case involving a patient with diplopia, the medial rectus of the right eye functions normally.

The **superior and inferior rectus muscles** move the eyeball from its primary position to orientations in which the cornea faces, respectively, superomedially and inferomedially. The superior and inferior oblique muscles move the eyeball from its primary position to orientations in which the cornea faces, respectively, inferolaterally and superolaterally. However, in testing the activities of the superior and inferior recti and the superior and inferior obliques, the patient is asked to look in directions that do not correspond to the actions of these muscles. With the cornea facing directly laterally (that is, with the patient looking directly to the side of the head), the activities of the superior and inferior rectus muscles are tested by asking the patient to look, respectively, upward and downward. With the cornea facing directly medially (that is, with the patient looking directly at the nose), the activities of the superior and inferior obliques are tested by asking the patient to look, respectively, downward and upward. **Figure 1.9** is a drawing of the superior view of the relationship of the superior oblique muscle (SO) to the right eyeball. Notice that if the cornea (C) faces directly medially, superior oblique is the only extraocular muscle whose actions can move the eyeball so that the cornea also faces inferiorly.

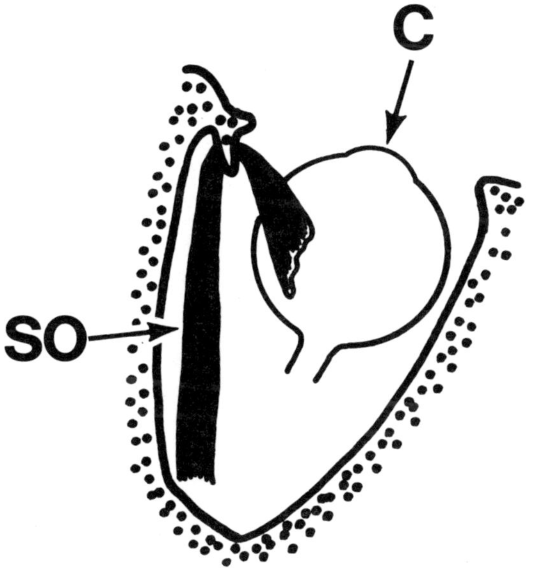

Figure 1.9

Answers and Tutorial on Items 5-6

The answers are: **5-C; 6-B. Pericardial tamponade** (accumulation of fluid within the pericardial cavity) broadens the region of cardiac dullness in the anterior chest wall, and thus shifts the right border of cardiac dullness to the right from its normal location at the right border of the sternum. The extracardiac pressure exerted by the pericardial fluid decreases intracardiac diastolic pressures, and thereby reduces venous return to the right atrium (as evidenced by bilateral distension of jugular veins) and systolic blood pressure. Sinus tachycardia occurs as a compensatory mechanism to maintain cardiac output. The pericardial fluid diminishes the intensity of S1 and S2.

The internal and external jugular (IJ and EJ) veins, subclavian (S) veins, brachiocephalic (B) veins and superior vena cava (SVC) are the major venous trunks which extend inferiorly through the neck and superior mediastinum to conduct blood into the right atrium of the heart (**Figure 1.10**). When a normal adult is standing or seated upright, blood fills these venous trunks up to a level about 2-3 cm above the sternal angle. In other words, under these conditions, blood fills the superior vena cava, brachiocephalic veins and subclavian veins but only the lowest parts of the jugular veins. The height to which the jugular veins are filled with blood is proportional to right atrial pressure. Accordingly, the jugular veins can serve as manometers of right atrial pressure. Right atrial pressure is frequently called central venous pressure, since the blood pressure of the right atrium approximates that of the large systemic veins converging upon the right atrium. The right internal jugular vein is the most appropriate jugular vein to select for the measurement of central venous pressure. This is because it is the only jugular vein which forms a straight-lined venous trunk with the right brachiocephalic vein and superior vena cava (**Figure 1.10**). The angular union of the left internal jugular vein with the left subclavian vein and the angular unions of the external jugular veins with the subclavian veins make the blood heights in these jugular veins less reliable monitors of central venous pressure.

During each heartbeat, there are three transient increases in right atrial pressure. The first pulsatile increase (the a wave) occurs when contraction of the atrial musculature increases atrial pressure. The second increase (the c wave) occurs during early systole, when the increasing pressure in the right ventricle bulges the tricuspid valve into the right atrium. The third pulsatile increase (the v wave) occurs as blood flowing into the right atrium during late systole begins to bulge the heart chamber. These pulsatile increases are transmitted in a retrograde fashion through the blood in the internal and external jugular veins. When these jugular venous pulses reach the meniscus (curved, upper surface) of the blood in each jugular vein, they produce fluctuations in the level of the meniscus, and these meniscal fluctuations, in turn, produce up-and-down movements of the overlying skin. These skin movements over each jugular vein are generally the best indicator of the height to which blood fills the vein.

Inspection of jugular pulses should begin with the patient in the supine position. In a normal individual, the jugular veins will be distended because the jugular veins and the right atrium now are all at about the same level. The patient's head, neck and trunk are next elevated above the horizontal plane sufficiently to lower the height of the jugular pulses to a level which is below the angle of the mandible but above the clavicle (a 30-45) degree elevation is generally sufficient). In a normal adult, pulsatile activity will be visible near the lower ends of the jugular veins, commonly up to a vertical distance of 2-3 cm above the level of the sternal angle. This is because the average central venous pressure in a normal individual is about 7-8 cm water, and the center of the right atrium is about 5 cm below the level of the sternal angle in an average adult.

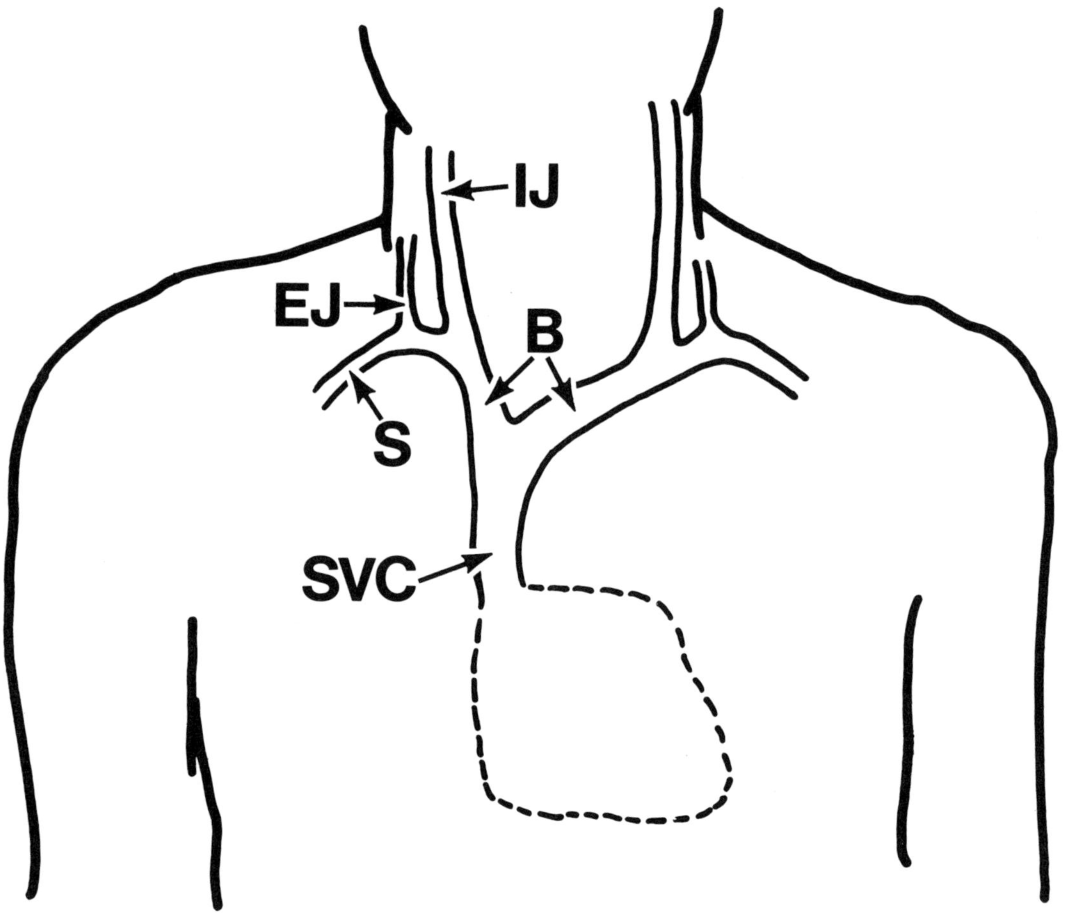

Figure 1.10

Answers and Tutorial on Items 7-8

The answers are: **7–C; 8-C.** Disease or injury of the sigmoid colon and other abdominal viscera supplied by the **inferior mesenteric artery** produces visceral pain that is most commonly localized to the **hypogastric region**. The terminal branches of the ileocolic (IC), right colic (RC) and middle colic (MC) branches of the superior mesenteric artery extend distally along the large intestine as far the border region between the middle and left thirds of the transverse colon (**Figure 1.11**). The terminal branches of the left colic (LC) and sigmoid (S) branches of the inferior mesenteric artery extend along the distal third of the transverse colon and the entire length of the descending and sigmoid colons. The anastomoses among the terminal branches of the colic branches of the superior and inferior mesenteric arteries form, in effect, an artery that runs along the medial margins of the ascending and descending colons and the mesenteric margins of the transverse and sigmoid colons. This artery is called the **marginal artery of Drummond**. The vagus nerves provide preganglionic parasympathetic innervation along the large intestine distally to the border between the middle and left thirds of the transverse colon. The pelvic splanchnic nerves provide preganglionic parasympathetic innervation to the remaining distal segments of the large intestine.

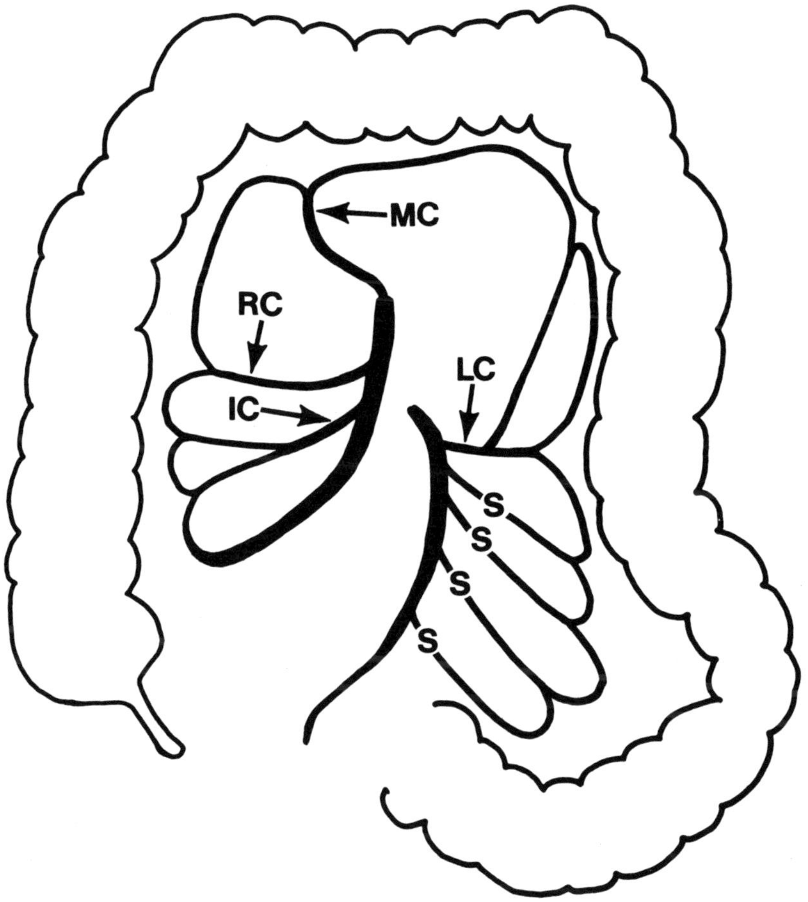

Figure 1.11

Answer and Tutorial on Item 9

The answer is: **9-B.** Disease or injury of the liver, gallbladder and other viscera supplied by the **celiac artery** produces visceral pain that is most commonly localized to the **epigastric region**. The left and right greater splanchnic nerves provide almost all the preganglionic sympathetic innervation for the viscera supplied by the celiac artery. Most of the sensory fibers that innervate the viscera supplied by the celiac artery enter the spinal cord at those spinal cord segments that give rise to the preganglionic sympathetic fibers for the greater splanchnic nerves (specifically, the sensory fibers enter at the T5-T9 levels). Some sensory fibers from the liver, gallbladder and the extrahepatic biliary ducts enter the spinal cord at the C3-C5 segments. The right phrenic nerve transmits these fibers to their cell bodies in the dorsal root ganglia of spinal nerves C3, C4 and C5. Disease or injury of any of the viscera supplied by the celiac artery may refer pain to parts of the T5-T9 dermatomes. The right upper quadrant of the anterolateral abdominal wall represents part of the T7-T10 dermatomes, the anterior chest wall overlying the 6th, 7th and 8th intercostal spaces represents part of the T6-T8 dermatomes, the posterior chest wall overlying the inferior angle of the scapula represents part of the T7 dermatome, and the posterior chest wall overlying the medial end of the spine of the scapula represents part of the T3 dermatome. Disease or injury of the liver, gallbladder and extrahepatic ducts may also refer pain to the shoulder (as it represents part of the C3-C5 dermatomes).

Percussion can be used to assess the size of the liver. As the patient lies supine and holds the breath at full expiration, the examiner percusses the anterior chest wall and anterolateral abdominal wall from the right 2nd intercostal space downward along the right midclavicular line. Normally, percussion resonance (due to percussion of the right lung) is encountered down to the highest level (which is typically that of the 4th intercostal space) at which the liver crosses the right midclavicular line. A thin wedge of the right lung's lower lobe anteriorly covers the diaphragm and the underlying liver down to the level of the 6th rib. Percussion of both the right lung and the liver between the levels of the 4th intercostal space and the 6th rib produces a zone of percussion dullness called hepatic dullness. A zone of percussion flatness called hepatic flatness is encountered from the level of the 6th rib down to that of the liver's anteroinferior margin. Percussion of bowel segments inferior to the liver produce percussion dullness, resonance or tympany below the zone of hepatic flatness. The combined heights of the zones of hepatic dullness and hepatic flatness are a measure of the size of the liver. The normal range for the combined adult heights is 6-12 cm. The presence of gas-filled bowel segments immediately posterior to the lower part of the liver's visceral surface can obscure determination of the lower limit of the zone of hepatic flatness and lead to a faulty underestimate of liver size.

The **left hepatic artery** supplies the left hepatic lobe, quadrate lobe and caudate lobe except for the caudate process. The right hepatic artery supplies the rest of the hepatic parenchyma. **Figure 1.12** shows the relationships of the left gastric artery (LGA), splenic artery (SA), left gastroepiploic artery (LGEA), gastroduodenal artery (GA) and right gastroepiploic artery (RGEA) to the stomach (S), pancreas (P) and 1st part of the duodenum (D). The **gastroduodenal artery** passes behind the first part of the duodenum before giving rise to the right gastroepiploic and superior pancreaticoduodenal arteries. Portal-systemic anastomoses are venous anastomoses between veins that are tributaries of the portal vein and veins that are tributaries of the superior vena cava or inferior vena cava. In the border region between the middle and lower thirds of the esophagus, tributaries of the left gastric vein (which drains toward the portal vein) anastomose with tributaries of the azygos system of veins (which drains toward the superior vena cava). In the border region between the upper and lower halves of the anal canal, tributaries of the superior rectal vein (which drains toward the portal vein) anastomose with tributaries of the inferior rectal vein (which drains toward the inferior vena cava). In the paraumbilical region, tributaries of the paraumbilical veins (which drain toward the portal vein) anastomose with tributaries of the lumbar veins (which drain toward the inferior vena cava). In the retroperitoneal region deep to the posterior abdominal wall, tributaries of the splenic vein (which drains toward the portal vein) anastomose with tributaries of the left renal vein (which drains toward the inferior vena cava).

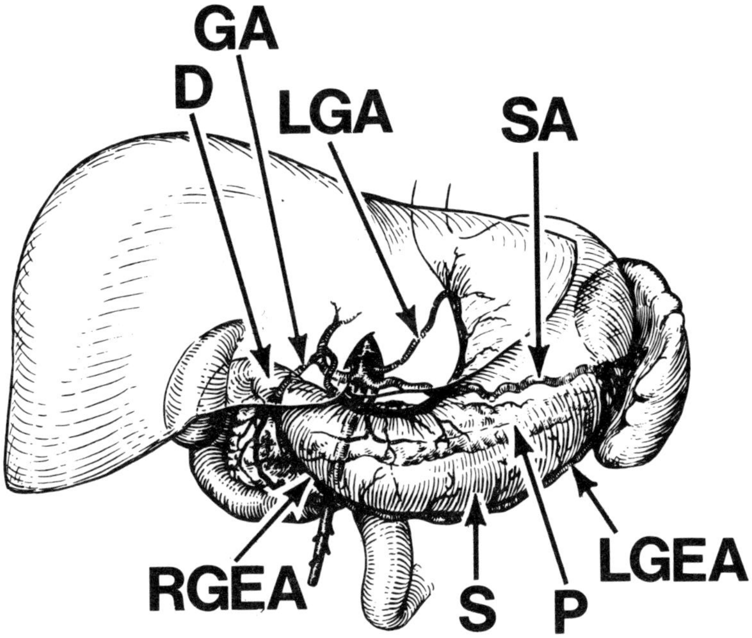

Figure 1.12

Answers and Tutorial on Items 10-12

The answers are: **10-E; 11-E; 12-B.** The **ulnar nerve** (UN) arises from the medial cord (MC) of the **brachial plexus (Figure 1.13)**. As the ulnar nerve extends across the elbow region, it passes directly posterior to the medial epicondyle (ME) of the humerus. The close relation of the ulnar nerve to the medial epicondyle of the humerus renders the ulnar nerve especially susceptible to injury from displaced fractures of the medial epicondyle.

Injury to the ulnar nerve from a displaced fracture of the medial epicondyle of the humerus may cause partial or complete denervation of the forearm muscles innervated by the ulnar nerve (flexor carpi ulnaris and the medial half of flexor digitorum profundus) and/or any of the intrinsic hand muscles innervated by the deep branch of the ulnar nerve (the palmar and dorsal interossei, the 3rd and 4th lumbricals, abductor digiti minimi, flexor digiti minimi, opponens digiti minimi and adductor pollicis). Weakness in holding a piece of paper between any two fingers may occur because of partial loss of action of one or more of the abductors and adductors of the fingers (the palmar and dorsal interossei and abductor digiti minimi). Weakness in flexing the distal phalanx of the little finger against resistance may occur because of partial loss of action of the only flexor of the distal phalanx of the little finger (the muscular part of flexor digitorum profundus that pulls upon the tendon that inserts onto the base of the distal phalanx of the little finger). Weakness in flexing the distal phalanx of the thumb against resistance will not occur because the sole flexor of the distal phalanx of the thumb (flexor pollicis longus) is innervated by the anterior interosseous branch of the median nerve.

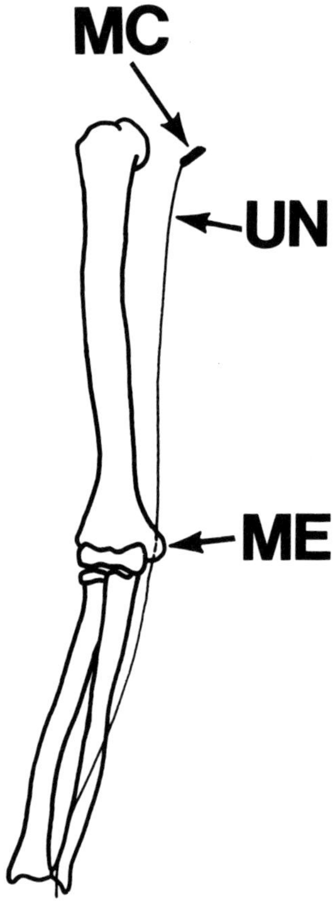

Figure 1.13

Answer and Tutorial on Item 13

The answer is **13-D.** If the leg is fully extended at the knee, the thigh can be passively flexed approximately 90° before tension in the hamstring muscles becomes painful and limits further flexion. Iliopsoas is the most powerful flexor of the thigh. Iliacus is innervated by the femoral nerve and psoas major is innervated by nerve fibers from L1, L2 and L3.

The **extensors of the thigh** and their innervation are as follows

Gluteus maximus—inferior gluteal nerve

Semitendinosus—tibial portion of the sciatic nerve

Semimembranosus—tibial portion of the sciatic nerve

Long head of biceps femoris—tibial portion of the sciatic nerve

Hamstring part of adductor magnus—tibial portion of the sciatic nerve

The chief **abductors of the thigh**, gluteus medius and gluteus minimus, are innervated by the superior gluteal nerve.

The adductors of the thigh and their innervation are as follows

Adductor part of adductor magnus—obturator nerve

Adductor longus—obturator nerve

Adductor brevis—obturator nerve

Pectineus—obturator and femoral nerves

Gracilis—obturator nerve

The **medial rotators of the thigh**, tensor fasciae latae, gluteus minimus and gluteus medius, are innervated by the superior gluteal nerve.

When an individual attempts to stand (or support the body) on one lower limb only, gluteus medius and minimus (the chief abductors of the thigh) on the side of the supporting lower limb tense to elevate the contralateral side of the pelvis. This tilting of the pelvis balances the body over the supporting lower limb. An inability to tilt the pelvis in this fashion is called a positive Trendelenburg sign. Any disorder which limits the capacity of gluteus medius and gluteus minimus to support and steady the body when standing on the ipsilateral lower limb or produces pain in the hip joint when it bears the weight of the upper body may produce a positive Trendelenburg sign. Ischial bursitis is inflammation of the ischial bursa. The ischial bursa lies directly superficial to the ischial tuberosity.

Answers and Tutorial on Items 14-15

The answers are: **14-E; 15-C. Legg-Calvé-Perthes disease** is a self-limiting hip disorder of children involving vascular compromise of the capital femoral epiphysis. Diminished vascularization in the anterolateral aspect of the capital femoral epiphysis is characteristic of the pattern of ischemic necrosis which occurs in Legg-Calvé-Perthes disease. The radiographic evidence of periarticular soft tissue swelling suggests that the patient is also suffering from inflammation of the synovial membrane and effusion of the hip joint.

The etiology of Legg-Calvé-Perthes disease is unknown. The anatomical basis of the disorder is believed to be related to the developmental changes in the blood supply to the hip during childhood. Branches of the medial and lateral circumflex femoral arteries form an extracapsular vascular ring around the base of the neck of the femur. Branches of the extracapsular vascular ring called the retinacular arteries ascend along the neck of the femur to penetrate the capsule of the hip joint and give rise within the joint to branches that supply the upper end of the femur. The retinacular arteries and their branches are believed to be the chief source of blood supply to the head of the femur at all ages. At birth, the cartilaginous femoral head is also supplied by arteries entering the head from the shaft of the femur. Establishment of an epiphyseal plate between the capital epiphysis and the metaphysis by about 4 years of age abolishes all blood supply from the metaphysis. This arrangement persists until about 9 years of age, at which time the arteries in the ligament to the head of the femur begin to become increasingly prominent in supplying the head of the femur. Medullary arteries of the metaphysis begin to supply the femoral head upon epiphyseal fusion in late adolescence or early adulthood. The childhood period from 4-9 years of age, when the retinacular arteries are the sole significant source of blood supply to the capital epiphysis, spans the years of the highest incidence of Legg-Calvé-Perthes disease.

Hip joint disease frequently refers pain to the groin, anteromedial aspects of the thigh and the medial aspect of the knee. Cutaneous branches of the obturator nerve supply the medial aspect of the thigh. Cutaneous branches of the femoral nerve supply the anterior aspect of the thigh and the anteromedial aspect of the knee. A major component of the patient's right hip pain is emanating from tension on the joint's inflamed synovial membrane. Synovial membrane tension in the hip joint is minimized when the thigh is flexed 90° and slightly externally rotated. Accordingly, patients with a painful hip joint effusion are generally most comfortable when seated with the painful thigh slightly externally rotated. Active and passive attempts at internal rotation or abduction of the thigh commonly exacerbate the lower limb pain of patients with Legg-Calvé-Perthes disease.

Answer and Tutorial on Item 16

The answer is **16-B.** The signs and symptoms of the patient's motor and sensory deficits in the right hand are characteristic of **carpal tunnel syndrome**. The carpal tunnel syndrome is produced by conditions which compress the median nerve as it passes through the carpal tunnel. The carpal tunnel is an osseofascial corridor in the wrist bordered anteriorly by the flexor retinaculum (FR) and posteriorly by the carpal bones (CB) (**Figure 1.14**). The **median nerve** (MN), the tendons of flexor digitorum superficialis and profundus and the tendon of flexor pollicis longus (FPLT) all cross the wrist through the carpal tunnel. In contrast, the ulnar nerve (UN), ulnar artery (UA), palmaris longus tendon (PLT) and the palmar cutaneous branch of the median nerve (PC) all cross the wrist anterior to the flexor retinaculum. The median nerve is susceptible to compression neuropathy by conditions which increase the pressure on the contents of the carpal tunnel.

The median nerve innervates five intrinsic muscles of the hand: the muscles of the thenar eminence (abductor pollicis brevis, flexor pollicis brevis and opponens pollicis) and the 1st and 2nd lumbricals. The median nerve also supplies cutaneous areas of the hand. The blocked areas of **Figures 1.15** and **1.16** respectively show the areas on the volar and dorsal surfaces of the hand innervated by cutaneous branches of the median nerve. However, it is important to note that the palmar cutaneous branch of the median nerve, which is the cutaneous nerve that provides sensory innervation for the radial two-thirds of the palmar surface of the hand, arises from the median nerve proximal to the carpal tunnel and crosses the wrist anterior to the flexor retinaculum. Severe compression neuropathy of the median nerve in the carpal tunnel can thus lead to atrophy of the muscles underlying the thenar eminence and weakness of thumb opposition. Opponens pollicis is the prime mover of thumb opposition. The little finger is the sole digit whose cutaneous innervation is completely spared in individuals suffering from carpal tunnel syndrome.

The digital pain and/or paresthesia associated with the carpal tunnel syndrome can be reproduced during physical examination by tapping a reflex hammer on the radial side of the palmaris longus tendon along the tendon's course over the flexor retinaculum (Tinel's sign). The median nerve (MN) in the carpal tunnel lies deep to the radial margin of the palmaris longus tendon (PLT) (**Fig. 1.14**). In individuals suffering from carpal tunnel syndrome, the light percussion momentarily increases the pressure upon an already compressed median nerve and thus may elicit pain and/or paresthesia in the areas of the lateral three and a half digits supplied by the digital cutaneous branches of the median nerve.

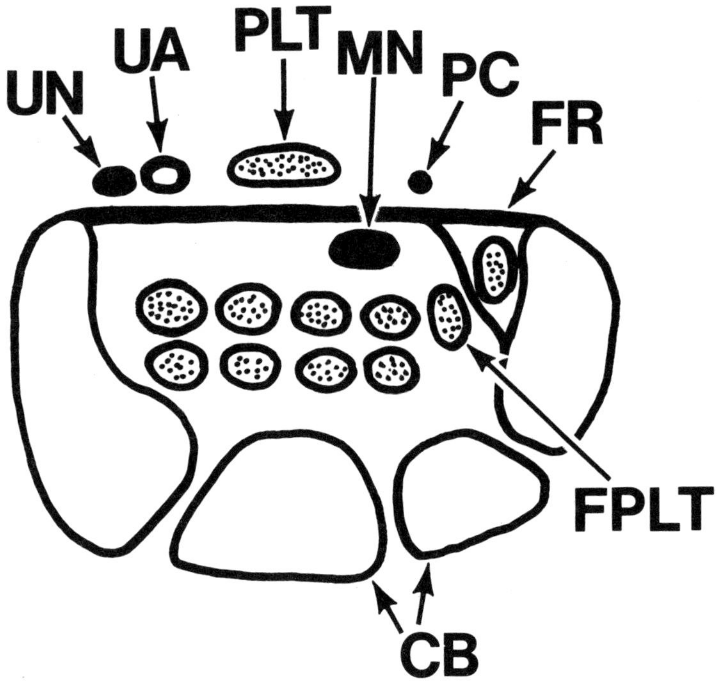

Figure 1.14

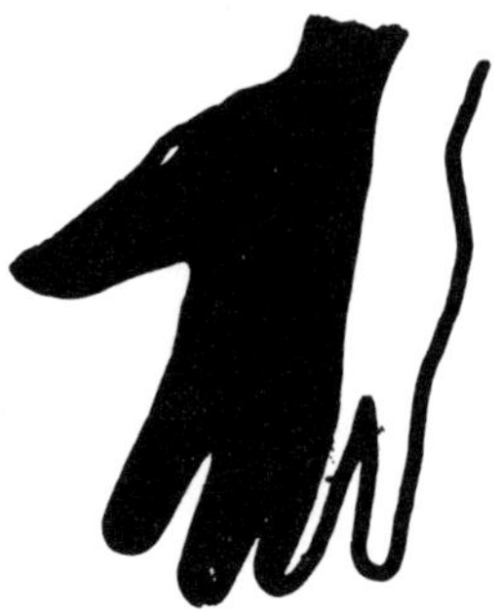

Figure 1.15

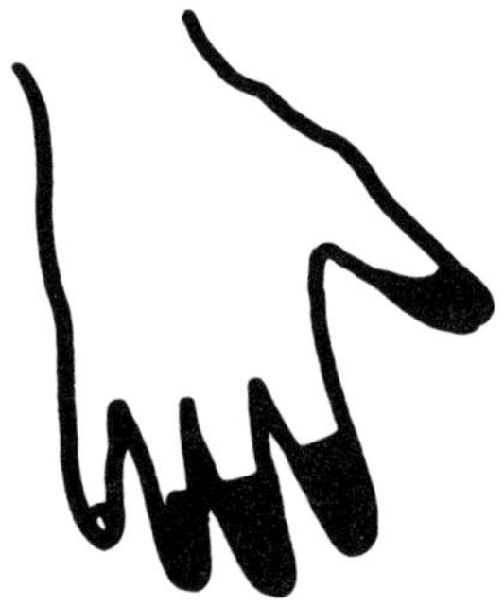

Figure 1.16

Answers and Tutorial on Items 17-18

The answers are: **17-A; 18-C.** The **upper trunk of the brachial plexus** is formed from the union of the C5 and C6 roots. A traction injury to the upper trunk chiefly affects those upper limb movements whose prime movers are muscles innervated exclusively by C5 and C6 fibers (supraspinatus, infraspinatus, teres minor and deltoid) or predominantly by C5 and C6 fibers (biceps brachii, brachialis, brachioradialis and supinator). Deltoid, infraspinatus and teres minor are the sole lateral rotators of the arm. Supraspinatus and deltoid initiate arm abduction from the anatomical position. Biceps brachii and brachialis are the chief flexors of the forearm. Biceps brachii and supinator are the sole supinators of the forearm. Trapezius is the chief retractor of the scapula and thus the prime mover for bracing the shoulder. Levator scapulae, rhomboid major and rhomboid minor assist trapezius in this action. Trapezius is innervated by the spinal part of the accessory nerve. Levator scapulae is innervated by C3 and C4 fibers and the dorsal scapular nerve. The rhomboids are innervated by the dorsal scapular nerve. The dorsal scapular nerve arises from the C5 root of the brachial plexus.

The **lower trunk of the brachial plexus** is formed from the union of the C8 and T1 roots. A traction injury to the lower trunk chiefly affects those upper limb movements whose prime movers are muscles innervated either exclusively or predominantly by C8 and/or T1 fibers (flexor carpi ulnaris, flexor digitorum superficialis, flexor digitorum profundus, flexor pollicis longus, pronator quadratus, extensor carpi ulnaris, abductor pollicis longus, extensor pollicis brevis, extensor pollicis longus, extensor indicis and all of the intrinsic muscles of the hand). A traction injury to the lower trunk of the brachial plexus can affect all movements of the hand and its digits. Flexor digitorum profundus is the sole flexor of the distal phalanx of the little finger. Abductor digiti minimi is the sole abductor of the little finger. Flexor pollicis longus is the sole flexor of the distal phalanx of the thumb. Abductor pollicis longus and abductor pollicis brevis are the sole abductors of the thumb.

Figures 1.17 and **1.18** show, respectively, the dermatomes on the anterior and posterior surfaces of the upper limb.

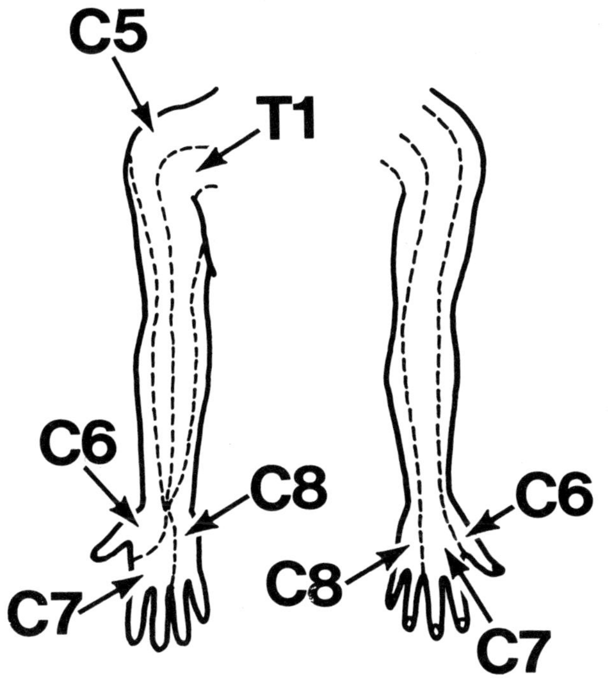

Figures 1.17 and 1.18

Answer and Tutorial on Item 19

The answer is **19-E.** The **supratrochlear lymph nodes** can be palpated along the medial side of the basilic vein immediately superior to the medial epicondyle of the humerus. The supratrochlear nodes drain superficial tissues of the medial aspect of the hand and forearm. The lateral group of axillary lymph nodes can be palpated along the humeral head. The lateral group of axillary nodes drains all of the deep tissues of the hand, forearm and arm.

Lymph nodes which are mounting an immunological response to infectious agents are enlarged but regularly shaped, tender, relatively mobile and firm. Normal superficial lymph nodes are frequently difficult to palpate because of their small size and are non-tender, relatively mobile and soft.

The deltopectoral group of **axillary nodes** drains superficial tissues on the lateral aspect of the hand, forearm and arm. The posterior (subscapular) group of axillary nodes drains superficial tissues of the posterior aspect of the trunk, down to the level of the iliac crest. The anterior (pectoral) group of axillary nodes can be palpated against the posterior aspect of the anterior axillary fold.

Answers and Tutorial on Items 20-22

The answers are: **20-B; 21-C; 22-E.** The structure labeled A in **Figure 1.1** is the right border of the right atrium, and the structure labeled D is the left border of the descending thoracic aorta.

Answers and Tutorial on Items 23-25

The answers are: **23-A; 24-C; 25-D.** The structure labeled B in **Figure 1.2** is the left brachiocephalic vein, and the structure labeled E is the left subclavian artery.

Answers and Tutorial on Items 26-32

The answers are: **26-B; 27-D; 28-A; 29-D; 30-D; 31-E; 32-C.** The **retroperitoneal viscera** of the abdomen include the abdominal aorta, inferior vena cava, kidneys, adrenal glands and ureters. The spleen is intraperitoneal. The **secondarily retroperitoneal viscera** of the abdomen include the head, neck and body of the pancreas; the distal half of the 1st part of the duodenum and the 2nd, 3rd and 4th parts of the duodenum; the ascending colon with the hepatic flexure at the upper end; and the descending colon with the splenic flexure at the upper end. The tail of the pancreas is **intraperitoneal**, lying sandwiched between the two peritoneal layers of the lienorenal ligament. The lesser sac of the peritoneal cavity is sealed off superiorly by the diaphragm, anteriorly by the lesser omentum, stomach and gastrocolic ligament, inferiorly by the transverse colon and transverse mesocolon, posteriorly by the upper posterior abdominal wall and on the left by the gastrophrenic, gastrosplenic and lienorenal ligaments. On the right, the lesser sac communicates with the greater sac via the epiploic foramen, which has four borders: superiorly the caudate process of the caudate lobe of the liver, anteriorly the free right margin of the lesser omentum (this margin transmits the portal vein, hepatic artery proper and bile duct), inferiorly the proximal half of the 1st part of the duodenum, and posteriorly the inferior vena cava. In the midline region, the peritoneum which covers the anterior surface of the uterus (U) is continuous anteriorly with the peritoneum that covers the superior surface of the urinary bladder (UB) (**Figure 1.19**).

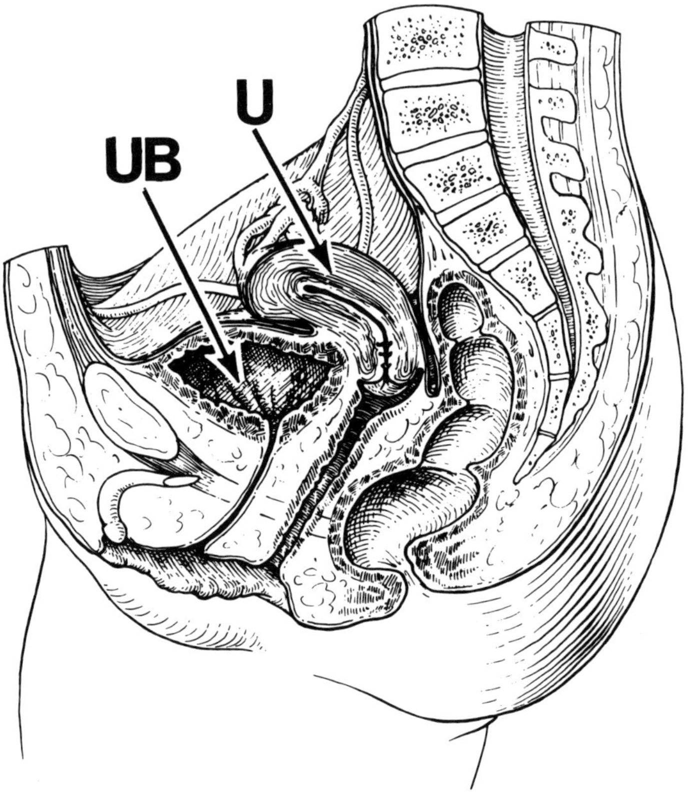

Figure 1.19

Answers and Tutorial on Items 33-35

The answers are: **33-C; 34-A; 35-D.** The structure labeled B in **Figure 1.3** is the right kidney, and the structure labeled E is the left psoas major muscle.

Answers and Tutorial on Items 36-38

The answers are: **36-E; 37-C; 38-A.** The space labeled B in **Figure 1.4** is the right ethmoid air cells, and the space labeled D is the left frontal sinus.

Answers and Tutorial on Items 39-42

The answers are: **39-D; 40-A; 41-A; 42-C**. This patient suffers from **myasthenia gravis** which is characterized by weakness and undue fatigability with exercise or muscular use. It most frequently affects the oculomotor, facial, laryngeal, pharyngeal, proximal limb and respiratory muscles. The facial muscle involvement gives rise to a characteristic smile call the "myasthenic snarl." Myasthenia gravis is an autoimmune syndrome that results in the loss of acetylcholine receptors from the postsynaptic membrane of the neuromuscular junction. It has been demonstrated that 85% of patients have circulating antibodies against human acetylcholine receptors. The thymus gland appears to play an as yet unidentified pathogenetic role in myasthenia gravis. While a CT scan of the mediastinum is not a diagnostic test, 65% of patients with this disease have thymic hyperplasia and 10% have thymomas.

Answers and Tutorial on Items 43-48

The answers are: **43-F; 44-J; 45-K; 46-C; 47-G; 48-H**. **Figure 1.5** is a magnetic resonance image (MRI) of a midsagittal section through the head (T1). Labeled structures are: A—third ventricle; B—thalamus; C—pineal gland; D—tectum of midbrain; E—4th ventricle; F—medulla; G—pons; H—tegmentum of midbrain. The roof of the cerebral aqueduct is known as the tectum and consists primarily of the corpora quadrigemina, the superior and inferior colliculi. Cerebrospinal fluid (CSF) circulates throughout the ventricular system of the brain. Three foramina in the roof of the 4th ventricle (foramen of Magendie and foramina of Luschka) allow the CSF to enter the subarachnoid space. A tumor of the pineal gland (C) may compress the anterior portion of the tectum and occlude the aqueduct of Sylvius causing an internal hydrocephalus. The thalamus (B) is the major sensory relay nucleus of the brain, receiving all sensory information except olfactory. The red nucleus and the substantia nigra are part of the extrapyramidal motor system and are large nuclei found within the tegmental region of the midbrain. The principle sensory nucleus of cranial nerve V (trigeminal nerve) lies within the pons and the fibers of the trigeminal nerve exit the brain stem from the lateral portion of the pons.

Answers and Tutorial on Items 49-53

The answers are: **49-C; 50-D; 51-B; 52-D; 53-A**. **Figure 1.6** is a cross-section through the rostral portion of the medulla. Structures found at this level include: A—restiform body; B—nucleus and tractus solitarius; C—vestibular nuclei; D—medial lemniscus; E—pyramids; F—inferior olive; G—nucleus ambiguus; and H—nucleus of cranial nerve XII (hypoglossal). The portion of the ventricular system seen at this level is the open portion of the 4th ventricle. The inferior olive (F) is probably the most distinctive structure seen in cross-section at this level of the brainstem. The pathway responsible for carrying proprioceptive information from the spinal cord is the medial lemniscus (D). The origin of most of the axons found in the pyramids (E) is from the motor and premotor cortices of the frontal lobes as well as from primary sensory cortex (postcentral gyrus). The nucleus ambiguus (G) provides axons that are carried by cranial nerve X (as well as cranial nerves IX and XI) for innervation of the muscles of the soft palate, pharynx and larynx.

Notes

CHAPTER 2

Histology and Cell Biology

DIRECTIONS (Items 1-92): For each of the numbered items that proceed, you must select the single best answer from among the lettered options listed.

Some of the numbered items will pose a question or incomplete sentence that is followed by a list of 4-5 lettered options. In all cases, select the ONE lettered option that best answers the question or completes the sentence given.

Some of the numbered items are preceded by 5-24 lettered options. In these sets, the lettered options will be preceded by a single instruction asking you to match one of the lettered options to each numbered item most closely associated with it. In all matching sets, you may use any of the lettered options once, more than once or not at all, but you should still only select ONE lettered option per numbered item.

If you wish to simulate actual USMLE testing conditions, you should aim to complete all the items in this chapter in ONE hour and 30 minutes.

Do NOT look at the answers and tutorials until you have completed all of the items in this chapter.

Good luck!

Item 1

1. You encounter a patient who is phenotypically female. Karyotype analysis reveals a normal-looking 46, XY karyotype. Molecular biological investigation of the Y chromosome DNA sequences shows a deletion of the testis-determining factor (TDF). If the patient had a 46, XX karyotype with the TDF region of the Y chromosome translocated into the X chromosome the patient would

    (A) be phenotypically female
    (B) be phenotypically male
    (C) be a hermaphrodite
    (D) exhibit Turner's syndrome
    (E) exhibit Klinefelter's syndrome

Items 2-4

Examine **Figure 2.1** below, a scanning electron micrograph, and then choose the correct answer.

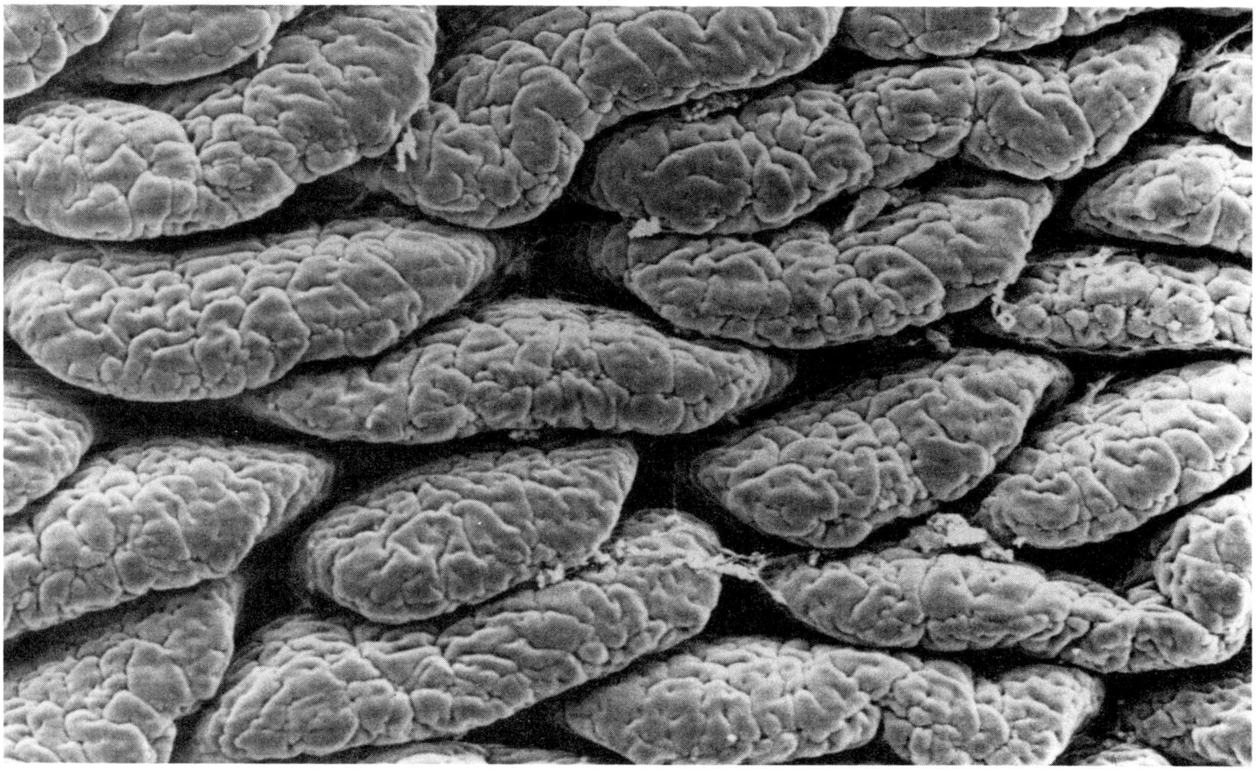

Figure 2.1

2. These structures have which major physiological function?

(A) taste perception
(B) nutrient absorption
(C) bile concentration
(D) gamete transport
(E) blood transport

3. These structures are characteristic of the mucosal surface of which organ?

(A) stomach
(B) jejunum
(C) uterine tube
(D) tongue
(E) gall bladder

4. The mucosal epithelium here consists of

(A) ciliated and secretory cells
(B) ciliated cells only
(C) absorptive cells and goblet cells
(D) a pseudostratified ciliated columnar epithelium with goblet cells
(E) transitional epithelium

Items 5-8

Examine **Figure 2.2** below, a labeled photomicrograph of a developing bone of the appendicular skeleton. Match the lettered structure in the photomicrograph with the most appropriate description of its developmental fate or role in endochondral bone formation in the questions.

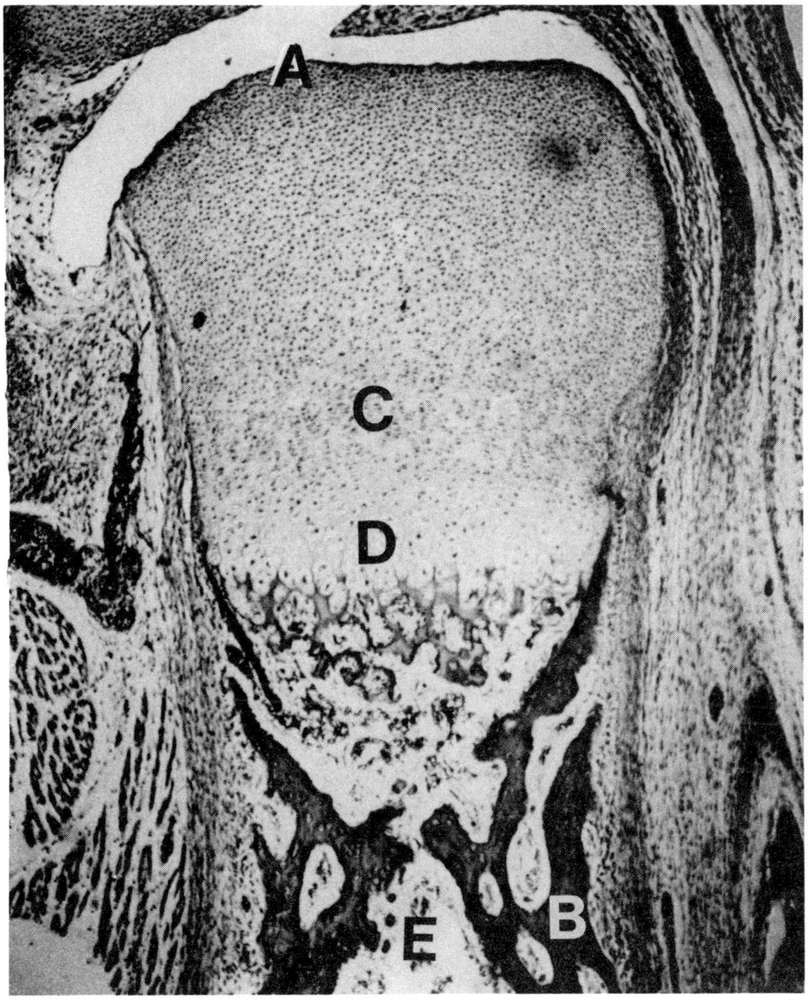

Figure 2.2

5. This structure represents a current site of osteoid deposition.

6. This region contains many chondrocytes actively involved in mitosis.

7. This region contains hypertrophic chondrocytes.

8. This region persists as hyaline cartilage even in the adult bone of the appendicular skeleton.

Items 9-10

Examine **Figure 2.3** below, a labeled light micrograph and then choose the most appropriate description of the morphology or functional role of the labeled structure.

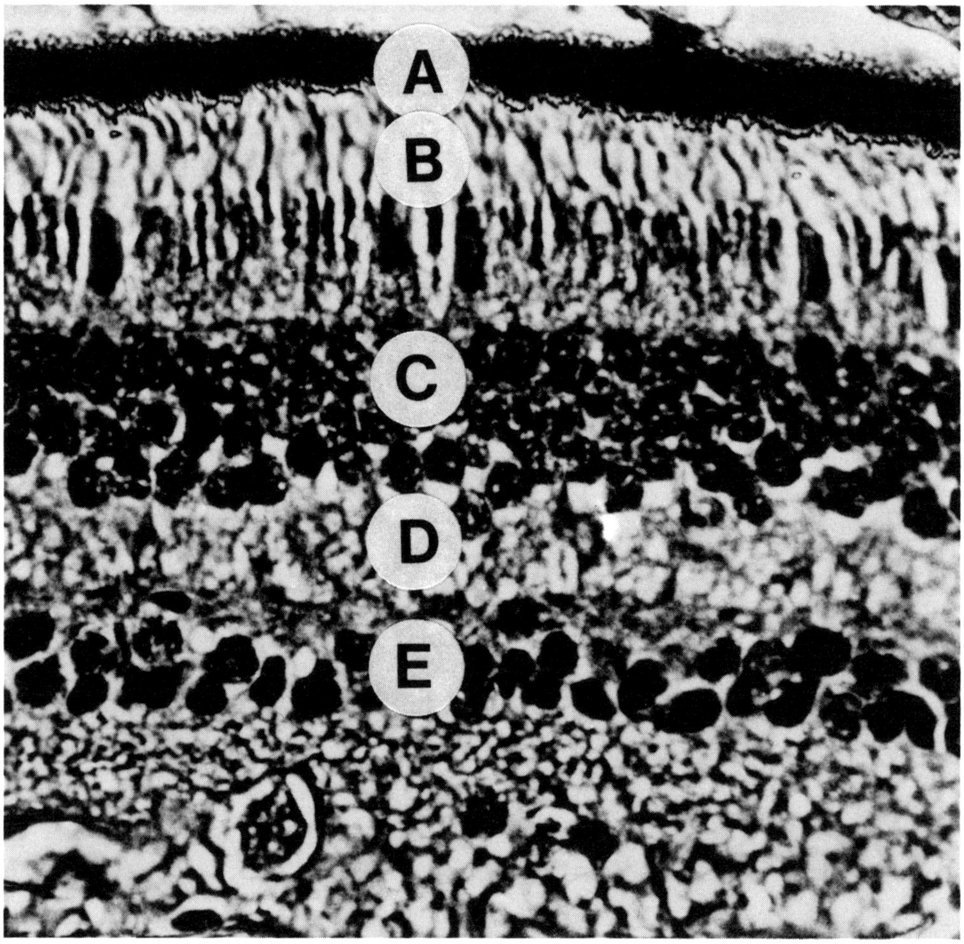

Figure 2.3

9. This structure is rich in melanin. The apical surfaces of epithelial cells here phagocytose the apical portion of effete rod and cone outer segments.

10. This structure contains neuronal processes connecting rods and cones to bipolar cell.

Items 11-14

Examine **Figure 2.4** below, a transmission electron micrograph, and then choose the correct answer.

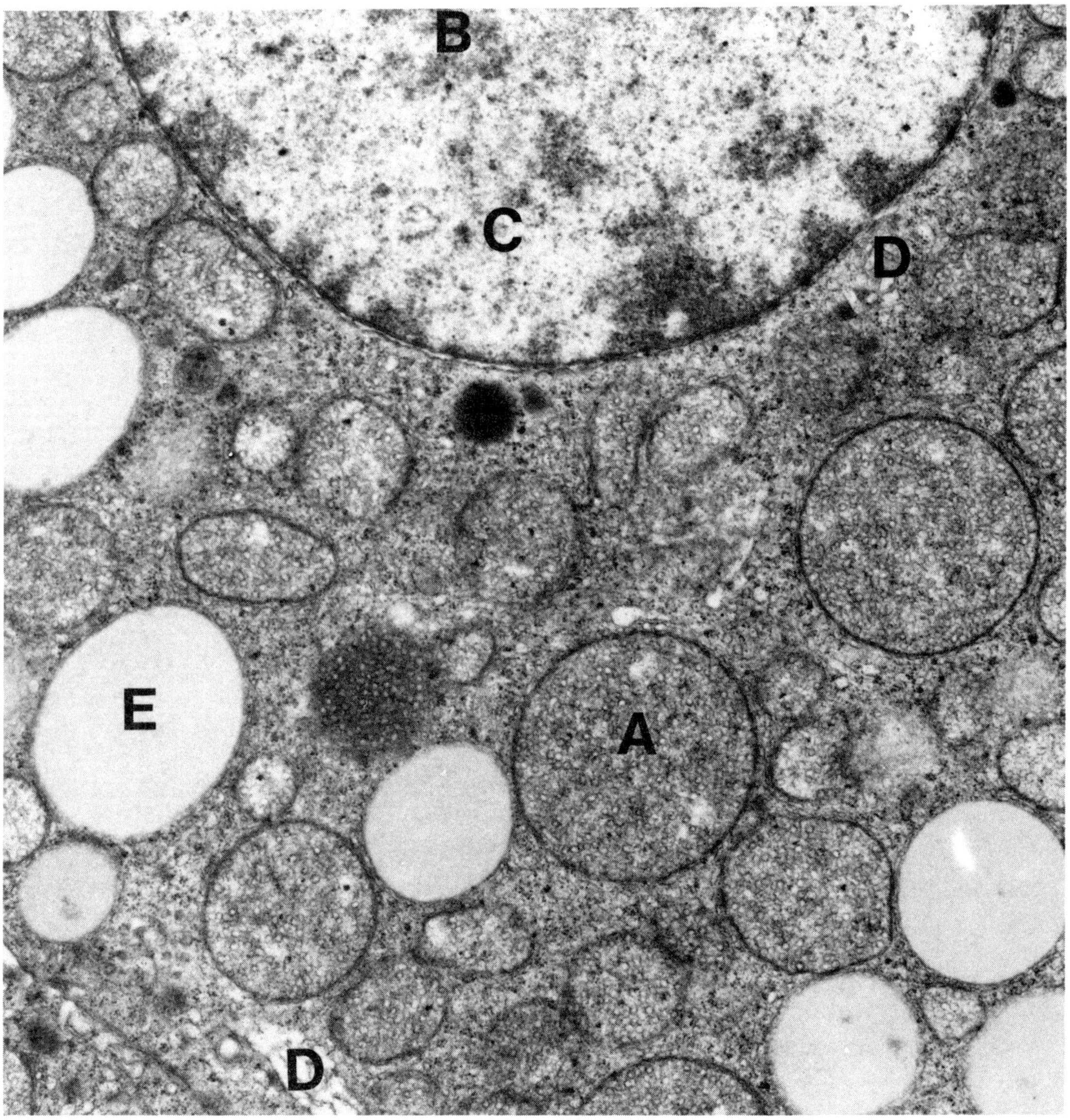

Figure 2.4

11. Which physiological function is most characteristic of a cell with this ultrastructure?

    (A) mucus secretion
    (B) zymogen granule production
    (C) steroid synthesis
    (D) glycogen storage
    (E) motility

12. This kind of a cell would be most prominent in which anatomical location?

    (A) gastric mucosa
    (B) pancreatic acini
    (C) adrenal cortex
    (D) liver parenchyma
    (E) wall of the urinary bladder

For each physiological function, select the corresponding labeled structure in **Figure 2.4**.

13. Site of storage of cholesterol esters, precursors for the steroid secretion products of this cell.

14. Produces ATP and is involved in steroid biosynthesis.

Items 15-17

A 55-year-old alcoholic male shows hemorrhages near the base of hair follicles and swollen gingivae around his teeth. He has cutaneous lesions that have healed poorly. A fractured toe has not healed properly after 3 months. Histological examination of the lesions reveals extensive granulation tissue with few collagen fibers. A diagnosis of scurvy is made.

15. The cells most affected in this patient are

    (A) liver parenchymal cells
    (B) osteoclasts
    (C) fibroblasts
    (D) plasma cells
    (E) eosinophils

16. This patient's condition is a defect in

    (A) elastin biosynthesis
    (B) tropocollagen biosynthesis
    (C) collagen cross-linking
    (D) laminin polymerization
    (E) fibronectin binding

17. The most accurate description of the fundamental lesion involved in the etiology of this dietary deficiency is

    (A) deficient synthesis of collagen alpha-chains
    (B) leakage of capillaries
    (C) decreased cross-linkage at desmosyl residues
    (D) increased hydrolysis of tropocollagen telopeptides
    (E) increased collagen turnover

Items 18-21

Examine **Figure 2.5** below, a scanning electron micrograph of a fractured specimen of liver. Match the labeled structure in the micrograph with the most appropriate microscopic anatomical or functional description of the labeled structure.

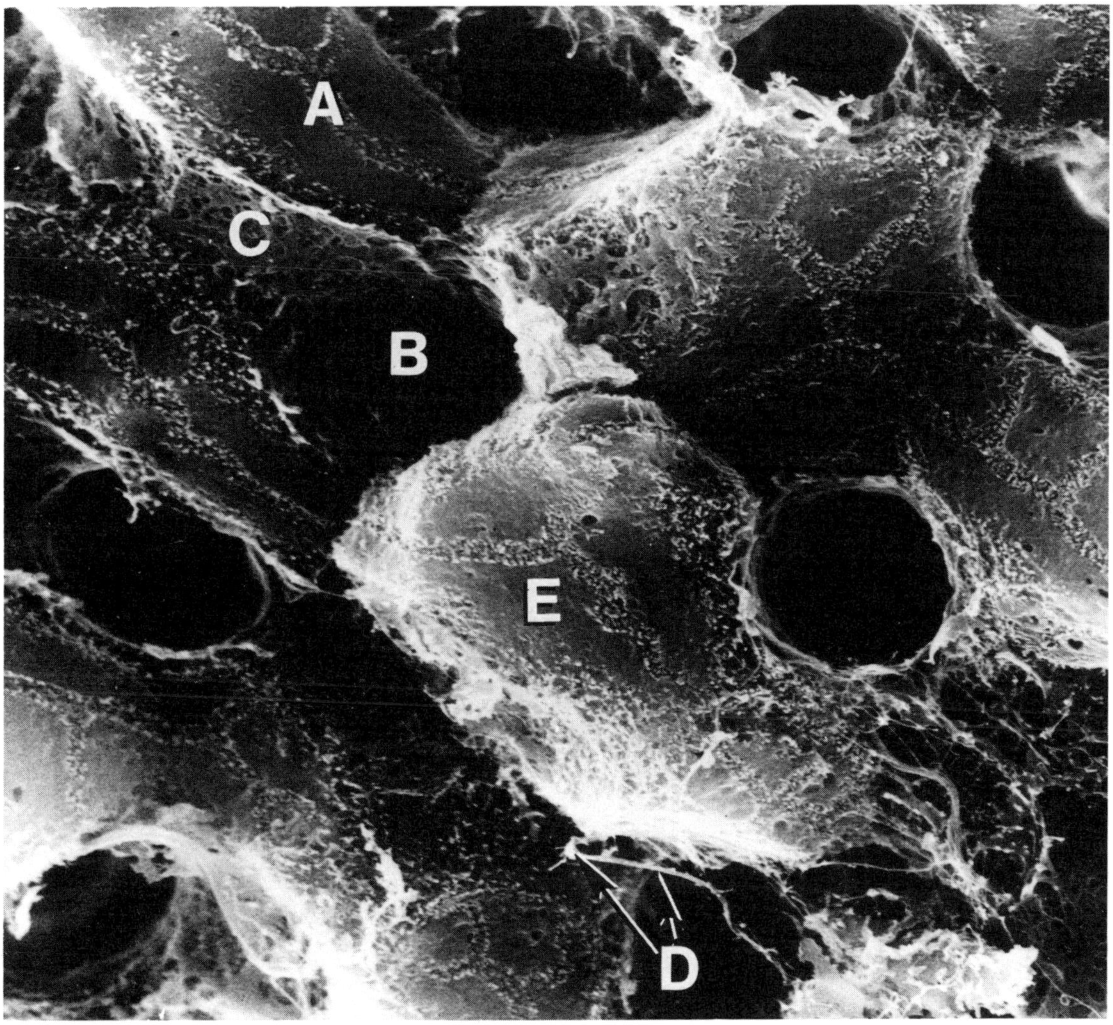

Figure 2.5

18. This structure receives blood from branches of the portal vein in the portal triads.

19. Liver parenchymal cells are joined by tight junctions at this structure to produce a blood-bile barrier.

20. This cell type is involved in synthesis of serum albumin and detoxification.

21. These endothelial cells form fenestrated and discontinuous capillaries.

Items 22-24

Examine **Figure 2.6** below, a high power transmission electron micrograph. It is an array of long hollow structures cut perpendicular to their long axis. The diameter of each hollow structure is 25 nm.

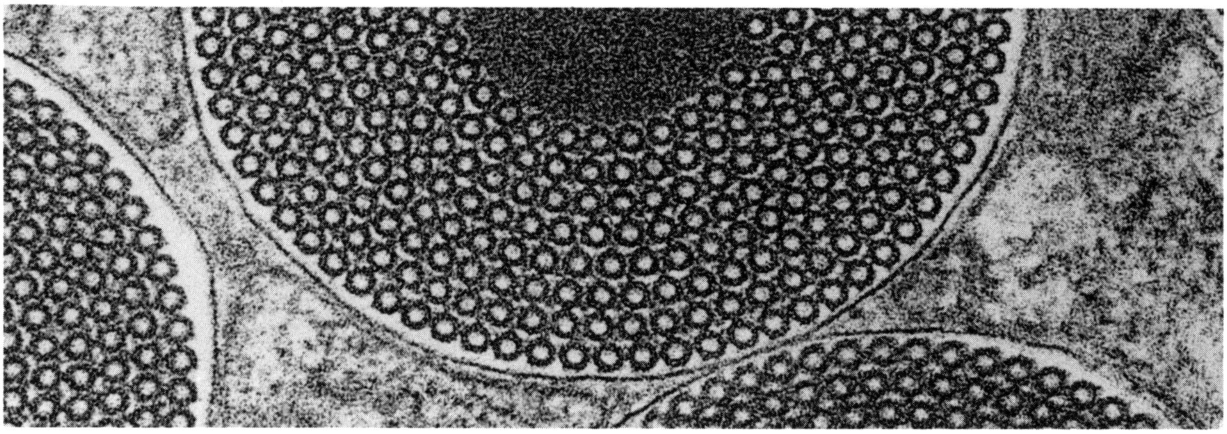

Figure 2.6

22. Each individual circular structure is a

(A) microfilament
(B) ciliary axoneme
(C) microtubule
(D) thick filament of muscle
(E) intermediate filament

23. The most abundant protein found in these structures is

(A) tubulin
(B) actin
(C) keratin
(D) desmin
(E) myosin

24. Which description is most appropriate for these structures?

(A) The thick filaments are composed of aggregates of myosin molecules.
(B) Dynein rich side-arms are involved in their movement.
(C) They consist of globular actin molecules arranged in two intertwined helices with troponin and tropomyosin molecules arrayed along the helix.
(D) They consist of 13 protofilaments composed of alternating α- and β-tubulin subunits arranged like a string of beads.
(E) They are abundant in the cores of microvilli.

Items 25-28

Examine **Figure 2.7** below, a labeled light micrograph, and then choose the most appropriate description of the morphology or functional role of the labeled structures.

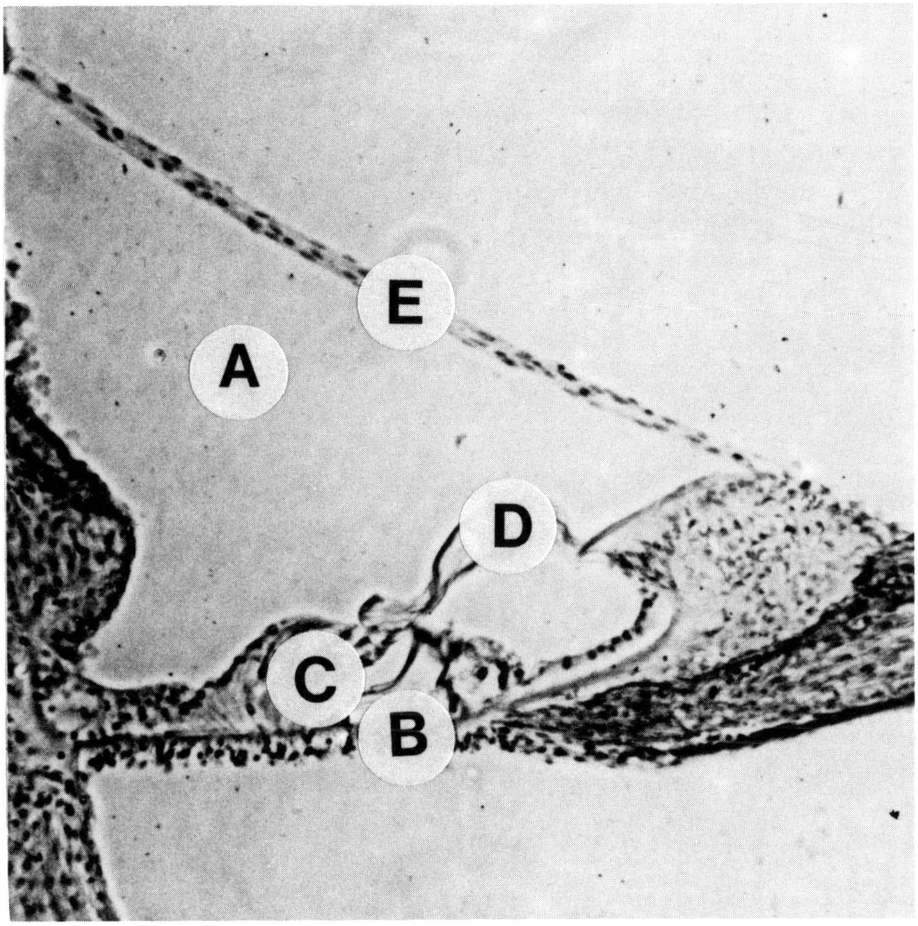

Figure 2.7

25. The apical surfaces of hair cells contact this structure.

26. This structure contains a blood filtrate which is produced in the stria vascularis and resorbed in the endolymphatic sac.

27. The apical projections from this structure are highly modified microvilli.

28. Basilar fibers are located in this structure.

Items 29-32

Examine **Figure 2.8** below, a scanning electron micrograph of fractured tissue, and then answer the questions.

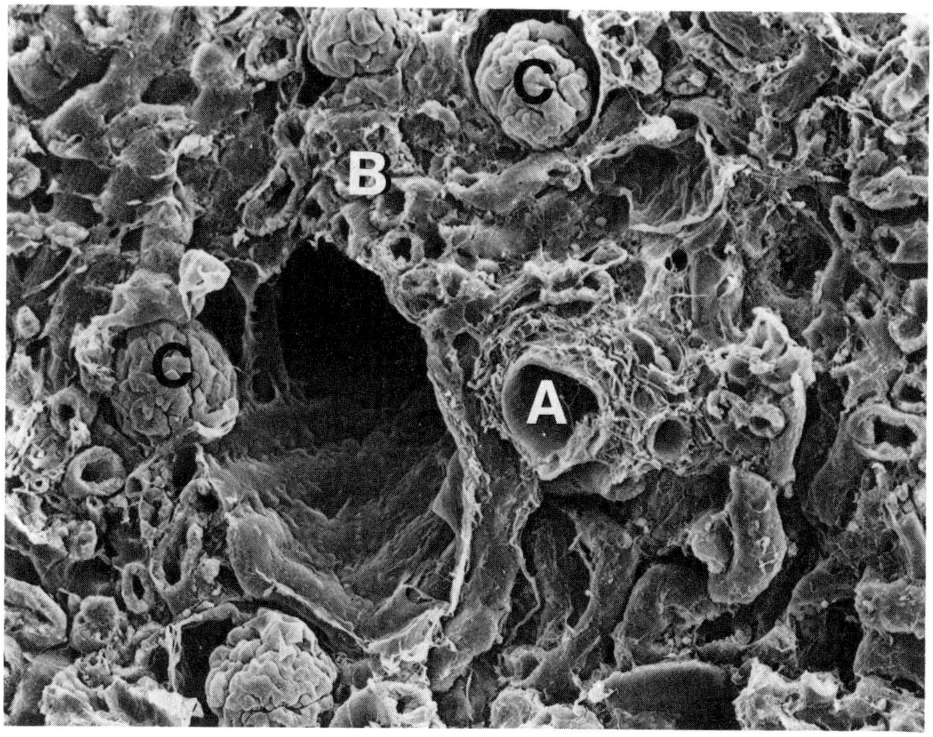

Figure 2.8

29. Structure A contains which of the following fluids?

    (A) blood
    (B) lymph
    (C) bile
    (D) dilute urine
    (E) cerebrospinal fluid

30. Structure B has which of the following physiological roles?

    (A) urine concentration
    (B) nutrient and waste transport
    (C) oxygen and CO_2 transport
    (D) bile transport
    (E) chylomicron transport

31. Structure C has which of the following physiological roles?

    (A) nutrient absorption
    (B) hormone synthesis
    (C) blood filtration to remove nitrogenous wastes
    (D) gas transport
    (E) lymphocyte transport

32. This morphological arrangement is found in the

    (A) adrenal cortex
    (B) liver parenchyma
    (C) brain parenchyma
    (D) thymic cortex
    (E) renal cortex

Items 33-35

Examine **Figure 2.9** below, a high power light micrograph of a mature ovarian follicle, and then choose the most appropriate labeled structure to match the functional role or morphological description of that structure.

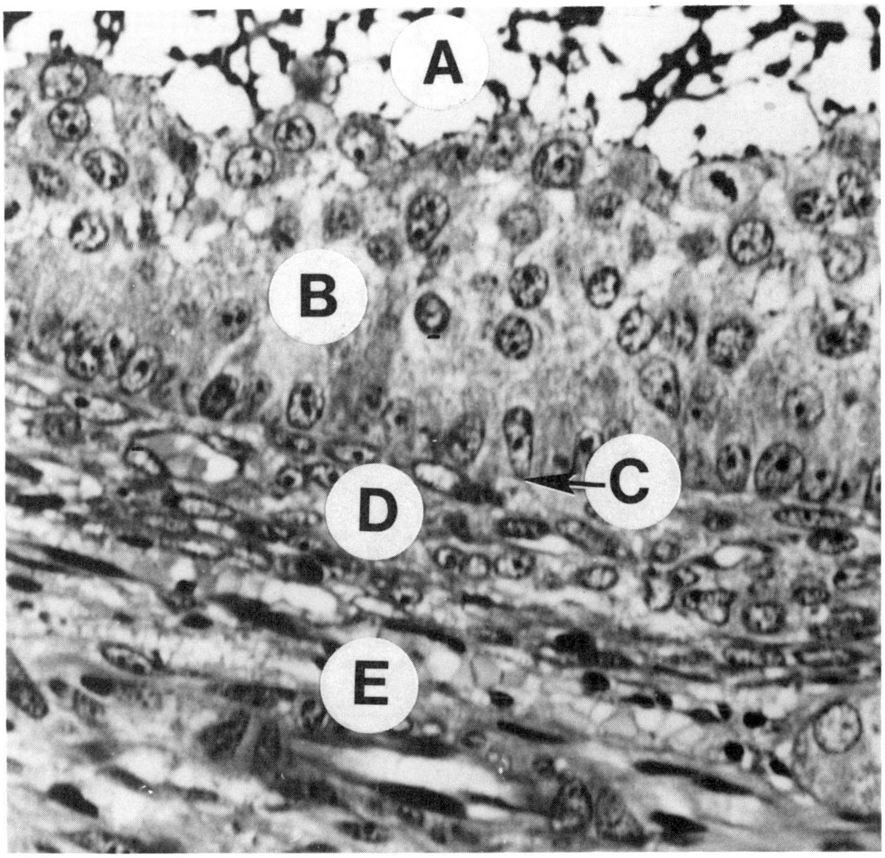

Figure 2.9

33. This structure is rich in laminin and is the outer boundary of the follicular epithelium.

34. These cells secrete androstenedione, an estradiol precursor.

35. These cells secrete liquor folliculi and the zona pellucida before ovulation and steroids after ovulation.

Items 36-39

For each statement of structure, function or embryological origin, select the most appropriate structure in **Figure 2.10** below, a photomicrograph.

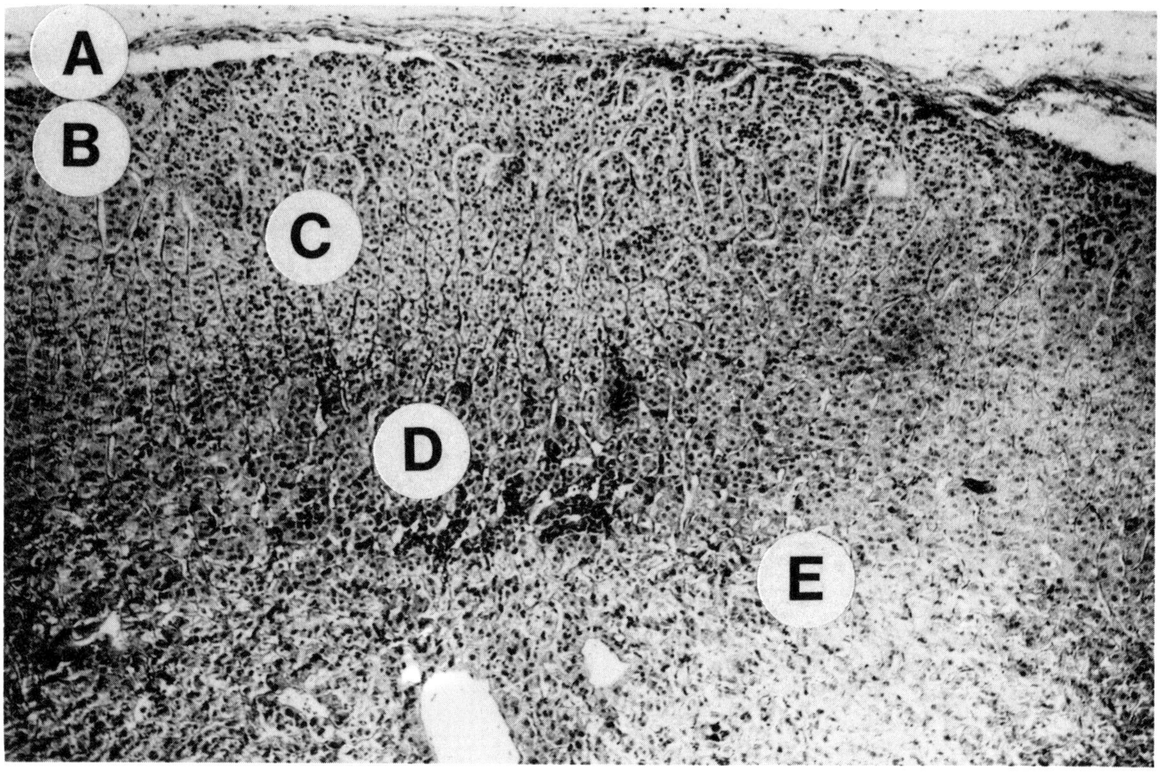

Figure 2.10

36. This structure is derived from the neural crest.

37. This structure has abundant smooth endoplasmic reticulum, mitochondria with tubular cristae and an abundance of large lipid droplets.

38. This structure secretes mineralocorticoids.

39. This structure secretes sex steroids and is derived from the lining of the primitive coelomic cavity.

Item 40

40. Which of the following membranes has the highest ratio of lipid-to-protein?

    (A) red cell membrane
    (B) myelin
    (C) Golgi membranes
    (D) rough endoplasmic reticulum
    (E) outer mitochondrial membrane

Items 41-48

For each numbered biochemical description of an extracellular matrix molecule or its receptor, choose the most appropriate lettered molecule. Answers may be used once, more than once, or not at all.

(A) Collagen
(B) Fibronectin
(C) Laminin
(D) Chondroitin sulfate
(E) Heparan sulfate
(F) Hyaluronic acid
(G) Integrin
(H) Elastin
(I) Fibrillin

41. This molecule is composed of subunits assembled into a cruciform aggregate. It binds to heparan sulfate, proteoglycan and type IV collagen. It is an essential structural component of many basement membranes.

42. This molecule is a glycosaminoglycan that has a MW = 1,000,000 or more. It forms the backbone of cartilage proteoglycan aggregates.

43. This molecule typically has approximately 1/3 of its amino acids as glycine and is also rich in proline. In some cases, it forms striated fibrillar aggregates.

44. This molecule forms anastomosing molecular chains. Upon hydrolysis, it releases the unusual amino acid desmosine.

45. This molecule is an important cell adhesion protein. It has a MW = 460,000 and contains two separate polypeptides chains of MW = 230,000 cross-linked by -S-S- bridges.

46. This molecule is a heterodimeric transmembrane glycoprotein. Different forms exist for recognition of fibronectin and laminin.

47. This molecule is a glycosaminoglycan with a repeating disaccharide containing N-acetyl-D-galactosamine and D-glucuronic acid.

48. This is the most abundant protein in the human body.

Items 49-54

For each numbered statement of function described in the items below, choose the most appropriate lettered component of the junctional complex or associated structure. Answers may be used once, more than once, or not at all.

(A) Tight junction (zonula occludens)
(B) Adhesive junction (zonula adherens)
(C) Desmosome (macula adherens)
(D) Hemidesmosome
(E) Gap junction (nexus)
(F) Microfilaments
(G) Tonofilaments
(H) Microtubules

49. This structure consists of a hexagonal array of aqueous channels between cells. These pores allow free passage of ions so that adjacent cells are electrically coupled. Small regulatory molecules such as cyclic nucleotides can also pass through these structures.

50. This structure is thought to hold cells together. It consists of paired electron-dense plaques on the cytoplasmic faces of apposed membranes. Anchoring intermediate filaments rich in keratin insert into these plaques.

51. The outer leaflets of the plasma membranes of adjacent cells come into direct contact. It forms a functional seal between a luminal and adluminal compartment.

52. F-actin is the most abundant and functionally important constituent of these structures.

53. These structures attach epithelial cells to their subjacent basement membranes.

54. The part of the junctional complex most directly responsible for minimizing fluid flow between epithelial cells.

Items 55-57

Examine **Figure 2.11** below, a transmission electron micrograph, and then choose the best response to the items below.

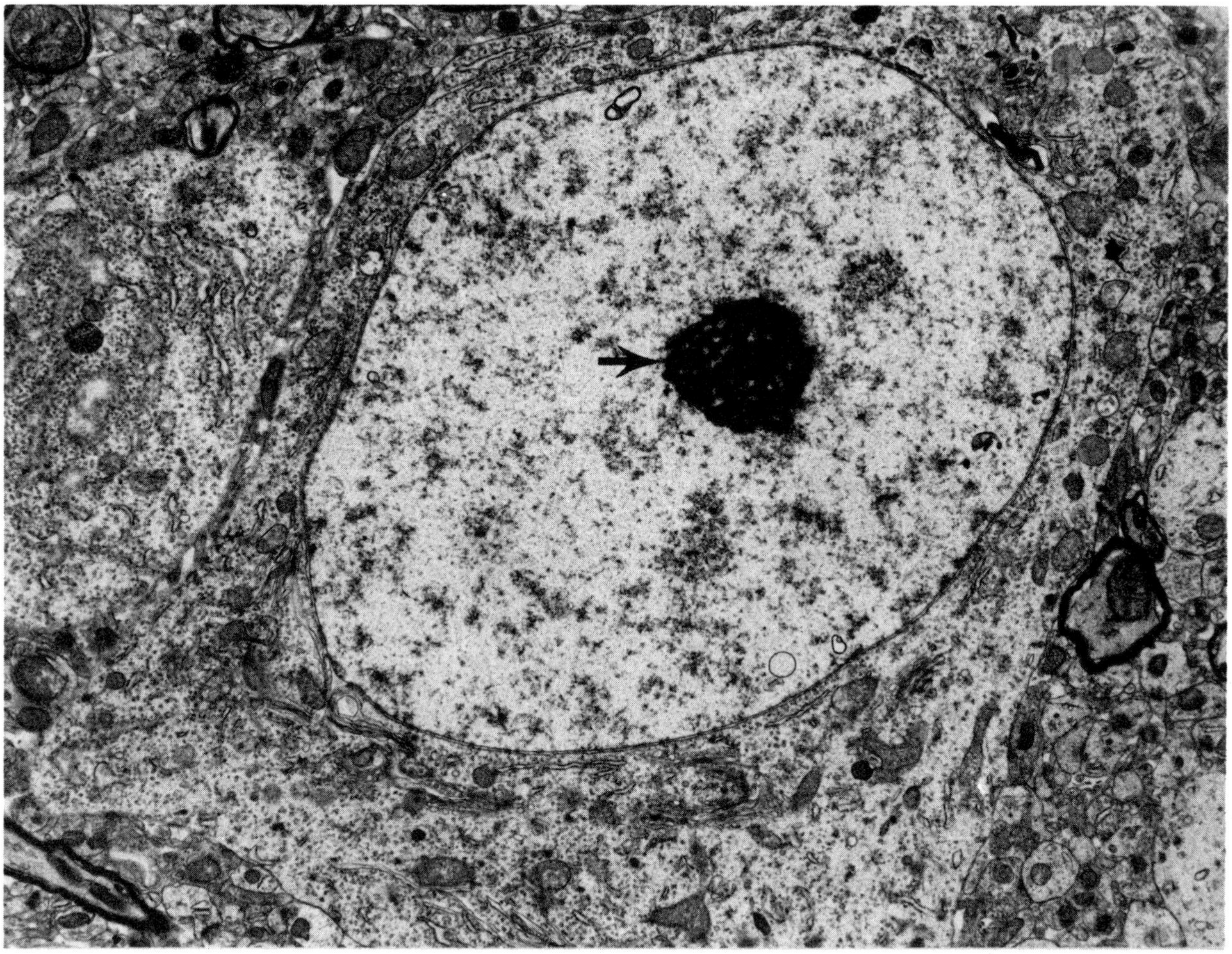

Figure 2.11

55. The chief function of the structure at the pointer is

(A) ribosomal RNA synthesis
(B) storage of inactive DNA
(C) transport of mRNA out of the nucleus
(D) boundary between nucleus and cytoplasm
(E) attachment site for spindle microtubules

56. This structure is most obvious during which portion of the cell cycle?

(A) interphase
(B) mitosis
(C) prophase
(D) telophase
(E) anaphase

57. This structure would be most metabolically active in which type of cell?

(A) one actively engaged in phagocytosis
(B) one actively engaged in steroid biosynthesis
(C) one actively engaged in protein synthesis
(D) one actively engaged in contraction
(E) an erythrocyte

Items 58-60

Examine **Figure 2.12** below, a transmission electron micrograph, and then choose the best response to the items that follow.

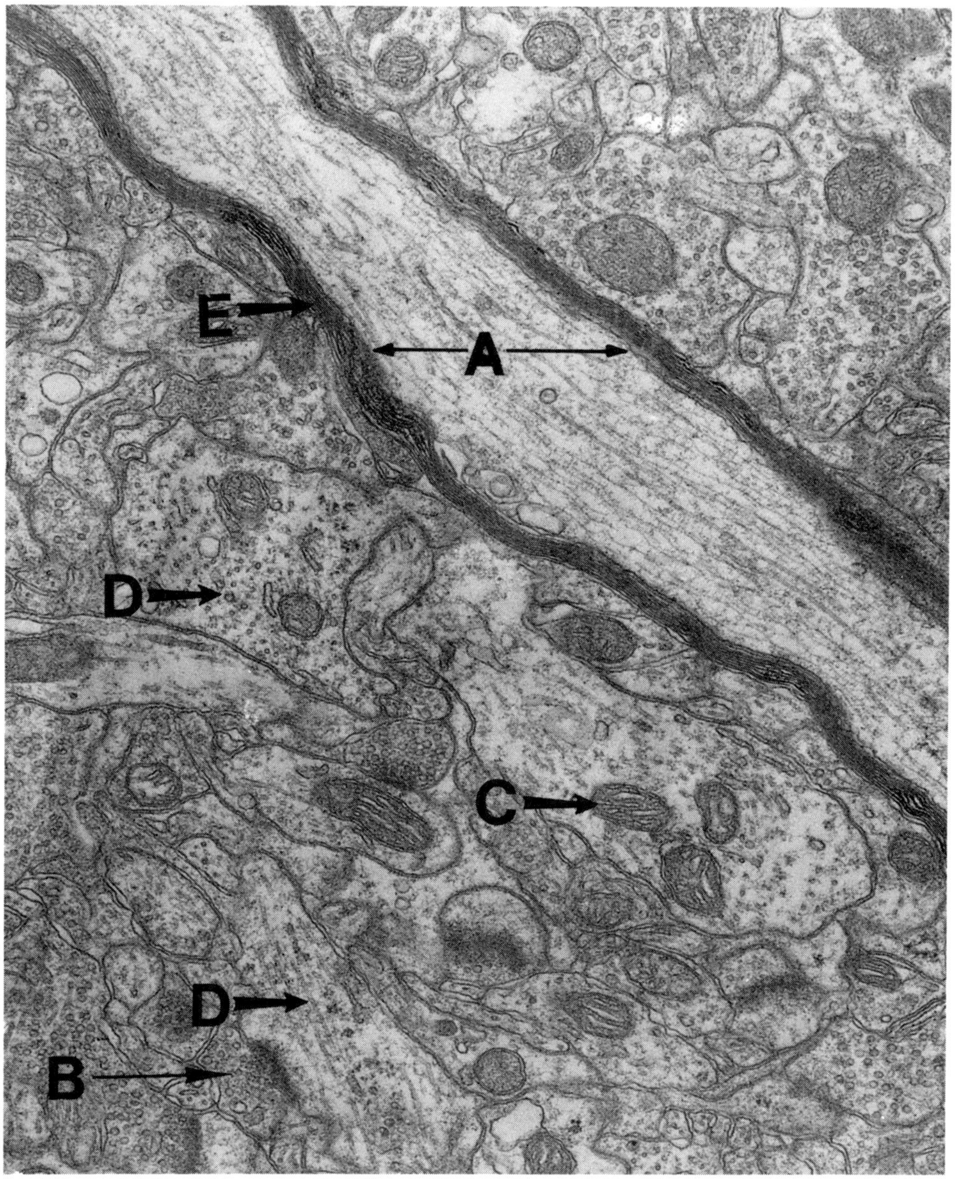

Figure 2.12

58. The elongate cellular projection labeled A is a

(A) flagellum
(B) nerve axon
(C) pseudopodium
(D) cilium
(E) microvillus

59. Structure labeled C is

(A) Golgi apparatus
(B) peroxisomes
(C) microtubules
(D) mitochondria
(E) secondary lysosomes

60. Structures labeled D are

(A) Golgi apparatus
(B) peroxisomes
(C) microtubules
(D) mitochondria
(E) secondary lysosomes

Items 61-62

Examine **Figure 2.13** below, a scanning electron micrograph of the apical surfaces on the epithelial cells lining the trachea. For each numbered item below, choose the one best answer.

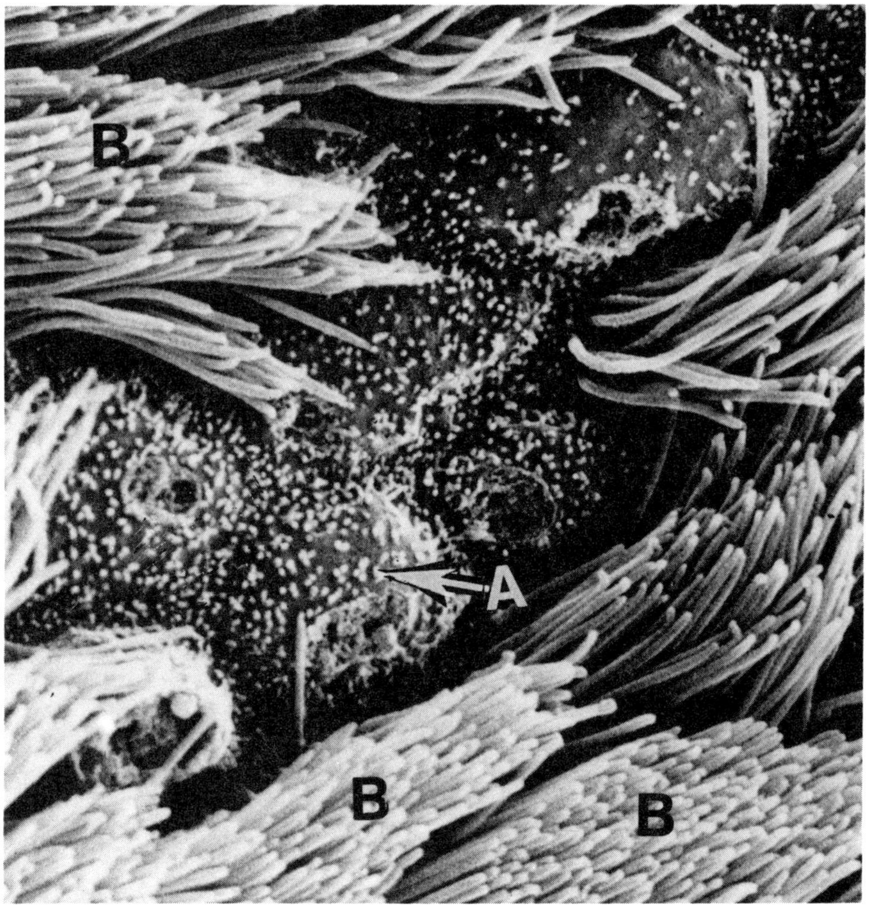

Figure 2.13

61. The structures labeled A are

    (A) cilia
    (B) flagella
    (C) microvilli
    (D) microtubules
    (E) collagen fibers

62. The structures labeled B are

    (A) cilia
    (B) flagella
    (C) microvilli
    (D) microfilaments
    (E) collagen fibers

Items 63-67

Examine **Figure 2.14** below, a transmission electron micrograph of skeletal muscle. Match the labeled structure in the micrograph with the most appropriate description of its microscopic anatomy or physiological role.

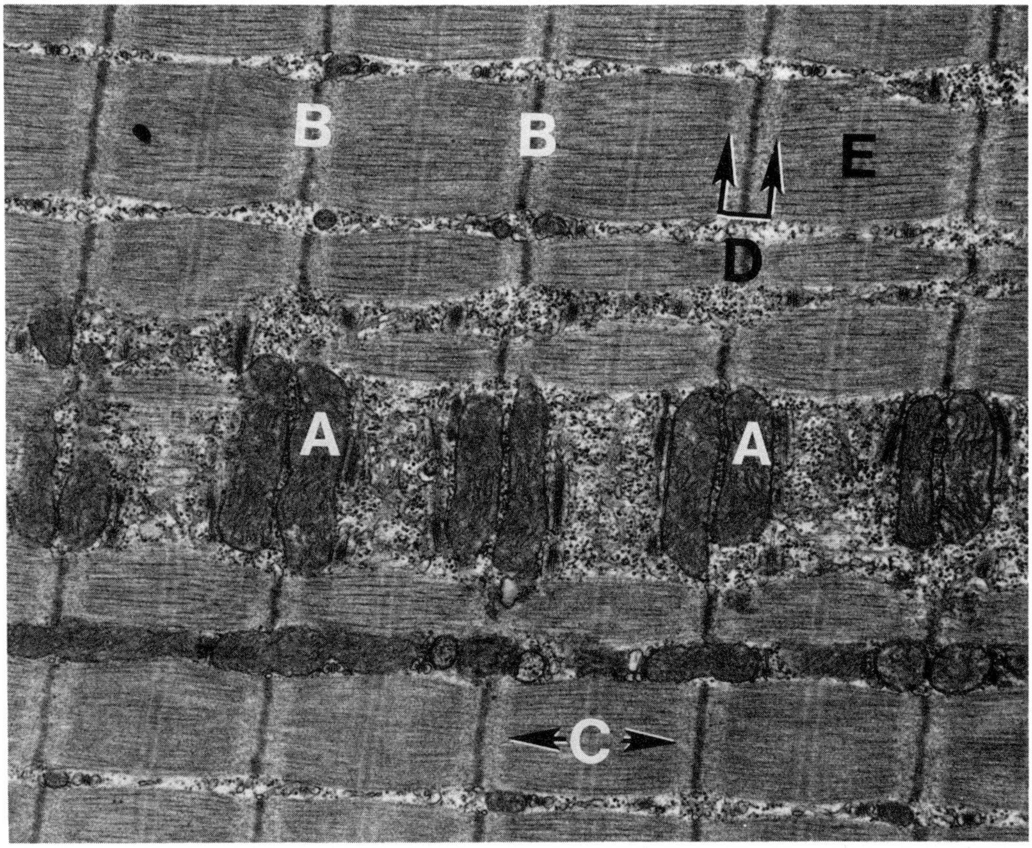

Figure 2.14

63. These structures are the ends of individual sarcomeres. They are regions rich in α-actinin.

64. These structures are regions of overlap between actin-rich thin filaments and myosin-rich thick filaments.

65. These structures produce ATP, which is hydrolyzed to provide the energy for muscle contraction.

66. These structures are regions rich in actin-containing thin filaments where there is no overlap between thin and thick filaments.

67. These structures are regions rich in myosin-containing thick filaments where there is no overlap between thick and thin filaments.

Items 68-70

The 8-year-old daughter of Jewish parents whose grandparents were born in Russia has hepatosplenomegaly and painful bone lesions. Urinalysis reveals high levels of the neutral sphingolipid, 1-β-glucoceramide.

68. The most likely diagnosis is

    (A) Tay-Sachs disease
    (B) Gaucher's disease
    (C) Fabry's disease
    (D) Niemann-Pick disease
    (E) Hurler's syndrome

69. The intracellular organelle most effected by this disease is the

    (A) mitochondrion
    (B) centriole
    (C) lysosome
    (D) rough endoplasmic reticulum
    (E) Golgi apparatus

70. Which enzyme is altered in this disease?

    (A) glucocerebrosidase
    (B) glucuronidase
    (C) gangliosidase
    (D) galactosyltransferase
    (E) chymotrypsin

Items 71-74

Examine **Figure 2.15** below, a diagrammatic view of a cell as seen in the transmission electron microscope. The black material in the upper left of the diagram is calcified extracellular matrix.

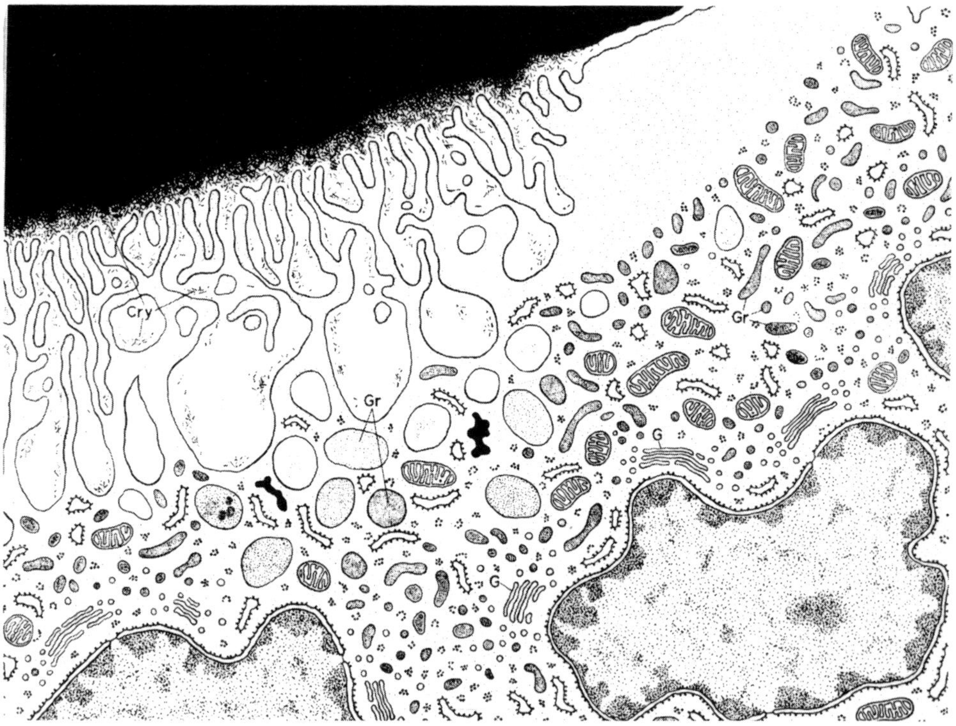

Figure 2.15

71. This cell is a/an

(A) bone marrow stem cell
(B) osteoblast
(C) fibroblast
(D) osteoclast
(E) nerve cell

72. The highly irregular surface of this cell is best described as

(A) microvilli
(B) stereocilia
(C) a ruffled membrane
(D) canaliculi
(E) fascia adherens

73. This cell is LEAST LIKELY to be involved in

(A) active transport of Cl^- out of the cell
(B) creation of an acidic environment to solubilize Ca^{2+} from mineralized matrix
(C) phagocytosis
(D) proliferation
(E) motility

74. Which of the following other cell types in the human body is most similar in structure and function to the cell shown in **Figure 2.15**?

(A) plasma cell
(B) erythrocyte
(C) goblet cell
(D) CNS neuron
(E) gastric parietal cell

Items 75-77

Various cytokines serve crucial roles in the maturation and stimulation of different cellular subpopulations. Match the cytokine in the answers with the most appropriate description of its primary function in the items below.

(A) IL-1
(B) IL-2
(C) IL-3
(D) IL-4
(E) IL-5
(F) IL-6
(G) IL-7
(H) IL-8
(I) IL-9
(J) IL-10
(K) Gamma interferon (INF- γ)
(L) Transforming growth factor- β

75. Produced by helper T cells, enhances both class I and class II MHC expression, also promotes immunoglobulin switching to IgG and IgE, in mice.

76. Produced by many cell types such as B cells, macrophages, and monocytes, enhances natural killer cell activation and stimulates helper T cell activation.

77. Produced by platelets, lymphocytes and macrophages, attracts other macrophages and monocytes, induces IL-1 production.

Items 78-81

A 7-year-old African-American girl is diagnosed with a kind of hemolytic anemia. **Figure 2.16** below shows a scanning electron micrograph (upper) and a transmission electron micrograph (lower) of her erythrocytes.

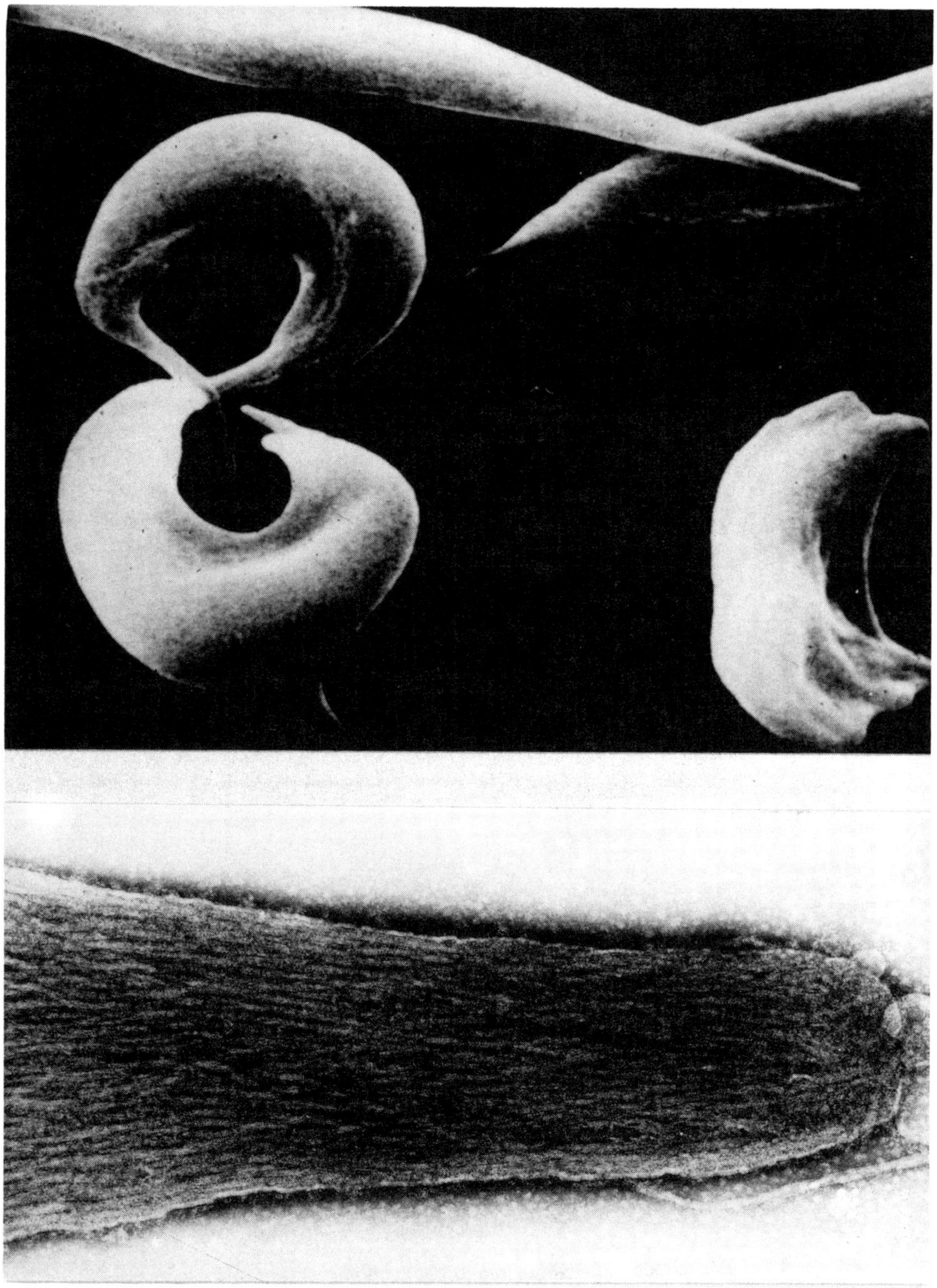

Figure 2.16

78. The most likely diagnosis of her condition is

(A) hereditary spherocytosis
(B) hereditary elliptocytosis
(C) sickle cell anemia
(D) α-thalassemia
(E) β-thalassemia

79. The fibrillar structures in the lower micrograph contain predominantly

(A) spectrin
(B) hemoglobin
(C) actin
(D) glucose-6-phosphate dehydrogenase
(E) glycophorin

80. The gene defect in this disease has what primary effect on Hb?

(A) increases catabolism
(B) increases solubility
(C) increases dissociation
(D) decreases solubility, especially of deoxyHb
(E) decreases catabolism

81. All of the following physiologic states would favor formation of fibrillar structures in her erythrocytes EXCEPT

(A) increase in Hb concentration
(B) decrease in serum P_{O_2}
(C) increase in concentration of deoxyHb
(D) respiratory acidosis
(E) hyperventilation

Items 82-84

An 18-year-old African-American from a small town in Alabama is seen at a rural clinic because of a broken radius, apparently suffered during a friendly bout of arm wrestling with his older sister. Physical examination reveals several poorly healed fractures. The young man confirms their occurrence and comments that a 40-year-old uncle has similar problems related to "clumsiness." Also, the youth has reduced hearing and his sclera are somewhat blue.

82. This patient is suffering from

(A) scurvy
(B) battered child syndrome
(C) chondromalacia
(D) osteogenesis imperfecta
(E) Marfan's syndrome

83. The most relevant finding upon analysis of a sample of bony tissue would likely be

(A) reduced levels of collagen type I in the extracellular matrix
(B) Haversian canals filed with crystals of hydroxyapatite
(C) numerous deposits of lead sulfate
(D) unusually high concentrations of elastin
(E) elevated concentrations of fibronectin

84. Testing of the uncle reveals the same defect as the patient. This is consistent with the diagnosis because

(A) the syndrome is linked to the Y chromosome
(B) such disorders are autosomal dominant
(C) the defect is usually found in men who play many sports
(D) impoverished families often have dietary deficiencies
(E) the condition only appears long after puberty

Items 85-88

The parents of a 6-year-old boy report that he has had repeated respiratory tract infections and persistent wheezing and coughing. The parents are of Swedish and German heritage and are healthy. The child shows elevated levels of salt in his sweat and thick respiratory mucous secretions. The child also shows pancreatic insufficiency due to obstruction of the pancreatic duct by mucus.

85. The most likely diagnosis of this child's condition is

    (A) cystic fibrosis
    (B) duodenal atresia
    (C) tetralogy of Fallot
    (D) biliary atresia
    (E) Tay-Sachs disease

86. This disease is caused by which genetic mechanism?

    (A) autosomal dominant gene
    (B) sex-linked recessive gene
    (C) autosomal recessive gene
    (D) translocation
    (E) deletion

87. The protein primarily altered by different alleles of the affected gene in this disease is

    (A) hexosaminidase A
    (B) β-glucuronidase
    (C) glucocerebrosidase
    (D) α-amylase
    (E) transmembrane conductance regulator

88. Cells from patients with this disease would show which response to elevated levels of adenosine 3′,5′-monophosphate?

    (A) normal increase in Na^+ efflux
    (B) lack of normal increase in Cl^- efflux
    (C) down regulation of steroid receptors
    (D) up regulation of steroid receptors
    (E) increase in gluconeogenesis

Items 89-92

A 12-year-old boy is seen by his pediatrician with numerous freckles and depigmented areas on his face and hands. Closer examination reveals numerous basal cell carcinomas on his face. This child also has a long history of photophobia and currently has severe conjunctivitis.

89. The most likely diagnosis of this disease is

    (A) malignant melanoma
    (B) vitamin D deficiency
    (C) xeroderma pigmentosum
    (D) shingles
    (E) psoriasis

90. The basic cellular mechanism that is DEFECTIVE in this disease is

    (A) excision repair of damaged DNA
    (B) activation of oncogenes by chemical carcinogens
    (C) collagen cross-linking
    (D) viral infection of epidermis, causing cell death
    (E) RNA transcription

91. Ultraviolet light induces which change in DNA?

    (A) excision of pyrimidines
    (B) formation of thymine dimers
    (C) substitution of purines for pyrimidines
    (D) frame shift mutations
    (E) nonsense mutations

92. The mutation causing this disease is

    (A) in enzymes for excision repair
    (B) autosomal dominant
    (C) sex-linked recessive
    (D) sex-linked dominant
    (E) pleiotropic

STOP.

YOU HAVE COMPLETED THIS SECTION.

Notes

Histology and Cell Biology

Answers and Tutorials

Layer's of Retina.

1. Pigment cell Layer
2. Photoreceptor Layer.
3. External limiting membrane
4. Outer nucleer layer
5. Outer plexiform layer
6. Inner nucleer layer
7. Inner plexiform layer
8. Ganglion cell layer
9. Optic nerve layer
10. Internal limiting membrane

ANSWER AND TUTORIAL ON ITEM 1

The answer is: **1-B.** The **testis-determining factor** is a gene product sharing significant homology with other zinc finger proteins, a class of transcription factors. Growth factors and oncogene products are also transcription factors. When the DNA sequence encoding the testis determining factor is deleted from the **Y chromosome**, sex reversal results. A male karyotype and a female phenotype will occur. Conversely, when the DNA sequence encoding for the testis determining factor is translocated from the Y chromosome to the X chromosome, sex reversal will result again. In this instance, a female karyotype and a male phenotype will be associated. The testis determining factor drives the differentiation of the indifferent gonad in the male direction. Differentiation of a testis then directs sexual differentiation in a male direction. Turner's syndrome is caused by a monosomy of the X chromosome (45, X). Klinefelter's syndrome is cause by aneuploidy of sex chromosomes (47, XXY).

ANSWERS AND TUTORIAL ON ITEMS 2-4

The answers are: **2-B; 3-B; 4-C**. **Figure 2.1** is a scanning electron micrograph of the mucosal surface of the **jejunum**, the second-longest component of the small intestine. While some digestion and nutrient absorption occurs in the stomach, most of the digestion and nutrient absorption occurs in the small intestine. The mucosa of the jejunum has a plethora of **villi**. Jejunal villi are long flat structures covered by a simple columnar epithelium consisting of many tall, thin columnar absorptive cells with an apical microvillous brush border. These cells are primarily responsible for absorption of digested nutrients from the lumen of the small intestine. In addition, the jejunal mucosal epithelium has goblet cells interspersed between columnar absorptive cells. Goblet cells secrete a thick coat of mucus that protects the jejunal mucosa from digestion.

ANSWERS AND TUTORIAL ON ITEMS 5-8

The answers are: **5-B; 6-C; 7-D; 8-A**. All bones of the appendicular skeleton as well as vertebrae, the base of the skull, ribs and the sternum are formed by the ossification of cartilaginous models of these bones. This type of bone formation is called **endochondral bone formation**. The bones of the vault of the skull and certain facial bones are formed spontaneously in mesenchyme without a pre-existing cartilaginous model by intramembranous bone formation. During endochondral bone formation, the cartilaginous model grows by mitotic proliferation of chondrocytes in the **zone of proliferation** (C, in **Figure 2.2**) or by addition of new chondrocytes to the outer surface of the growing cartilaginous model. Certain mesenchymal cells in the future metaphysis of the bone differentiate into osteoblasts. These cells secrete an extracellular matrix characteristic of bone which calcifies rapidly, forming a **bony collar** (B) around the cartilage. The nutrient supply of chondrocytes is restricted by the bony collar and they therefore undergo **hypertrophy** (D) and then degenerate and die, leading to the formation of a **marrow cavity** (E). Meanwhile, growth continues in the zone of proliferation. New cartilage is rapidly converted into bone. Once the final size of the bone has been established at puberty, further proliferation of the cartilage is not possible. The hyaline cartilage on the articular surface (A) of these bony models persists as the articular cartilage.

ANSWERS AND TUTORIAL ON ITEMS 9-10

The answers are: **9-A; 10-D**. **Figure 2.3** is a photomicrograph of the photoreceptive portion of the **neural retina**. The innermost layer here consists of the **pigmented retina** (A). This is a simple cuboidal epithelium of melanin-containing pigmented cells. It functions to absorb stray light and also phagocytoses the apical portions of the outer segments of the **rods and cones** (B). The nuclei of the rods and cones are contained in the **outer nuclear layer** (C). Axons of these rods and cones project through the **outer plexiform layer** (D) and synapse with dendrites of bipolar cells, the nuclei of which are found in the **inner nuclear layer** (E) along with the nuclei of Müller cells, horizontal cells and amacrine cells. Müller cells are supportive, tall columnar cells that span much of the thickness of the neural retina. Horizontal cells integrate signals from multiple photoreceptors. Amacrine cells establish contacts between ganglion cells. Their function is poorly understood. Processes extending between the inner nuclear layer and the ganglion cell layer are found in the inner plexiform layer. Ganglion cells have their nuclei in the ganglion cell layer and project axons toward the optic nerve through the optic nerve fiber layer.

Answers and Tutorial on Items 11-14

The answers are: **11-C; 12-C; 13-E; 14-A**. **Figure 2.4** is a transmission electron micrograph of a cell from the **adrenal cortex**. It has an ultrastructure characteristic of cells secreting steroids including an abundance of **smooth endoplasmic reticulum** (D) (not well illustrated here), numerous **lipid droplets** (E), large round **mitochondria** with **tubulovesicular cristae** (A) and small dense bodies. The **nucleolus** (B) in a **nucleus** (C) is prominent. This cell synthesizes cortisol from cholesterol esters stored in lipid droplets (E). Cholesterol is released from the lipid droplets and enters mitochondria where it is converted into pregnenolone. In the smooth endoplasmic reticulum, pregnenolone is converted to progesterone and then 17-deoxycorticosterone, which is finally converted into cortisol by mitochondrial enzymes. The factors controlling the shuttling of different intermediates from lipid droplets to mitochondria to smooth endoplasmic reticulum and back to mitochondria are not well understood. Also, the mechanism of steroid secretion is controversial with most authors favoring direct release of steroids by diffusion. Steroid secreting cells are abundant in the adrenal cortex, in the corpus luteum, in the placenta and in the interstitium of the testis (Leydig cells).

Answers and Tutorial on Items 15-17

The answers are: **15-C; 16-C; 17-E**. **Vitamin C deficiency** results in a disease called **scurvy**. This disease is especially common in alcoholics because of dietary deficiency. Rupture of capillaries leads to follicular and gingival hemorrhages. Wound healing and fracture repair are also unusually slow in scorbutic patients. The granulation tissue at poorly healed wounds would have many fibroblasts, a cell type primarily involved in collagen biosynthesis. Vitamin C is an essential co-factor in enzymatic reactions catalyzing the hydroxylation of prolyl and lysyl residues of collagen. Procollagen molecules without hydroxyproline residues have significant instability in their triple helices and are therefore more susceptible to degradation. In addition, extracellular collagen molecules have few hydroxylysine residues. Their poor cross-linkage renders them more susceptible to turnover. Also, fibroblasts secrete collagen more slowly in the vitamin C deficient state. Bone growth and fracture repair are also abnormal in scurvy.

Answers and Tutorial on Items 18-21

The correct answers are: **18-B; 19-A; 20-E; 21-C**. **Figure 2.5** is a scanning electron micrograph of fractured **liver tissue**. It consists of numerous liver parenchymal cells (E) held together by delicate collagen fibers (D). Liver parenchymal cells are the main, functional, organ-specific cell type of the liver. They are involved in serum protein synthesis, metabolism of lipids and bile salts and detoxification of drugs. Individual liver parenchymal cells are joined together by tight junctions on surfaces facing the bile canaliculi (A). These minute channels convey bile toward the portal canal where they join with hepatic ducts. Cords of liver parenchymal cells are surrounded by sinusoids (B) which convey blood from the portal triads to the central vein of a liver lobule. The endothelial cells (C) lining these sinusoids are arranged in a fenestrated and discontinuous layer and have some phagocytic capacity.

Answers and Tutorial on Items 22-24

The answers are: **22-C; 23-A; 24-D**. **Figure 2.6** is a high power transmission electron micrograph of an array of **microtubules** cut perpendicular to their long axis. Microtubules are long hollow structures with an outside diameter of 25 nm. They consist of 13 protofilaments. Each protofilament consists of alternating subunits of **α- and β-tubulin**. Tubulins have similar molecular weights (55 kD) but are distinct due to subtle chemical differences. In addition to tubulin, microtubules have microtubule associated proteins that are involved in the interaction of microtubules with other cytoskeletal elements. Microtubules are important cytoskeletal structures that are involved in maintenance of cell morphology. They are also important constituents of cilia, flagella, centrioles and the mitotic spindle. Microtubules are important for moving entire cells as well as chromosomes within cells during mitosis.

Answers and Tutorial on Items 25-28

The answers are: **25-D; 26-A; 27-C; 28-B**. **Figure 2.7** is a light micrograph of **the organ of Corti**, the mechanoreceptor in the inner ear responsible for converting vibrations into electrical impulses for sound perception. The organ of Corti resides within an endolymph-filled cavity called the **cochlear duct**

↳ High in K^+

(scala media) (A). Endolymph is a blood filtrate secreted into the cochlear duct at the stria vascularis and resorbed in a diverticulum of the membranous labyrinth called the endolymphatic sac. The organ of Corti rests on the **basilar membrane** (B). Basilar fibers reside in the basilar membrane. Traveling waves of deflection are produced in the basilar membrane by vibrations in the oval window. These waves are damped out at different locations along the basilar membrane depending upon the frequency of the traveling waves, resulting in stimulation of different **hair cells** (C) depending upon the frequency of the sound. Hair cells have long apical microvilli that contact the relatively stationary **tectorial membrane** (D). When the basilar membrane moves the hair cells, their apical microvilli are deformed because they move with respect to the relatively fixed tectorial membrane. These deformations lead to the initiation of action potentials from hair cells. Subsequently, these action potentials are conducted into the brain where they are perceived as sounds. The **vestibular membrane** (E) is the boundary between the cochlear duct and the scala vestibuli. The basilar membrane is the boundary between the cochlear duct and the scala tympani. The scala vestibuli and the scala tympani are continuous with one another. Both are filled with perilymph.

Answers and Tutorial on Items 29-32

The answers are: **29-A; 30-A; 31-C; 32-E**. **Figure 2.8** is a low power scanning electron micrograph of the **renal cortex**. The cortical portion of the kidneys consists of large numbers of **blood vessels** (A), **renal corpuscles** (C) and **tubules** (B). Large branches of the renal arteries carry blood rich in nitrogenous wastes into the afferent arterioles which supply a glomerular capillary tuft in the renal corpuscles. The glomerular capillary tuft resides in a deep invagination of Bowman's capsule, the other portion of the renal corpuscle. Bowman's capsule has a visceral epithelial layer consisting of podocytes and a parietal layer consisting of simple squamous epithelial cells that are continuous with the cuboidal epithelial cells of the proximal convoluted tubule. The glomerular blood filtrate crosses the glomerular basement membrane, passes between the foot processes of podocytes and enters the urinary space of the renal corpuscle. The urinary pole of Bowman's capsule conveys dilute urine into the proximal convoluted tubules where the complex process of recovery of proteins and salts from the blood filtrate begins. As the filtrate passes through the proximal convoluted tubules, loop of Henle, distal convoluted tubules and collecting tubules, the blood filtrate is modified further by recovery of most of the protein that crosses the glomerular basement membrane and by changes in salt and urea concentrations to produce urine.

Answers and Tutorial on Items 33-35

The answers are: **33-C; 34-D; 35-B**. **Figure 2.9** is a high magnification light micrograph of a portion of a mature ovarian follicle and the adjacent thecal and stromal cells associated with this follicle. The follicle is bounded by a **basement membrane** (C). Inside the basement membrane, there are several layers of **granulosa cells** (B). Not shown in this photograph is the oocyte surrounded by a group of granulosa cells known collectively as the cumulus oophorus. The granulosa cells are thought to be involved in supporting the development of the follicle in several ways. First, they proliferate and contribute to the growth of the follicle. Second, they secrete a viscous **liquor folliculi** (A) into a growing follicular antrum. Third, they secrete estradiol synthesized from androstenedione derived from the cells of the **theca interna** (D). After ovulation, the follicle is converted into a steroid secreting corpus luteum. The granulosa cells differentiate into granulosa lutein cells of the corpus luteum. The theca interna cells also contribute to the formation of the corpus luteum by differentiating into theca lutein cells. The steroids secreted by the developing follicle prior to ovulation stimulate the growth of endometrial glands. After ovulation, hormones of the corpus luteum stimulate the secretory activity of endometrial glands in preparation for implantation of the conceptus in the wall of the uterus.

Answers and Tutorial on Items 36-39

The answers are: **36-E; 37-C; 38-B; 39-D**. **Figure 2.10** is a photomicrograph of the human adrenal gland. It is surrounded by a thin **connective tissue capsule** (A). The adrenal cortex (B-D) is derived from proliferation of the mesodermally derived coelomic epithelium and consists of three layers of cells. The outer layer is the **zona glomerulosa** (B). It is a source of mineralocorticoids. The middle and thickest layer is the **zona fasciculata** (C). It consists of long, straight epithelial cords of epithelial cells arranged between long sinusoids. The cortical cells all have an abundance of smooth endoplasmic reticulum and mitochondria with tubular cristae, ultrastructural features common to all steroid secreting cells. The cells of the zona fasciculata have a foamy appearance in the light microscope due to a profusion of large lipid rich vacuoles. They secrete glucocorticoids. The cells of the **zona reticularis** (D) secrete sex steroids. The **adrenal medulla** (E) is derived from the neural crest and consists of two populations of secretory cells, one secreting epinephrine and the other secreting norepinephrine.

Answer and Tutorial on Item 40

The answer is: **40-B**. **Cellular membranes** are **lipid-protein bilayers**, consisting of a core bilayer of lipids with which various proteins are associated. The **hydrophobic** tails of the **amphipathic** lipids forming the core of the bilayer associate with one another by hydrophobic interactions. These core lipids are weakly associated with one another within the plane of the membrane; hence, while the bilayer membrane strongly resists separation in a direction perpendicular to the membrane plane, lipid-lipid and lipid-protein associations are relatively labile (fluid) within the plane of the membrane.

Proteins that are specifically associated with membranes may be loosely bound, bound firmly via electrostatic interactions, or so tightly bound that they can only be released by treatment with detergents that completely dissolve the membrane. Proteins that can only be released by detergent treatment are referred to as **integral membrane proteins.** In many cases, such integral membrane proteins extend from one side of the membrane to the other side. Such **transmembrane proteins** are frequently responsible for selective transport of specific hydrophilic molecules across the membrane, thus facilitating passage of such molecules through the hydrophobic lipid bilayer core. The plasma membrane surrounds each cell and is the boundary between the external and the internal environments of the cell.

Deep within cells, there are other (intracellular) membranous systems, including the **rough and smooth endoplasmic reticulum**, the **Golgi apparatus** and the **nuclear envelope**. Individual intracellular organelles such as **lysosomes** are also surrounded by membranes. **Mitochondria** have an **outer membrane** which compartmentalizes the organelle from the cytoplasm. The outer mitochondrial membrane surrounds an **inner mitochondrial membrane**.

The **red cell membrane** is one of the most well characterized plasma membranes. In general, integral membrane proteins span the entire thickness of the plasma membrane and can not be released from their associated lipids without strong detergent treatment or solvent extraction of membranes. They often have a carbohydrate rich portion on the external surface, a middle region rich in hydrophobic amino acids which interact strongly with the hydrophobic domain of membrane lipids and a second hydrophilic domain on the internal (cytoplasmic) surface. The inner hydrophilic domain often interacts with cytoskeletal proteins in the cytoplasmic domain. In the red blood cell, **glycophorin** is an integral membrane glycoprotein of unknown function. **Band 3** is a another integral membrane protein. It interacts strongly with the cytoskeletal protein ankyrin and may be involved in facilitating diffusion of anions across the plasma membrane. **Glucose translocase** is an integral membrane protein that actively transports glucose into red blood cells. **Spectrin** is a cytoplasmic protein that interacts with both glycophorin and band 3 protein; spectrin is thought to have a cytoskeletal function, strengthening the cortex of erythrocytes. **Ankyrin** stabilizes the interaction between spectrin and band 3 protein.

Membrane lipids consist largely of **phosphoglycerides**, **sphingomyelin**, **cholesterol** and "other" lipids, e.g., carbohydrate-containing **glycolipids** such as cerebrosides and gangliosides. The phosphoglycerides, sphingomyelin and glycolipids, are extended amphipathic molecules with hydrophilic charged portions containing phosphate and other water soluble moieties such as choline, ethanolamine, serine and inositol esterified to long, hydrophobic, aliphatic hydrocarbon chains. The **amphipathic membrane lipids** form a bilayer where the polar heads of one layer interact with the aqueous external milieu and the polar heads of the other half of the bilayer interact with the aqueous cytoplasmic environment. The hydrophobic portions of each half of the bilayer face one another and interact strongly with one another, with cholesterol and with the hydrophobic portions of integral membrane proteins.

Cholesterol is a compact, hydrophobic, planar compound. It is an important constituent of many membranes even though it is less abundant that phosphoglycerides in the plasma membrane. Cholesterol plays a significant role in determining membrane fluidity. At physiological concentrations, cholesterol limits membrane fluidity. Abnormally high plasma membrane cholesterol levels significantly decrease membrane fluidity. In red blood cells, when the membrane fluidity decreases, these cells become more susceptible to splenic destruction, leading to anemia.

Different cellular membranes have striking differences in their chemical composition. For example, the **myelin sheath** of nerve fibers (a highly modified plasma membrane) is about 80% lipid and 20% protein. The high lipid content of myelin relates to its insulation function in nerve conduction. In contrast, the **inner mitochondrial membrane** is about 80% protein and 20% lipid. Here, there are large numbers of enzymes dedicated to electron transport. Most other plasma membranes are just under 50% lipid and just over 50% protein. Similarly, the lipid composition of different intracellular membranes varies considerably.

Answers and Tutorial on Items 41-48

The answers are: **41-C; 42-F; 43-A; 44-H; 45-B; 46-G; 47-D; 48-A**. **Collagen** (A) is the most abundant protein in the human body. It exists in fibrous, laminar and amorphous forms. Collagen consists of subunit molecules with three helically intertwined α chains of many different types and combinations of chains. Each α chain is a polypeptide with 1/3 of the residues as glycine; it is relatively rich in proline and lysine.

Fibronectin (B) is a MW = 460,000 glycoprotein composed of two similar subunits bound together by -S-S- bridges. It exists in two forms. The cellular form is widely distributed in cells of the connective tissues and on cell surfaces. It has several distinct domains that are involved in binding cells to the collagenous extracellular matrix of connective tissues. The plasma form is dissolved in blood and is involved in the clotting mechanism because of its ability to bind to platelets and to the serum protein fibrin.

Laminin (C) is an important component of the basement membrane under many epithelial cells. This molecule, a large glycoprotein, is composed of two different polypeptide chains with MW = 220,000 and 440,000 assembled into a cruciform aggregate. It binds to heparan sulfate, proteoglycan and type IV collagen.

Chondroitin sulfate (D) is a glycosaminoglycan composed of a repeating disaccharide unit with D-glucuronic acid and N-acetyl-D-galactosamine sulfated at the 4 or 6 positions. It is abundant in hyaline and elastic cartilage where it forms a key component of cartilage proteoglycan.

Heparan sulfate (E) is a glycosaminoglycan composed of a repeating disaccharide unit with D-glucuronic acid (or iduronic acid) and N-acetyl-D-glucosamine (or glucosamine). It is sulfated, but less so than the closely related compound heparin. It is found in blood vessel walls, associated with reticular fibers, in the brain and on the surface of many cells.

Hyaluronic acid (F) is a glycosaminoglycan composed of a repeating disaccharide unit with D-glucuronic acid and N-acetyl-D-glucosamine. Unlike other glycosaminoglycans, it can be found free in the extracellular matrix. It is also an important component of cartilage proteoglycan. It is an extended polymer, often with a MW > 1,000,000.

The **integrins** (G) form a complex family of integral membrane proteins. Each distinct integrin contains different types of α and β subunits which are assembled in many different combinations to confer ligand specificity on the integrin. It is a cell surface receptor for many different extracellular matrix glycoproteins including fibronectin and laminin. Integrins are transmembrane proteins involved in signal transduction from the exterior to the interior of many cells.

Elastin (H) is a complex polypeptide found in abundance in elastic fibers. About 30% of its amino acids are glycine and it is also rich in proline and lysine. Several different lysine residues are chemically modified and then covalently bound together to form cross-links which, when hydrolyzed, yield the unusual amino acids desmosine and isodesmosine.

Fibrillin (I) is a glycoprotein with MW = 350,000. It forms a major component of 8-10 nm beaded extracellular fibrils. These are often closely associated with elastic fibers of the basement membrane.

Answers and Tutorial on Items 49-54

The answers are: **49-E; 50-C; 51-A; 52-F; 53-D; 54-A.** Epithelial tissues define boundaries and establish compartments in the human body. For example, the lumen of the small intestine contains a complicated mixture of digestive enzymes capable of digesting the wall of the small intestine. The contents of the lumen of the GI tract are isolated from the sensitive wall of the gut by a membrane specialization known as the junctional complex.

At the most apical portion of the junctional complex there is a **tight junction** where the outer leaflets of the membranes fuse into a belt-like occluding junction called the **zonula occludens** (A). This structure extends around the apex of the columnar epithelial cells and makes a seal between the lumen and the lateral extracellular fluid environment. In freeze-fracture-etch electron microscopy, the zonula occludens sometimes occurs as an anastomosing network of ridges (points of membrane fusion) representing multiple barriers to movement of molecules from the lumen to the lateral extracellular compartment. Below the zonula occludens there is a divergence of the plasma membrane with a clear separation of 10 to 15 nm. This structure is called the **adhesive junction** (zonula adherens) (B). Here there is simple membrane apposition with variable amounts of electron dense material in the intervening 10-15 nm gap. Numerous actin-rich 6 nm **microfilaments** (F) radiate away from the zonula adherens into the cytoplasm of apposed cells. This structure is usually described as an adhesive junction. The **desmosome** (macula adherens) (C) is found below the zonula adherens, as well as at numerous other points of membrane apposition between adjacent cells. At the desmosome, the plasma membranes diverge to 25-30 nm. There is an intermediate dense line running between the cells. On the inner face of each apposed plasma membrane there is a plaque of electron dense material. Long bundles of keratin-rich 10 nm intermediate filaments (called **tonofilaments**) (G) radiate away from the plaque of electron dense material. The macula adherens is thought to be a structure that holds cells together; it is sometimes likened to a "spot weld." **Hemidesmosomes** (D) are often found on the basal surface of epithelial cells where they anchor these cells firmly to the underlying basement membrane.

The **gap junction** (nexus) (E) is also commonly near the junctional complex. In the gap junction, the outer leaflets of the membranes of adjacent cells approach to within 2 nm, but a small, definite gap remains. Gap junctions are composed of hexagonal arrays of barrel-shaped structures with six protein subunits (**connexons**) arranged around an electron lucent central core. This core is an aqueous channel between closely apposed cells, allowing the free passage of ions and other small molecules between epithelial cells.

Answers and Tutorial on Items 55-57

The answers are: **55-A; 56-A; 57-C**. **Figure 2.11** is a transmission electron micrograph of a neuronal cell body in the central nervous system. The arrow points to the **nucleolus**. In interphase nuclei, especially in cells actively engaged in protein synthesis, the nucleolus is often a prominent feature easily seen in the light microscope. Electron microscopy of the nucleolus reveals a central region with fibrous DNA and a granular component which consists of recently transcribed rRNA being assembled into ribosomes by combination with ribosomal proteins. The variability in the size of the nucleolus is primarily due to variations in the amount of granular component, a reflection of variations in rate of assembly of ribosomes.

The assembled ribosomes are then transported through the nuclear pores and into the cytoplasm where they either remain free in the cytoplasm for the synthesis of proteins for internal utilization (e.g., hemoglobin) or become bound to membranes to form the rough endoplasmic reticulum for the synthesis of secretory proteins (e.g., digestive enzymes).

Answers and Tutorial on Items 58-60

The answers are: **58-B; 59-D; 60-C**. **Figure 2.12** is a transmission electron micrograph of neural tissue, showing a large **axon** (A) with its **myelin sheath** (E). The surrounding structures are axons and dendrites of other neurons, as well as portions of supportive—or glial—cells. One of the most prominent membranous organelles are the **mitochondria** labeled (C) which produce the ATP required to power the various synthetic and motile events occurring in these cells. Nerve axons are long slender extensions reaching from the neuronal cell bodies (not shown) to the receptor cell (also not shown) receiving a signal from the nerve cell. The activation of a neuron cell body leads to the passage of a membrane depolarization that propagates along the nerve cell plasma membrane, as an **action potential**, to the axon terminus. Axons contain a variety of organelles, but—having no ribosomes (either free or bound to rough ER)—are unable to synthesize proteins. All proteins required for the establishment and maintenance of the axon are synthesized in the nerve cell body and carried to the nerve terminus by **axoplasmic transport**.

ANSWERS AND TUTORIAL ON ITEMS 61-62

The answers are: **61-C; 62-A. Figure 2.13** is a scanning electron micrograph, showing that the apical surfaces of the epithelial cells lining the trachea may have two distinct types of apical projections. The shorter ones (A) are **microvilli**; although not as numerous as the microvilli in the brush border of intestinal epithelial cells, these microvilli have a similar structure and function. They are maintained as elongate extensions of the plasma membrane by a core of actin microfilaments and serve to provide extra membrane surface to house a variety of proteins that play a role in transfer of substances across the apical surface of the epithelium. The longer projections (B) are **cilia**; they contain a core complex of microtubules called the axoneme and serve, by their coordinated "beating" to move fluids over the surfaces of the epithelium, in this case in a direction towards the lumen of the oral cavity. Because they contain a bundle of microfilaments, microvilli can be probed by agents specific for actin. They will bind the fungal toxin **phalloidin** and, if a fluorescent derivative (rhodamine-phalloidin) of that toxin is applied, the microfilaments (and thus the microvilli) will be strongly and selectively labeled. Another probe that is nearly, but not absolutely, specific for actin is the family of drugs called **cytochalasins**. Cytochalasins (the most specific of which is cytochalasin D) bind to actins in such a way as to bring about their breakdown, hence causing large scale shortening (collapse) of the microvilli.

ANSWERS AND TUTORIAL ON ITEMS 63-67

page 18 physiology

The answers are: **63-B; 64-C; 65-A; 66-D; 67-E. Figure 2.14** is a high magnification transmission electron micrograph of skeletal muscle cut in longitudinal section. Skeletal muscle fibers contain many **myofibrils**, each consisting of many **sarcomeres**. Each sarcomere is formed by a regular array of thick (myosin-rich) and thin (actin-rich) filaments. Myofibrils are composed of many sarcomeres. Individual sarcomeres extend from **Z line** (B) to Z line. Sarcomeres have central **A bands** (C) where there is extensive overlap between **thin, actin-rich filaments** and **thick, myosin-rich filaments**. When a muscle fiber (cell) contracts, the width of the **I bands** (D) and **H bands** (E) decrease because the thin and thick filaments increase their overlapping due to sliding of thin filaments past thick filaments. The H bands are regions of no overlap between thin and thick filaments. H bands contain no thin filaments. The length of the A bands remains constant during muscle contraction; however, the I bands and H bands decrease in length and the Z lines move closer together, leading to a shortening of the sarcomere. When many sarcomeres shorten, the entire muscle cell shortens. Muscle contraction is driven by the energy rich compound ATP which is produced in **mitochondria** (A).

Contractile force in muscle is generated by a change in the position of **actin** and **myosin**, which is regulated by intracellular calcium concentration. Energy for muscle contraction is derived from the hydrolysis of ATP. Under appropriate conditions, the actin-myosin complex has ATPase activity. Release of energy from ATP hydrolysis causes conformational changes in the muscle proteins resulting in useful movement. A sarcomere has a variable total length depending on the contractile status of the cell. When a muscle contracts, thick and thin filaments slide past one another. During a contraction and relaxation cycle, calcium concentration around the myofibrils increases suddenly. This causes a conformational change in the **troponin** molecule, which exposes the S-1 (cross-bridge) binding site of actin, and a myosin-actin complex forms. Another conformational change occurs, and the S-1 fragment, still in association with the actin-containing thin filament, swings like an oar in an oarlock and causes the thin filament to slide relative to the thick filament. When this occurs at millions of cross-bridges, the entire sarcomere is shortened. The calcium concentration falls rapidly, following hydrolysis of ATP and the swinging of cross-bridges. The drop in calcium severs the association between actin and myosin and the contraction stops. ATP is hydrolysed to adenosine diphosphate (ADP), which subsequently is phosphorylated to form ATP. Skeletal and cardiac muscle cells have large numbers of mitochondria, which synthesize the large amounts of ATP required for the work done by muscle cells contracting against and external load.

ANSWERS AND TUTORIAL ON ITEMS 68-70

The answers are: **68-B; 69-C; 70-A**. This child suffers from **Gaucher's disease**. There are many different mutations including point mutations, deletions and crossover events that lead to this disease. Gaucher's disease is most common in Ashkenazi Jews. The secretion of **glucocerebroside**, a neutral sphingolipid formed by the covalent coupling of glucose to ceramide, is characteristic of Gaucher's disease. This disease is due to congenital abnormalities in the function of a **lysosomal enzyme** for degradation of glucocerebroside, **glucocerebrosidase**. Lysosomes are used to degrade endogenous molecular components of cells. They are particularly abundant in macrophages. Although the mutant genotype is present in all cells of the body, it is most often expressed only in macrophages, leading to hepatosplenomegaly and erosion of long bones.

Tay-Sachs disease, caused by a deficiency in **hexosaminidase A**, leads to the accumulation of **ganglioside G_{M2}**. **Fabry's disease**, caused by a deficiency in **α-galactosidase A**, leads to the accumulation of **ceramide trihexoside**. **Niemann-Pick disease**, caused by a deficiency in **sphingomyelinase**, leads to the accumulation of **sphingomyelin**. **Hurler's syndrome**, caused by a deficiency in **α-L-iduronidase**, leads to the accumulation of **dermatan sulfate** and **heparan sulfate**.

Answers and Tutorial on Items 71-74

The answers are: **71-D; 72-C; 73-D; 74-E. Figure 2.15** shows a large multinucleate cell called an **osteoclast**. Osteoclasts reside on the surfaces of bone spicules and, under the stimulus of parathyroid hormone, they break down the bone. This degradative activity involves the formation of an extensively folded surface (ruffled membrane) in contact with the bone surface. The osteoclasts secrete hydrogen ions across this folded surface, coupled to the release of chloride ions. The acidification of the immediate environment of the bone matrix leads to the decalcification of the matrix, thus increasing the calcium level in the blood stream. Osteoclasts also break down the proteinaceous bone matrix, by phagocytosing (also across the ruffled membrane border) chunks of the matrix and degrading them using the hydrolytic enzyme contents of lysosomes. Osteoclasts are end-stage cells and do not proliferate. There are other cells in the body that have functions (and thus structures) that are similar to those of the osteoclasts. Of the list of cells in Item 74, the one with the greatest such similarities to osteoclasts is the **gastric parietal cell**; this cell also has an extensively folded surface (the apical surface in the case of the parietal cell, which is an epithelial cell) across which hydrogen ions are actively secreted, thus acidifying the adjacent extracellular space (the lumen of the stomach).

Answers and Tutorial on Items 75-77

The answers are: **75-D; 76-A; 77-L**. The efficiency of the immune response mechanism is dependent upon direct cell-to-cell contact and indirect chemical signaling by cytokines. A large array of cytokines are produced by leucocytes. They are called **interleukins** (IL); and, along with **gamma interferon** (INF-γ), are the major soluble mediators of immunological function. An evaluation of the interleukins demonstrates multiple regulatory functions. Interleukins are designated by IL- followed by a number. All are proteins and many are glycosylated. They have molecular weights ranging from 15,00 to 60,000. Most have mitogenic properties and each is antigenically unique. Functionally different interleukins share similar roles in stimulating certain B cell or T cell populations.

IL-1 (A) is produced by many cells and has both T cell and B cell activating functions. It also induces IL-2 receptor expression. IL-1 stimulates the cytocidal actions of cytotoxic T cells, macrophages and natural killer cells. **IL-2** (B) up-regulates lymphokine production and cytotoxic activity of different leucocytes. **IL-3** (C) helps to maintain the growth of mast cells and differentiation of monocytes. **IL-4** (D) enhances both class I and II MHC expression, stimulates IgG4 and IgE production and stimulates IgE receptor expression on B cells. **IL-5** (E) stimulates B cell growth, induces differentiation of eosinophils, stimulates IgA secretion and stimulates B cell growth. **IL-6** (F) stimulates IgG secretion, induces the growth of plasma cells and activates B cells. **IL-7** (G) stimulates B cell differentiation and increases IL-2 receptor expression. **IL-8** (H), produced by macrophages, is a neutrophil chemoattractant. **IL-9** (I) stimulates helper T cells. **IL-10** (J) suppresses production of certain other lymphokines produced by helper T cells. **Transforming growth factor-β** (L) is produced by macrophages, lymphocytes and platelets. It acts to attract other macrophages and monocytes and stimulates IL-1 production. It may also down-regulate the inflammatory response. It is important to realize that cytokines usually have multiple roles which may change under different immunological conditions. Many cytokines also act **synergistically**.

Answers and Tutorial on Items 78-81

The answers are: **78-C; 79-B; 80-D; 81-E. Figure 2.16** shows erythrocytes as they appear in **sickle cell anemia**. This disease is caused by a substitution of valine for glutamic acid in the chain of hemoglobin. Under normal circumstances, the hemoglobin concentration in erythrocytes is extremely high. The point mutation for sickling decreases the solubility of HbS, especially when deoxygenated, leading to the formation of semi-rigid fibrillar aggregates in cells and significant deformation of the normally biconcave discs of erythrocytes. These abnormal erythrocyte shapes and excessive rigidity lead to hemolytic anemia.

Answers and Tutorial on Items 82-84

The answers are: **82-D; 83-A; 84-B**. The patient has **osteogenesis imperfecta** (type I). This is an inherited defect (**autosomal dominant**) that leads to reduced production of **type I collagen**. The collagen present in bone matrix is of type I and is produced by osteoblasts. The mechanism of collagen synthesis (by ribosomes of the rough ER), processing, and secretion is closely similar to that occurring in fibroblasts. Individuals with osteogenesis imperfecta have a deletion in one of the genes for the α(I) chain of collagen (I). The deletion leads to production of a shortened α(I) chain. The shortened α(I) chains associate with normal α1(I) and α2(I) chains causing formation of defective triple helices that are especially sensitive to proteolytic degradation. Victims have numerous fractures and resulting bone deformities. Other associated effects are dental problems, hearing loss and a bluish tint to the sclera.

Answers and Tutorial on Items 85-88

The answers are: **85-A; 86-C; 87-E; 88-B**. This child suffers from **cystic fibrosis** (CF), a common serious disease especially prevalent in Caucasians originating in Northern Europe. It is caused by an **autosomal recessive gene**. Many parents are asymptomatic heterozygous carriers. Approximately 1 in 2,500 newborns suffer from cystic fibrosis.

Typically, the respiratory and digestive tracts are most severely affected in cystic fibrosis. The airways of the respiratory system and ducts of exocrine glands in the digestive system are blocked by viscous mucus. This thick mucus impedes ciliary clearance of the respiratory system, leading to repeated infections (most commonly with *Pseudomonas*) and can compromise digestive function by limiting secretion of enzymes. Sweat glands are also affected in cystic fibrosis, leading to the secretion of sweat with increased salt concentration. This feature of the disease has been exploited for simple screening procedures.

Recently, the gene for cystic fibrosis has been identified and mapped to **chromosome 7**. The CF gene is large, containing about 250,000 base pairs, and encodes a protein of 1480 amino acids called the **cystic fibrosis transmembrane conductance regulator** (CFTR), a member of a large family of proteins involved in active transport of molecules across cell membranes. CFTR has two hydrophobic domains, each with six loops that span the cell membrane. It also has two nucleotide binding folds that bind and cleave ATP to release the energy required for active ion transport. This gene product also has a serine rich regulatory domain (R), thought to be the target of protein kinase activity. The most recent theory on how CFTR works involves several steps. When the R component is not phosphorylated, the Cl^- channel in the transmembrane domain of the molecule is closed. Cyclic AMP-dependent protein kinase activity leads to the phosphorylation of the R domain at the expense of ATP conversion to ADP. After phosphorylation of the R domain, the nucleotide binding folds are prepared to bind ATP. Binding and subsequent hydrolysis of ATP then causes a conformational change, leading to the opening of the Cl^- channel and a release of ADP and P_i. After release of bound nucleotide, the channel decays back to a closed state. Defects in the CFTR lead to decreased Cl^-efflux from cells and a generalized dehydration of mucous secretions in the body, especially in the respiratory and gastrointestinal systems. Dehydrated mucus has a higher viscosity and is thus more difficult to clear from the lungs, leading to blockage of airways and repeated respiratory infections.

Answers and Tutorial on Items 89-92

The answers are: **89-C; 90-A; 91-B; 92-A**. This patient suffers from **xeroderma pigmentosum**. This rare malady occurs in approximately 1/250,000 people worldwide. It is caused by an **autosomal recessive mutation** found in all races of the human population. It is primarily manifested as an extreme sensitivity of the skin and other exposed portions of the body to ultraviolet light. In some varieties of xeroderma pigmentosum, systemic effects, e.g., damage to the central nervous system, are also observed.

One mechanism for ultraviolet light-induced damage to DNA is the formation of thymine dimers between adjacent thymine residues of one strand of the DNA double helix. Several mechanisms for repair of damage to DNA have been discovered in bacterial systems. For example, excision repair utilizes a endonuclease which recognizes abnormal DNA near the 5′ side of the thymine dimer, causing the damaged strand to separate from the double helix. Next, a DNA polymerase forms a new polynucleotide to replace the damaged sequence. Finally, a 5′-exonuclease removes the damaged sequence and a DNA ligase closes the break, resulting in the formation of a repaired duplex. In some cases of xeroderma pigmentosum, a genetic defect in **excision repair of damaged DNA** has been reported.

Notes

CHAPTER 3

Embryology

DIRECTIONS (Items 1-96): For each of the numbered items that proceed, you must select the single best answer from among the lettered options listed.

Some of the numbered items will pose a question or incomplete sentence that is followed by a list of 4-5 lettered options. In all cases, select the ONE lettered option that best answers the question or completes the sentence given.

Some of the numbered items are preceded by 5-24 lettered options. In these sets, the lettered options will be preceded by a single instruction asking you to match one of the lettered options to each numbered item most closely associated with it. In all matching sets, you may use any of the lettered options once, more than once or not at all, but you should still only select ONE lettered option per numbered item.

If you wish to simulate actual USMLE testing conditions, you should aim to complete all the items in this chapter in ONE hour and 35 minutes.

Do NOT look at the answers and tutorials until you have completed all of the items in this chapter.

Good luck!

Items 1-2

During a routine obstetrical examination, you find that your patient has an abnormally small abdominal girth for her 30-week pregnancy. Ultrasonographic examination reveals a normal fetus, a posterior fundal placenta and oligohydramnios.

1. The decreased volume of amniotic fluid (oligohydramnios) would most likely be caused by which of the following?

    (A) renal agenesis
    (B) bladder extrophy
    (C) anencephaly
    (D) tracheoesophageal fistula
    (E) duodenal torsion

2. The most likely fundamental developmental defect leading to this clinical case is

    (A) failed ureteric bud induction
    (B) failed cloacal membrane septation
    (C) failed neural tube closure
    (D) failed secondary canalization
    (E) failed mid-gut loop rotation

Items 3-5

A 15-year-old adolescent presents with a chief complaint of amenorrhea. She is 5'9" tall and weighs 130 pounds. Her temperature is 98.7 F., pulse is 64 beats/minutes, and blood pressure is 120/60. Physical examination reveals a normal female body habitus except for scant axillary and pubic hair. Pelvic examination reveals a shallow vagina with no cervix. A mobile mass can be palpated in the left labium majorum. Ultrasonographic examination reveals a complete lack of uterus and adnexal structures.

3. Which of the following chromosomal complements would you be most likely to find with this patient after karyotype analysis?

   (A) 45, X
   (B) 47, XX, +21
   (C) 47, XXY
   (D) 46, XY
   (E) 69, XXY

4. The most appropriate diagnosis is

   (A) Turner's Syndrome
   (B) Down Syndrome
   (C) Klinefelter's Syndrome
   (D) testicular feminization syndrome
   (E) triploidy

5. This patient would lack paramesonephric duct derivatives because

   (A) testes produce müllerian inhibiting substance
   (B) their differentiation is testosterone dependent
   (C) the patient is genetically female
   (D) the patient is genetically male
   (E) no testis determining factor is produced

Items 6-10

Examine **Figure 3.1** below, a karyotype, and then answer each of the questions following.

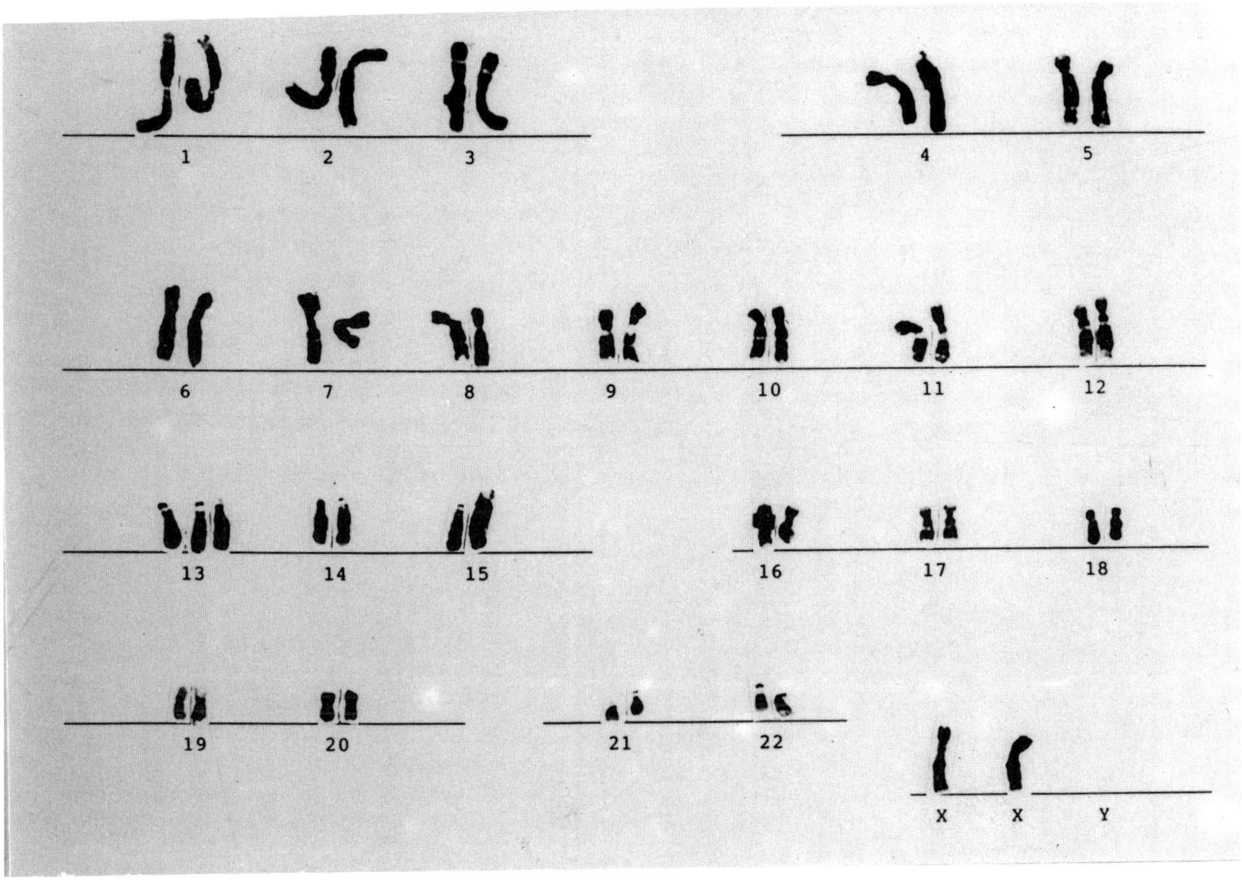

Figure 3.1

6. The developmental process whose disruption leads to the cause of this karyotype is

   (A) meiotic disjunction
   (B) block to polyspermy
   (C) polar body formation
   (D) crossing over
   (E) zona pellucida formation

7. The best shorthand notation describing this karyotype is

   (A) 46, XX
   (B) 47, XY, +18
   (C) 47, XX, +13
   (D) 48, XXXY
   (E) 46, XY

8. The most appropriate diagnosis of a child with this karyotype is

   (A) Down syndrome
   (B) Edwards' syndrome
   (C) Patau's syndrome
   (D) fetal alcoholism syndrome
   (E) Turner's syndrome

9. Which of the following symptoms is most characteristic of this aneuploid disorder?

   (A) death soon after birth
   (B) cardiovascular anomalies
   (C) cleft palate
   (D) normal mental function
   (E) prominent occipital region of skull

10. The most predictive maternal characteristic for occurrence of this congenital birth defect is

(A) heroin abuse
(B) age greater then 40 years
(C) pelvic inflammatory disease
(D) eclampsia
(E) cytomegalovirus infection

Items 11-14

A fetus is delivered at 32 weeks since the mother's last menstrual period. At birth, the fetus weighs 1500 gm but otherwise appears normal. Soon after birth, however, the fetus becomes cyanotic and breathes with a grunting noise. Chest x-rays reveal dense lungs with significant atelectasis.

11. The most likely diagnosis associated with these symptoms is

(A) congenital diaphragmatic hernia
(B) coarctation of the aorta
(C) tetralogy of Fallot
(D) renal agenesis
(E) respiratory distress syndrome

12. The most significant predictive prenatal test for this disease would be

(A) ultrasonography
(B) x-rays
(C) measurement of amniotic fluid lecithin/sphingomyelin ratio
(D) karyotype analysis
(E) measurement of maternal serum α-fetoprotein

13. The cell type most directly involved in etiology of this condition is

(A) type II pneumocyte
(B) macrophage
(C) ciliated cell
(D) goblet cell
(E) erythrocyte

14. In threatened premature delivery, the most useful drug class for treatment of the mother to accelerate fetal lung maturation is

(A) antibiotic
(B) antimetabolite
(C) neuroleptic
(D) steroid
(E) diuretic

Items 15-17

A 37-year-old, 148-lb woman is found to be carrying monoamnionic twins. In spite of complete continuous bed rest from 28 weeks after conception, she is found to have ruptured membranes at 34 weeks. Two days after rupture of membranes, maternal temperature is 103°F. and her white blood count is 20,000/mm_3 with a predominance of neutrophils. Your diagnosis is chorioamnionitis.

15. The chief morphological change in the fetal lymph nodes as a result of this intrauterine infection would be

(A) ingression
(B) increase in T cells
(C) infiltration by neutrophils
(D) appearance of eosinophils
(E) appearance of germinal centers

16. These morphological changes are a reflection of which immunological process?

(A) T-cell proliferation
(B) activation of memory B cells
(C) delayed hypersensitivity
(D) plasma cell phagocytosis
(E) B-cell activation and differentiation

17. Which mechanism is most important for passive immunization of the fetus against antigenic exposure of the mother prior to birth?

(A) placental transport of maternal IgGs
(B) synthesis of secretory IgAs
(C) placental transport of maternal IgMs
(D) colostrum formation
(E) placental transport of IgEs

Item 18

18. In a second pregnancy, a 25-year-old woman delivers a hydropic fetus with severe edema, jaundice and hepatosplenomegaly. Her blood type is O negative and her husband's blood type is O positive. The blood type of the fetus is

    (A) A negative
    (B) A positive
    (C) O negative
    (D) O positive
    (E) B positive

Items 19-20

You are a Public Health Service pediatrician working on an Indian reservation in Montana. An obese woman with hepatomegaly and facial spider angiomas visits your clinic with her 4-year-old son. The mother admits to drinking whiskey on a regular basis but denies alcohol consumption during her pregnancy. The child is short for his age and shows significant mid-facial hypoplasia, including ocular ptosis and a flat nasal bridge. The child seems lethargic and there is a significant deficit in his social interactions.

19. The most likely diagnosis of the maternal-child disease is

    (A) healthy-Down syndrome
    (B) healthy-Treacher-Collins syndrome
    (C) alcoholism-fetal alcohol syndrome
    (D) alcoholism-vitamin B_{12} deficiency
    (E) alcoholism-pellagra

20. The most likely defective developmental process that lead to the child's symptoms is

    (A) neural crest cell migration
    (B) bone formation
    (C) ocular induction
    (D) cartilage proliferation
    (E) endochondral ossification

Items 21-22

A newborn infant fails to defecate for 3 days after birth in spite of normal feeding without excessive vomiting. Rectal examination reveals a normal rectum but a fecal mass retained in the colon. There is an explosive release of feces following cessation of rectal examination. Barium enema and x-rays reveals a narrowed distal segment of the colon and a dilated proximal segment.

21. The most likely diagnosis of this condition is

    (A) sprue
    (B) colic
    (C) colonic aganglionosis
    (D) imperforate anus
    (E) gastric atresia

22. The most likely developmental abnormality leading to this condition is

    (A) gluten allergy
    (B) abnormal gastric rotation
    (C) abnormal neural crest cell migration
    (D) failure of proctodeal membrane degeneration
    (E) situs inversus

Items 23-24

Contrast media can be injected into blood vessels to reveal by x-ray the blood flow from one vessel to another. In the hemochorial human placenta, a contrast dye is injected into either the uterine artery or the umbilical vein and 10 seconds later, the dye is located by radiography.

23. The vascular space most intensely labeled immediately after injection of contrast medium into the uterine artery is

    (A) the umbilical artery
    (B) the umbilical vein
    (C) capillaries in the chorionic villi
    (D) the intervillous space
    (E) the uterine vein

24. The vascular space most intensely labeled immediately after injection of contrast medium into the umbilical vein is the

    (A) inferior vena cava
    (B) ductus venosus
    (C) ductus arteriosus
    (D) umbilical artery
    (E) superior vena cava

Items 25-29

Examine **Figure 3.2** below, a karyotype, and then answer each of the questions following.

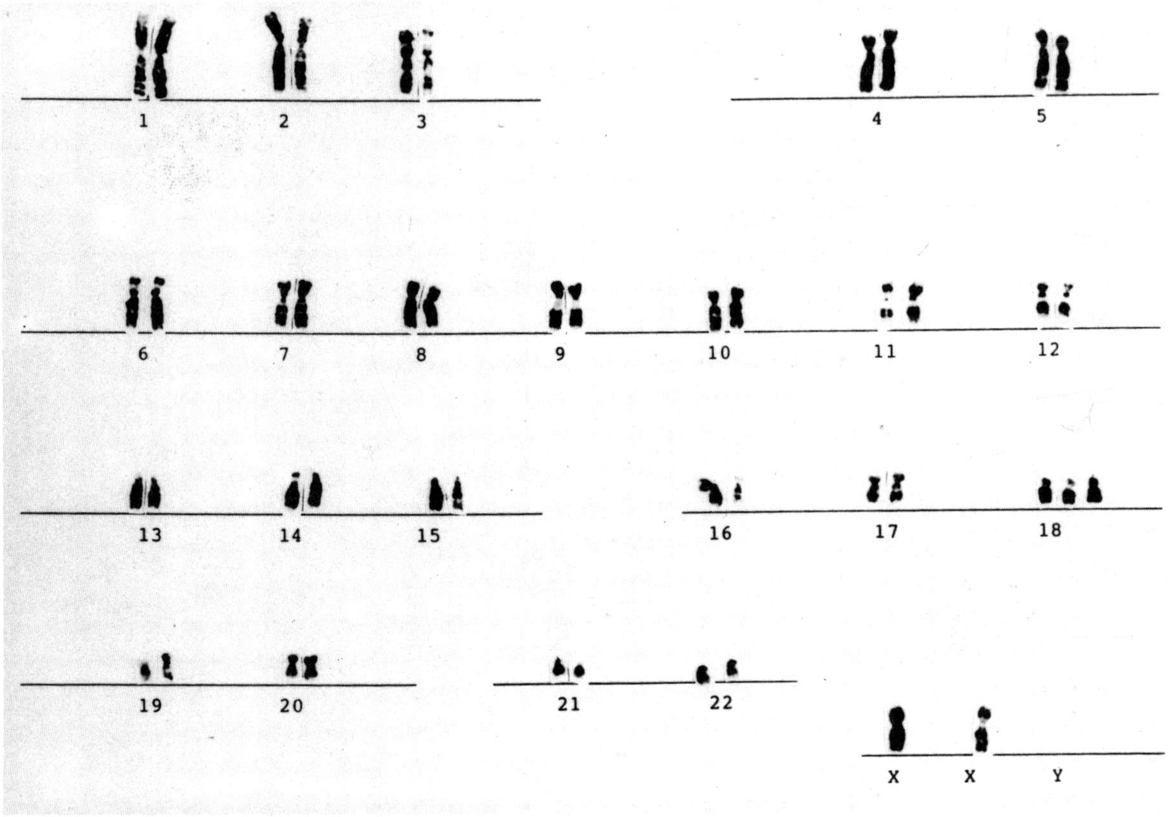

Figure 3.2

25. The developmental process whose disruption leads to the cause of this karyotype is

(A) mitosis
(B) synapsis
(C) differentiation of primordial germ cells
(D) meiotic disjunction
(E) migration of primordial germ cells

26. The best shorthand notation describing this karyotype is

(A) 46, XY
(B) 47, XX, +18
(C) 47, XY, +21
(D) 47, XXY
(E) 45, X

27. The most appropriate diagnosis of a child with this karyotype is

(A) Down syndrome
(B) Edwards' syndrome
(C) Marfan's syndrome
(D) Klinefelter's syndrome
(E) Turner's syndrome

28. Which of the following symptoms is most characteristic of this aneuploid disorder?

(A) death soon after birth
(B) cardiovascular anomalies
(C) cleft palate
(D) normal mental function
(E) prominent occipital region of skull

29. The most predictive maternal characteristic for occurrence of this congenital birth defect is

(A) age greater then 40 years
(B) cocaine abuse
(C) hypertension
(D) high fever during pregnancy
(E) alcoholism

Items 30-34

Examine **Figure 3.3** below, a karyotype, and then answer the questions following.

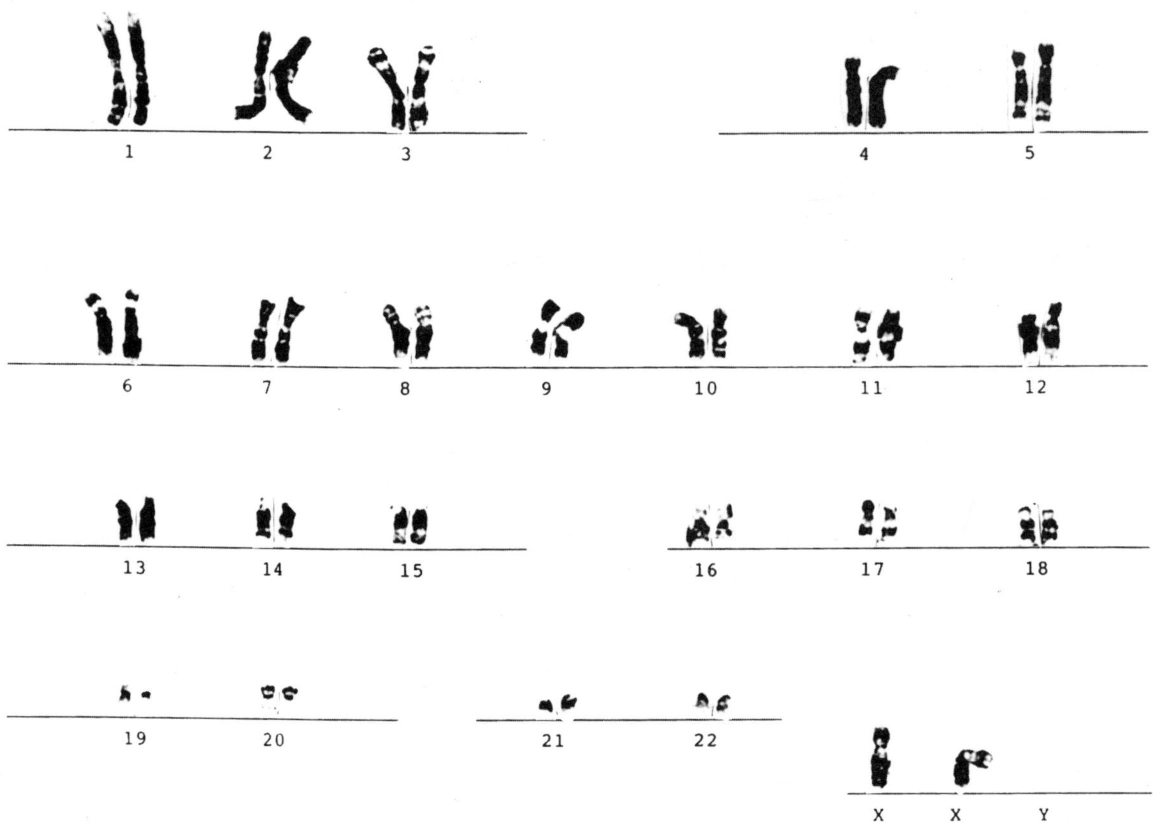

Figure 3.3

30. Which prenatal diagnostic technique is most commonly used in karyotype analysis?

(A) ultrasound
(B) amniocentesis
(C) fetal heart monitoring
(D) measurement of maternal serum α-fetoprotein
(E) urinalysis

31. Which drug is most commonly used in karyotype analysis?

(A) steroids
(B) β-blockers
(C) colchicine
(D) ACTH
(E) prolactin

32. Which shorthand notation is most appropriate for describing the karyotype?

(A) 46, XX
(B) 47, XXY
(C) 46, XY
(D) 45, X
(E) 45, Y

33. Which statement best characterizes this karyotype?

(A) aneuploidy with numerical anomalies in sex chromosomes
(B) aneuploidy with numerical anomalies in autosomes
(C) euploidy
(D) monosomy
(E) trisomy

34. Which of the following disorders would be associated with this karyotype?

(A) testicular feminization syndrome
(B) Klinefelter's syndrome
(C) sickle cell anemia
(D) Turner's syndrome
(E) Down syndrome

Item 35

35. A mother and her 2-year-old son come to your office. The mother complains that the child is not acting normally. After a brief period of active play, her son becomes exhausted, breathes rapidly and squats or lies down. On physical examination, you find that the child's pulse and blood pressure are normal. His oral mucosa, fingernails and toenails are cyanotic. You also detect a significant systolic murmur best heard along the left sternal border at the level of the second intercostal space. A PA (posteroanterior) chest film shows a concavity on the left border of the heart, diminished pulmonary vascularity and a rounded heart apex located slightly higher than normal above the diaphragm. The most likely diagnosis of the boy's problem is

    (A) isolated ventricular septal defect
    (B) isolated atrial septal defect
    (C) isolated aortic stenosis
    (D) transposition of the great vessels
    (E) tetralogy of Fallot

Items 36-37

36. Which statement best describes the acrosomal reaction?

    (A) occurs in epididymis
    (B) required for capacitation
    (C) aids in degradation of extracellular matrix between corona radiata cells
    (D) causes block to polyspermy
    (E) prevents zona penetration

37. Fertilization is thought to occur normally in which location in women?

    (A) uterus
    (B) cervix
    (C) interstitial uterine tube
    (D) ampullary uterine tube
    (E) vagina

Items 38-40

38. Human chorionic gonadotrophin (hCG) is secreted by which tissue?

    (A) syncytiotrophoblast
    (B) cytotrophoblast
    (C) epiblast
    (D) hypoblast
    (E) endometrial epithelium

39. Which statement best describes the most direct role of hCG in the female reproductive cycle?

    (A) It stimulates completion of meiosis.
    (B) It stimulates endometrial proliferation.
    (C) It maintains the progestational state.
    (D) It causes regression of the corpus luteum.
    (E) It stimulates endometrial secretion.

40. Decidual cells are best described as

    (A) partially fetal and partially maternal in origin
    (B) completely derived from maternal endometrial epithelium
    (C) derivatives of maternal blood vessels
    (D) derivatives of syncytiotrophoblast
    (E) derivatives of maternal endometrial stroma

Items 41-44

41. Which of the following are ectodermal derivatives?

    (A) dermal fibroblasts
    (B) sweat glands
    (C) skeletal muscle
    (D) erythrocytes
    (E) endothelium

42. Which of the following are mesodermal derivatives?

    (A) dermis
    (B) epidermis
    (C) enamel
    (D) neurons in brain
    (E) retina

43. Which of the following are endodermal derivatives?

    (A) endothelium
    (B) endometrium
    (C) tracheal epithelium
    (D) melanocytes
    (E) macrophages

44. Which of the following are neural crest derivatives?

    (A) oligodendroglia
    (B) adrenal cortex
    (C) lymphocytes
    (D) Schwann cells
    (E) glucagon-secreting cells in islets of Langerhans

Items 45-46

Match the embryonic structure from the list of answers below with the most accurate description of its developmental fate in the items below. Answers may be used once, more than once, or not at all.

(A) Head fold of the amnion
(B) Tail fold of the amnion
(C) Somatopleuric intraembryonic mesoderm
(D) Splanchnopleuric intraembryonic mesoderm
(E) Intermediate mesoderm
(F) Somite
(G) Stomodeum
(H) Proctodeum
(I) Yolk sac
(J) Vitelline duct
(K) Septum transversum

45. Source of primordial germ cells

46. Makes a major contribution to diaphragm and connective tissue of liver

Items 47-48

For each description of the development of an adult brain structure, select the most appropriate lettered adult brain structure in **Figure 3.4** below.

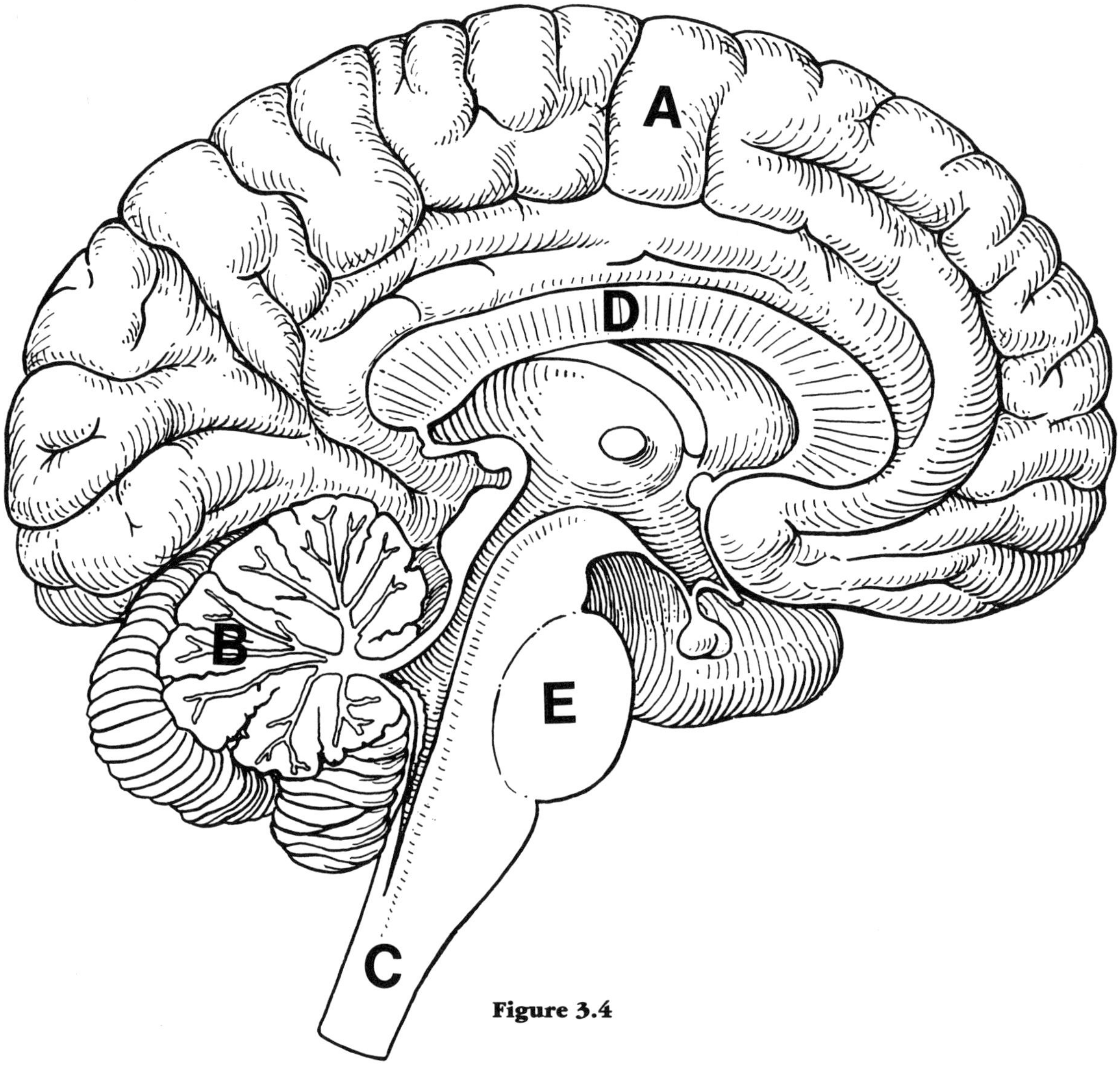

Figure 3.4

47. This structure develops from the myelencephalon of the rhombencephalon.

48. This structure contains Purkinje cells, Golgi neurons, and cortical grey matter.

Items 49-52

Examine the photograph of an autopsy specimen in **Figure 3.5** below and then answer the items, choosing the best response.

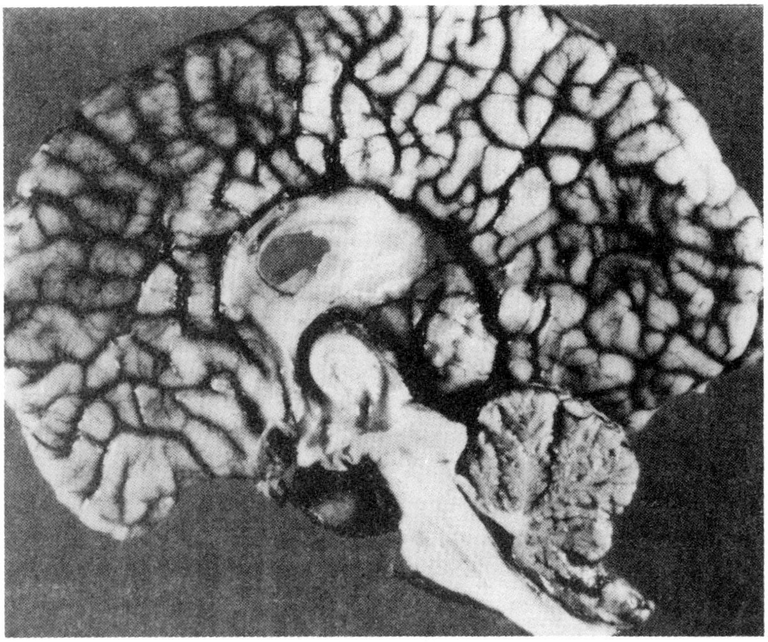

Figure 3.5

49. This brain represents and example of which specific clinical entity?

    (A) myelomeningocele
    (B) spina bifida cystica
    (C) Arnold-Chiari malformation
    (D) anencephaly
    (E) acrania

50. The etiology of this condition is

    (A) virally induced
    (B) strictly genetic
    (C) multifactorial
    (D) drug induced
    (E) none of the above

51. This malformation is often associated with

    (A) hydrocephalus
    (B) blindness
    (C) cleft palate
    (D) conductive hearing loss

52. This malformation in also associated with

    (A) spina bifida occulta
    (B) lumbosacral myelomeningocele
    (C) rachischisis
    (D) maternal diabetes mellitus
    (E) maternal hypertension

Items 53-54

A 28-year-old woman of Irish ethnic background in the 30th week of her first pregnancy reports a lack of fetal movements. Maternal serum α-fetoprotein levels are significantly elevated. Ultrasonography in **Figure 3.6** reveals the following: (FC = fetal cranium; FCS = fetal cervical spine)

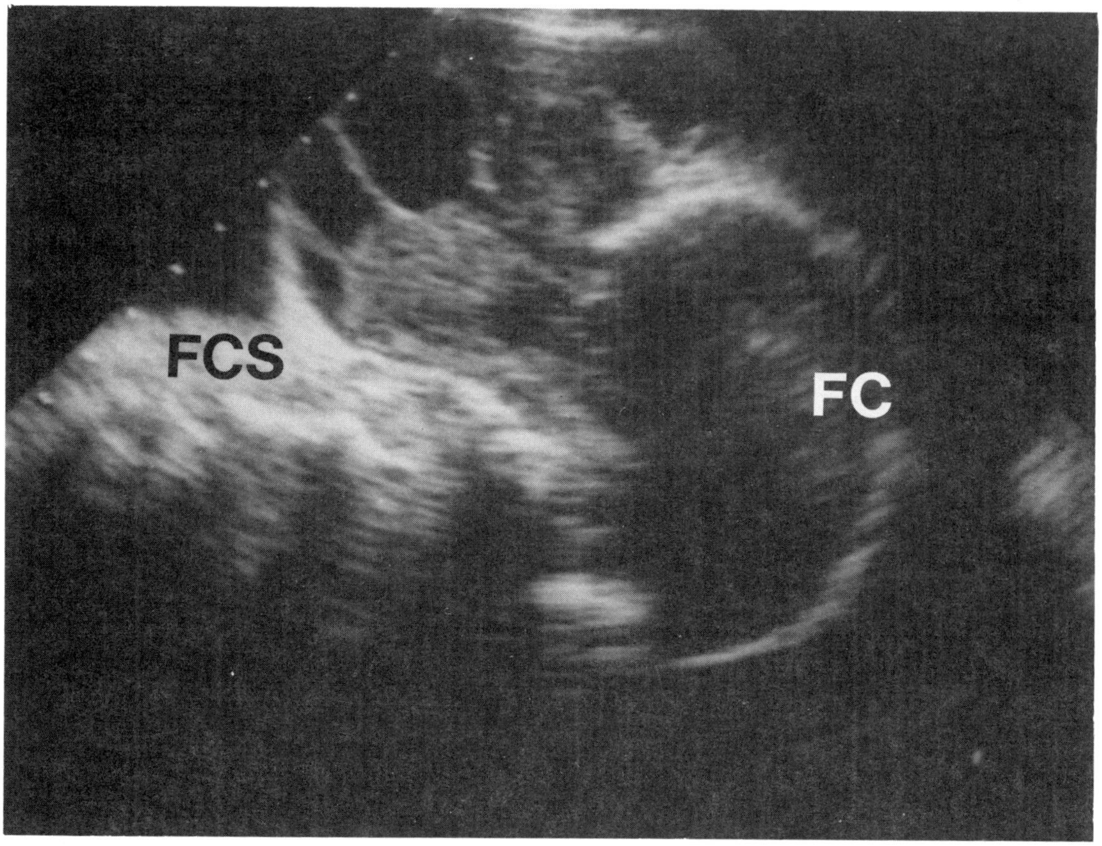

Figure 3.6

53. The most accurate diagnosis of this anomaly is

(A) anencephaly
(B) spina bifida
(C) respiratory distress syndrome
(D) spina bifida occulta
(E) encephalocele

54 The most likely developmental process causing the congenital anomaly shown in **Figure 3.6** is

(A) failure of neural tube closure
(B) failure of lung differentiation
(C) duodenal atresia
(D) breakage of chromosomes
(E) nondisjunction during meiosis

Items 55-60

Examine the diagram in **Figure 3.7** showing various endocrine organs with labels for answers and then match the most appropriate description of the embryonic development of the labeled organ in the items below. Answers may be used once, more than once, or not at all.

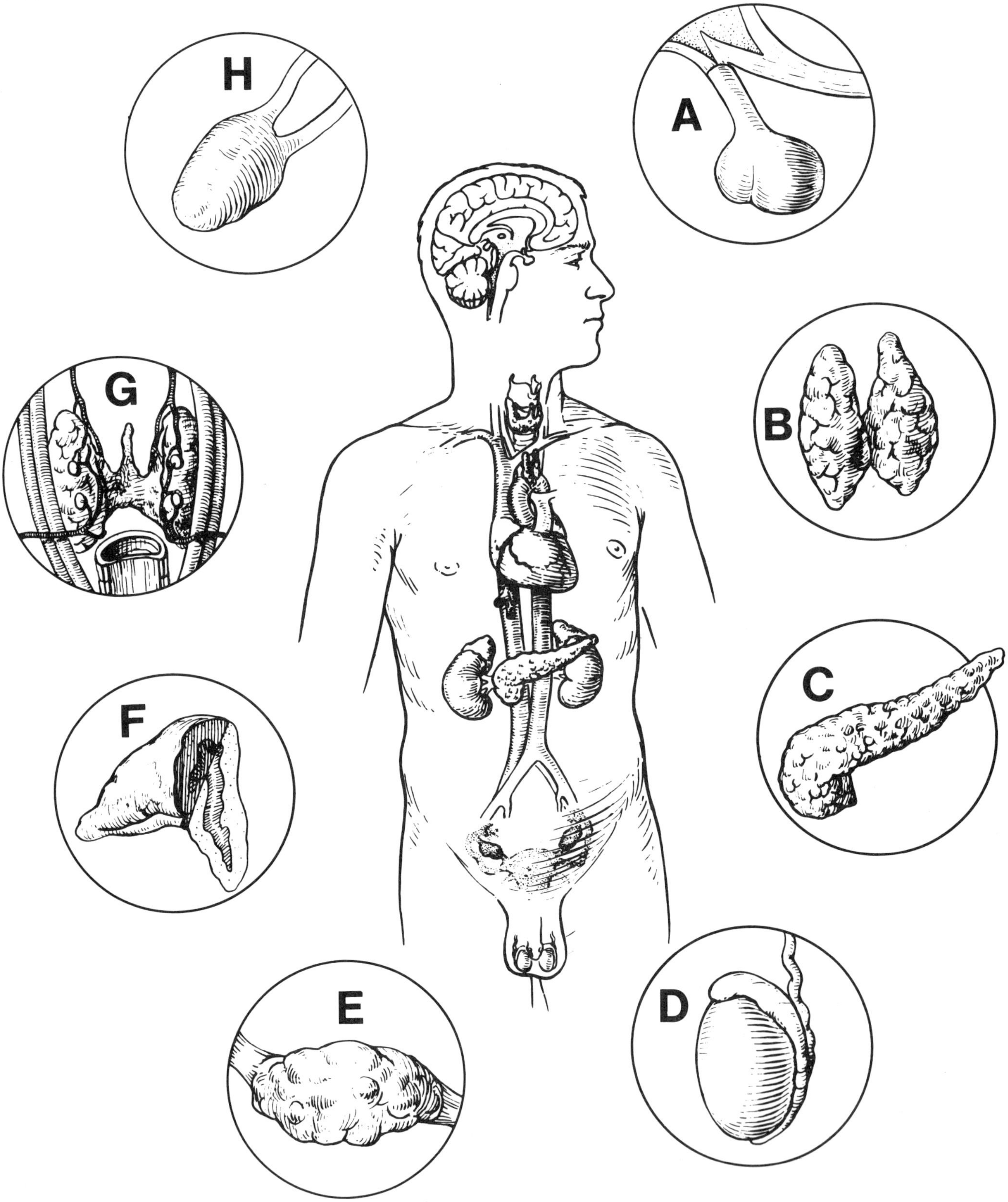

Figure 3.7

55. This organ contains a neural crest and coelomic epithelial derivative.

56. This organ is formed from a diverticulum of the foregut. Developmental defects can result in formation of ectopic functional tissue at the root of the tongue. It is not a pharyngeal apparatus derivative.

57. This organ is formed from two rudiments, one arising in the roof of the mouth and the other arising in the floor of the diencephalon.

58. The endocrine cells of this organ arise from a diverticulum of the inferior portion of the foregut.

59. This organ contains derivatives from the yolk sac, coelomic epithelium, and mesenchyme of Wolffian body. At birth, gametogenic portion contains only gametogenic with 46 chromosomes and the somatic diploid amount of DNA.

60. Endocrine cells here are derived from the third or fourth pharyngeal pouch.

Item 61

61. Many congenital birth defects are caused by aneuploidy. Abnormalities in the development of the ocular system are most severe in which clinical syndrome due to aneuploidy?

(A) trisomy 21 (Down syndrome)
(B) trisomy 13 (Patau syndrome)
(C) trisomy 18 (Edwards syndrome)
(D) Klinefelter syndrome
(E) Turner syndrome

Item 62

62. Prior to the bone marrow, which organ is the most important site of hematopoiesis?

(A) dermis
(B) yolk sac
(C) spleen
(D) liver
(E) thymus

Item 63

63. In a new born infant, the majority of their circulating IgG molecules are derived from

(A) fetal B cells
(B) fetal plasma cells
(C) maternal T cells
(D) fetal T cells
(E) passive immunization via placental transport of maternal IgGs

Items 64-66

You are a neonatologist on-call for a busy obstetric service. You examine a new born male infant with tetany, cyanosis, and unusual craniofacial features including mandibular hypoplasia, a reduced philtrum, and low-set ears. Laboratory findings reveal hypocalcemia, decreased parathormone levels, but a nearly normal immunoglobulin profile.

64. The most likely diagnosis of this patient's condition is

(A) Down syndrome
(B) DiGeorge syndrome
(C) Bruton's agammaglobulinemia
(D) mandibulofacial dysostosis
(E) fetal alcohol syndrome and AIDS

65. Agenesis of which embryonic structures usually produces which one of the following conditions?

(A) thyroglossal duct
(B) first pharyngeal arch mesenchyme
(C) second pharyngeal pouch
(D) third and fourth pharyngeal pouches
(E) septum transversum

66. In many cases of DiGeorge syndrome, minor deletions have been detected in short arm of which chromosome?

(A) 20
(B) 22
(C) X
(D) 13
(E) Y

Items 67-69

In a second pregnancy, a 25-year-old woman delivers a hydropic fetus with severe edema, jaundice, and hepatosplenomegaly. Her first child was delivered at home by her aunt without any other medical intervention. Her blood type is O negative and her husband's blood type is O positive.

67. The blood type of the fetus is

(A) A positive
(B) A negative
(C) O positive
(D) O negative
(E) B positive

68. The most appropriate description of the cause of fetal hepatosplenomegaly is

(A) maternal IgGs stimulate hepatic parenchymal cell proliferation
(B) extramedullary hematopoiesis
(C) increased conjugation of heme degradation products
(D) increase in fetal blood volume
(E) compensation for reduced placental function

69. The primary cause of Rh isoimmunization is

(A) abnormal hepatic morphogenesis
(B) mixing of fetal and maternal blood
(C) accumulation of maternal IgGs at placenta
(D) failure of transplacental transport of maternal IgGs
(E) maternal formation of anti-spermatozoa IgGs

Item 70

A 6 month-old female infant is referred to you because of an abnormality in her upper lip and roof of her oral cavity. Upon examination you observe the defect shown in **Figure 3.8**.

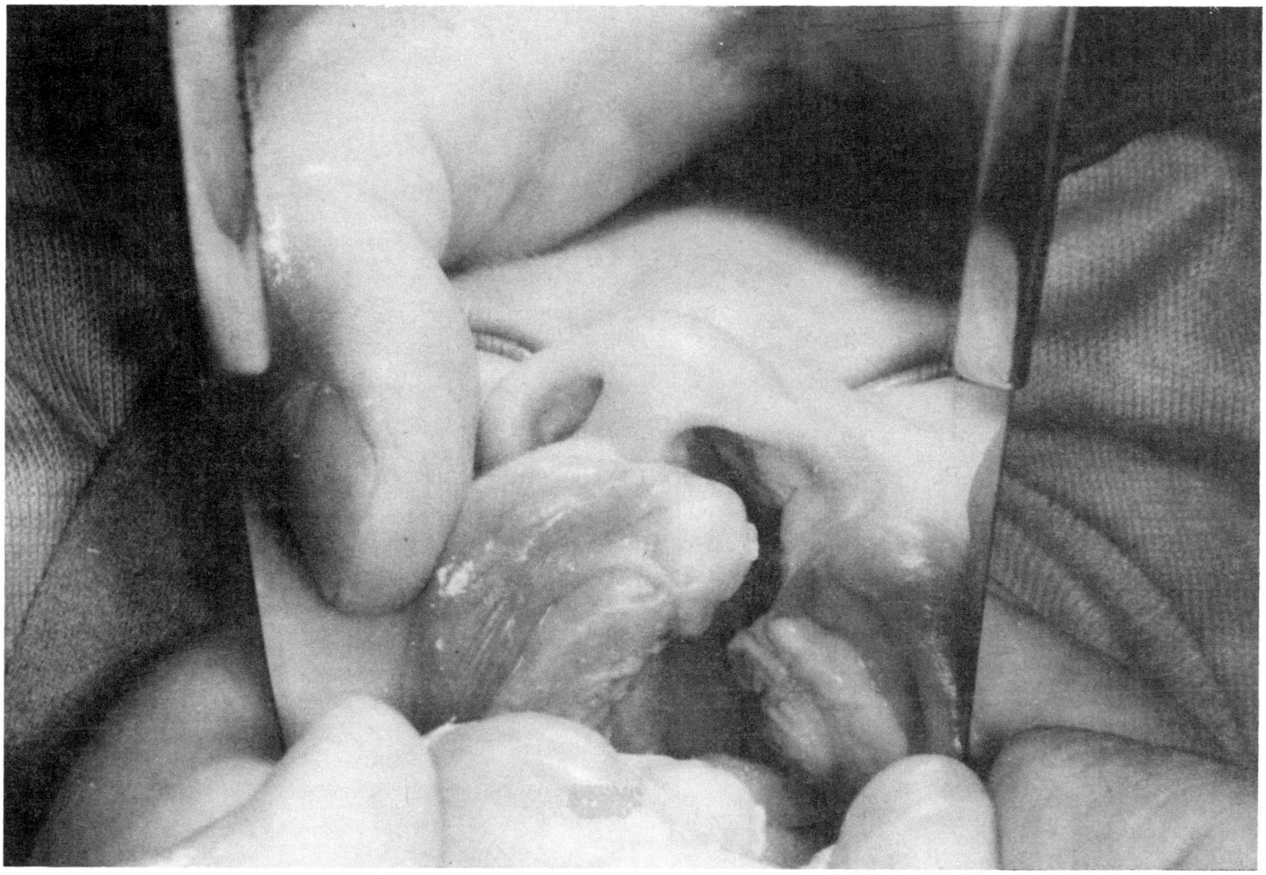

Figure 3.8

70. Which of the following is a true statement about clefts of the lip and palate?

(A) Most cases of cleft lip and palate are of multifactorial inheritance and not associated with other anomalies.
(B) Cleft lip and palate can be prevented by folic acid supplementation during pregnancy.
(C) Most children with cleft lip and palate will have below normal intelligence.
(D) Cleft palate results from a breakdown of the previously formed hard and soft palate junction.
(E) Repair of cleft lip and palate is difficult and usually not performed until a child is 2 years of age.

Items 71-72

Examine the child shown in **Figure 3.9**. Then choose the best response to the items below.

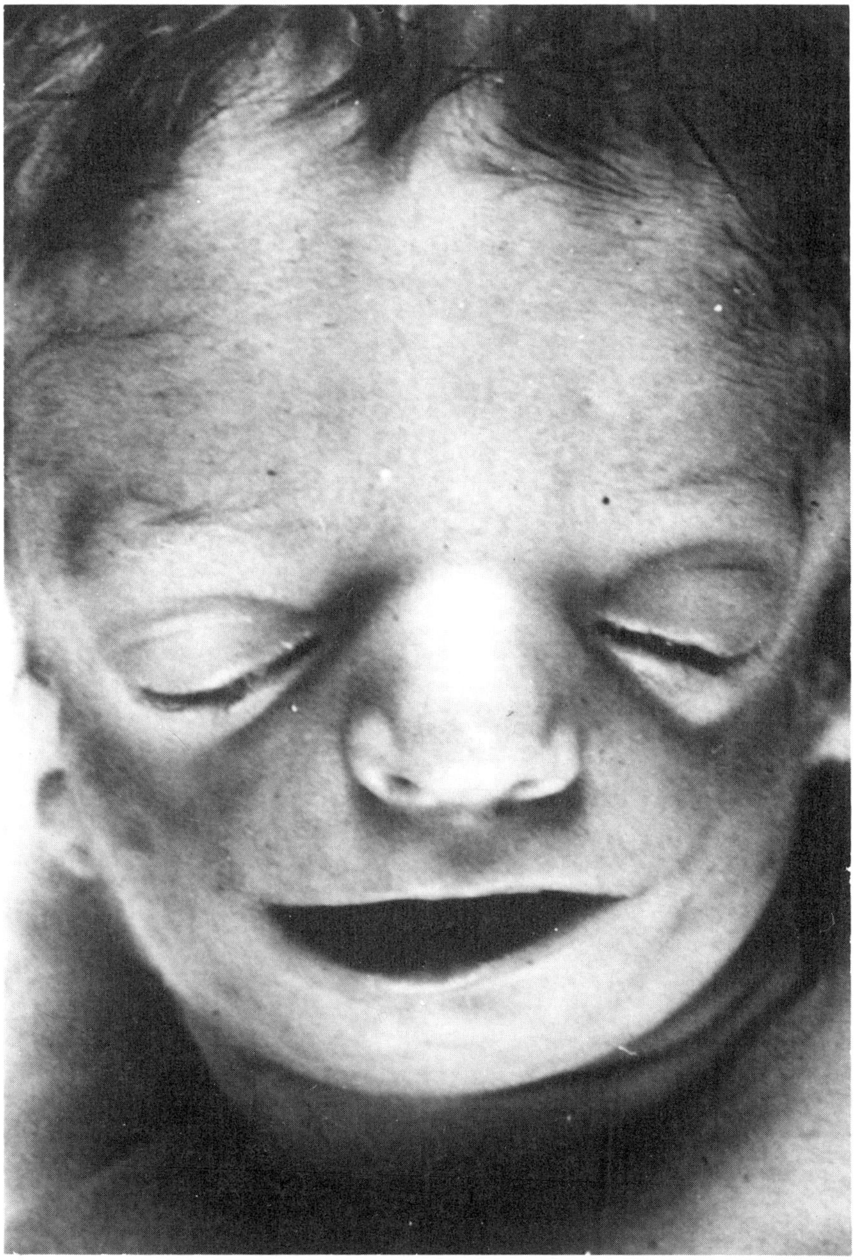

Figure 3.9

71. This child is most likely afflicted with which condition?

(A) fetal alcohol syndrome
(B) trisomy 21
(C) DiGeorge syndrome
(D) Treacher Collins syndrome
(E) trisomy 18

72. Individuals with this condition

(A) exhibit maldevelopment of mainly 2nd pharyngeal arch components
(B) rarely exhibit irregular tooth eruption even through the mouth is often large
(C) often exhibit hypoplasia of the hyoid apparatus resulting in swallowing difficulties
(D) typically exhibit mandibulofacial dysostosis
(E) probably produced supernumerary neural crest cells during the embryonic period

Item 73

73. The thyroid gland primordium

(A) appears shortly after the appearance of the pituitary gland primordium
(B) begins as a down growth of endoderm from the second pharyngeal (branchial) pouch
(C) may form ectopic thyroid tissue in the tongue
(D) does not form thyroid follicles until near term
(E) is non functional in the first trimester

Item 74

74. A poorly formed stapes in the tympanic cavity may result from inadequate development of

(A) lst pharyngeal arch mesenchyma
(B) 1st pharyngeal pouch endoderm
(C) 1st pharyngeal groove ectoderm
(D) 2nd pharyngeal arch mesenchyma
(E) 2nd pharyngeal pouch endoderm

Item 75

75. Which embryonic structure is most responsible for formation of the umbilical cord?

(A) extraembryonic coelom
(B) amnion
(C) chorion
(D) connecting stalk
(E) vitelline duct

Items 76-78

Match the placental secretion product in the list of answers below with its most appropriate functional role in the items below. Answers may be used once, more than once, or not at all.

(A) Chorionic gonadotrophin
(B) Somatomammotropin
(C) Progesterone
(D) Estriol
(E) Prostaglandins

76. Structurally and functionally similar to luteinizing hormone

77. High levels inhibit uterine smooth muscle contraction

78. Increased synthesis late in term initiates labor

Items 79-80

Examine the karyotype in **Figure 3.10** and then choose the best response to the items below.

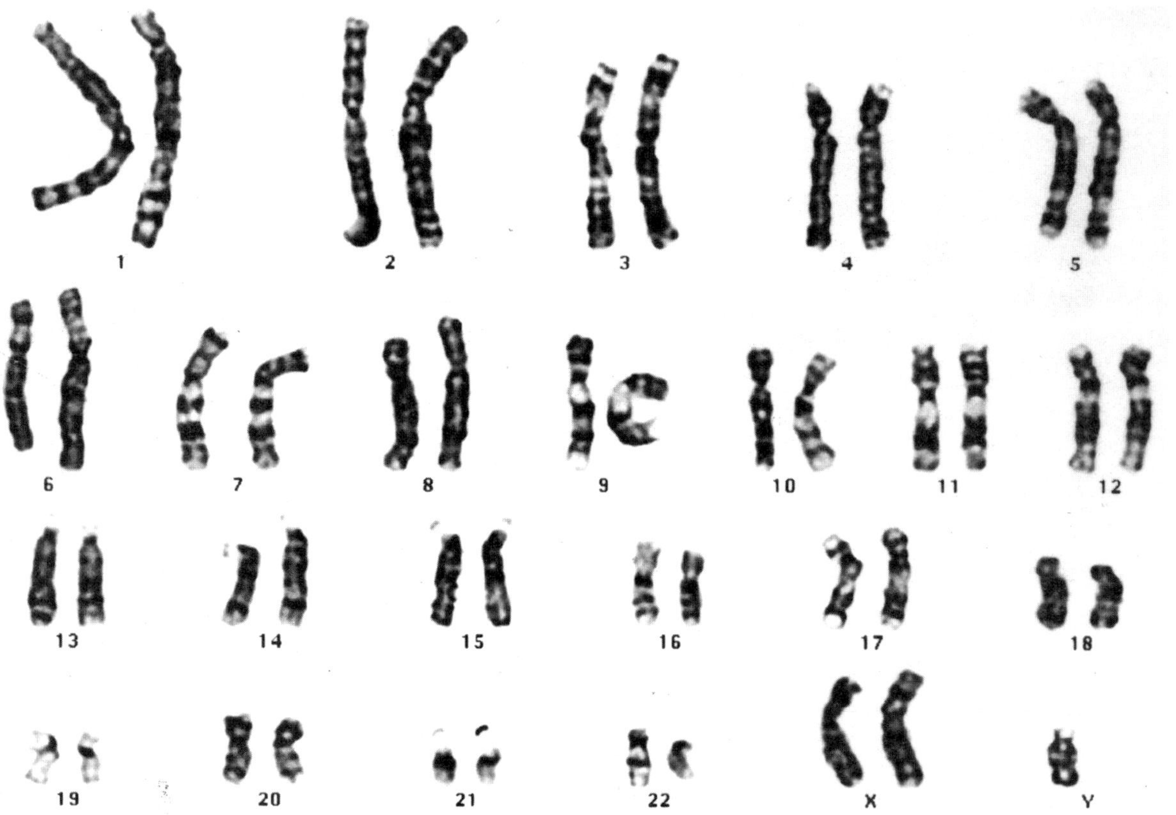

Figure 3.10

79. Which clinical syndrome is associated with this karyotype?

(A) Down syndrome
(B) Klinefelter's syndrome
(C) Turner's syndrome
(D) Edwards' syndrome
(E) Patau's syndrome

80. Which phrase would most appropriately describe the testis of such a person?

(A) hypertrophied
(B) absent
(C) frequently undescended with hyalinization of seminiferous epithelium
(D) lacking Leydig cells
(E) hermaphroditic

Items 81-82

Match the set of symptoms in the items below with the most appropriate teratogenic agent in the list of answer. Answers may be used once, more than once, or not at all.

(A) Thalidomide
(B) Alcohol
(C) Cocaine
(D) Heroin
(E) Rubella virus
(F) Herpes simplex virus
(G) *Toxoplasma gondii*
(H) Organic mercurial compounds
(I) Synthetic progestins
(J) High doses of ionizing radiation

81. Spontaneous abortion, often soon after acute exposure

82. Chorioretinitis, microcephaly, and calcifications around the choroid plexus

Item 83

A 34-year-old woman who is a severe, chronic alcoholic gave birth 5 years ago to the child shown in **Figure 3.11**. The child exhibits a pattern of defects associated with fetal alcohol syndrome (FAS).

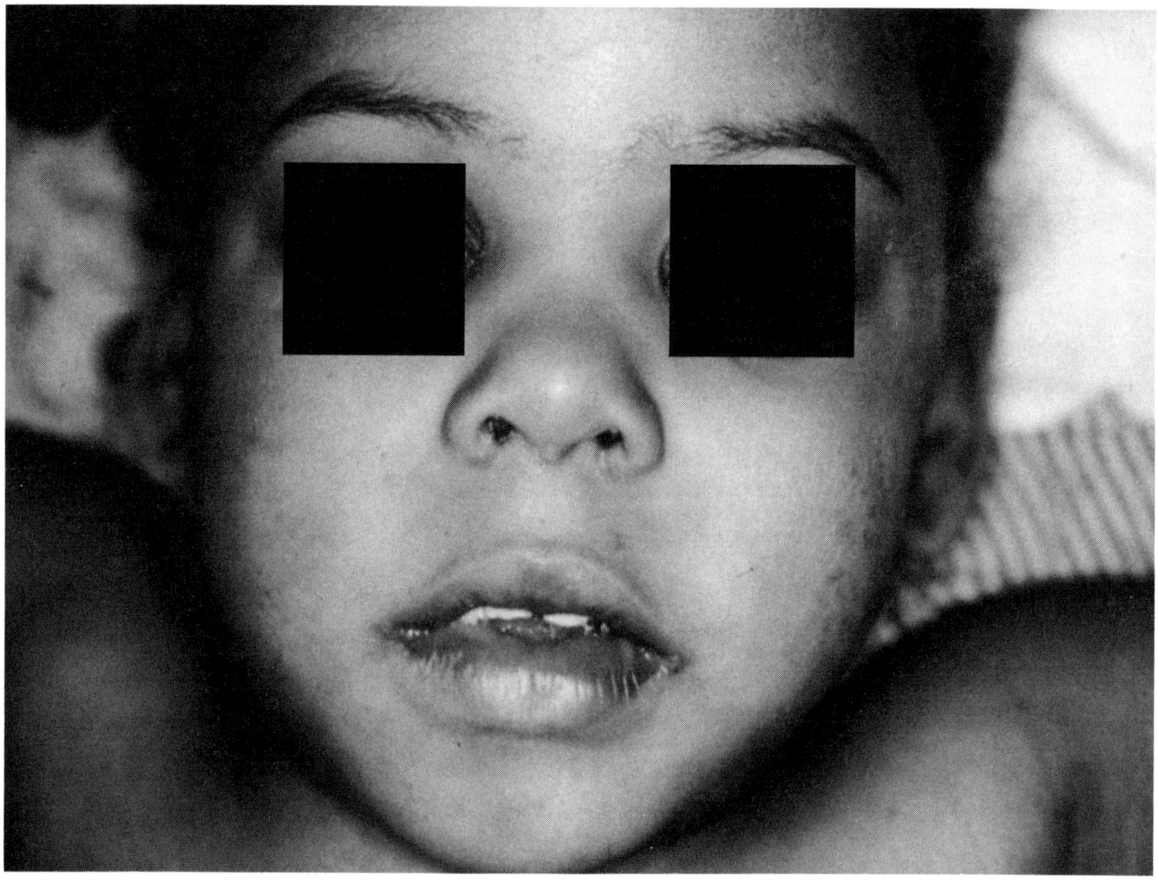

Figure 3.11

83. Which of the following statements concerning the fetal effect of maternal alcohol consumption during pregnancy is true?

(A) Moderate maternal alcohol consumption has no effect.
(B) Maternal alcohol abuse is thought to be the most common cause of mental retardation.
(C) Heavy alcohol consumption limited to a few days during pregnancy is thought to have no effect.
(D) The susceptible period of brain development is limited to the first trimester.
(E) Fetal alcohol effects (FAE) usually do not involve brain functions

Item 84

84. The period during pregnancy most sensitive to teratogens is

(A) preimplantation
(B) first trimester
(C) second trimester
(D) third trimester
(E) fetal

Items 85-87

Match the clinical entity or situation caused by a structural defect in the items below with the portion of the embryonic mesoderm responsible for this abnormality. Answers may be used once, more than once, or not at all.

(A) Somatopleuric mesoderm
(B) Splanchnopleuric mesoderm
(C) Sclerotome
(D) Dermatomyotome
(E) Intermediate mesoderm
(F) Notochord
(G) None of the above

85. Meckel's diverticulum

86. Congenital absence of vertebral body

87. Horseshoe kidney

Items 88-89

A child born to apparently normal parents is unusually short with a depressed nasal bridge, a prominent forehead, and significant bowing of the lower limbs. Further tests reveal that the child is affected by achondroplasia.

88. In most cases, this developmental defect is caused by which fundamental underlying genetic mechanism?

(A) aneuploidy
(B) autosomal dominant mutation
(C) autosomal recessive mutation
(D) trisomy
(E) sex-linked mutation

89. Which developmental process is most disrupted in the patient's anomaly?

(A) somitogenesis
(B) osteoid secretion
(C) neural crest cell migration
(D) chondrocyte proliferation at epiphyseal plate
(E) intramembranous ossification

Items 90-91

A newborn male infant is delivered prematurely and alive. The infant had a beak-like nose, small thorax, and numerous fractures in the limbs. One day after birth, the child died from respiratory failure.

90. The most likely diagnosis here is

(A) osteogenesis imperfecta, type I
(B) osteogenesis imperfecta, type II
(C) achondroplasia
(D) Marfan's syndrome
(E) Hurler's syndrome

91. The biochemical lesion in this disease affects which important constituent of the extracellular matrix of connective tissue in limbs?

(A) hyaluronic acid
(B) type I collagen
(C) type IV collagen
(D) chondroitin sulfate
(E) heparan sulfate

Items 92-93

92. In a normal 25-year-old adult, growth in length of long bones is normally precluded because

  (A) epiphyseal plates have reduced sensitivity to growth hormone
  (B) epiphyseal plates stop growing and become completely ossified
  (C) osteolysis outstrips osteogenesis
  (D) osteoclastic activity becomes more intense
  (E) osteoblasts disappear

93. In the repair of a simple fracture of the radius, which cell type is most active in the secretion of osteoid in the repairing callus?

  (A) osteoclast
  (B) fibroblast
  (C) monocyte
  (D) osteoblast
  (E) osteoprogenitor cell

Item 94

94. Which of the following are neuroblast derivatives?

  (A) oligodendrocytes in the spinal cord
  (B) astrocytes in the spinal cord
  (C) Schwann cells in a peripheral nerve fiber
  (D) rods in the retina
  (E) pigmented epithelium in retina

Items 95-96

95. Which of the following are alar plate or alar lamina derivatives?

  (A) spinal cord sensory neurons
  (B) spinal cord motor neurons
  (C) general visceral efferent nuclei
  (D) dorsal root ganglia
  (E) intermediate horn interneurons

96. Which of the following are basal plate or basal lamina derivatives?

  (A) spinal cord intermediate neurons
  (B) spinal cord motor neurons
  (C) rhombencephalic general visceral efferent nuclei
  (D) rhombencephalic special visceral afferent nuclei
  (E) mesencephalic tectal nuclei

STOP.

YOU HAVE COMPLETED THIS SECTION.

Notes

Embryology

Answers and Tutorials

Answers and Tutorial on Items 1-2

The answers are: **1-A; 2-A**. Complete **renal agenesis** most likely results from a failure of development of the metanephric (definitive) kidney. The fundamental process leading to formation of the metanephros is a reciprocal inductive interaction between the **ureteric bud** (a branch of the mesonephric duct) and the **metanephric blastema** (the caudal portion of the urogenital ridge). The ureteric bud grows into the metanephric blastema and is induced to branch many times leading to the formation of the ureters, major calyces, minor calyces and collecting ducts of the definitive kidney. The ureteric bud induces the formation of nephrons in the metanephric blastema. Derivatives of the metanephric blastema include the renal glomerulus and other blood vessels, connective tissue, Bowman's capsule, proximal convoluted tubule, loop of Henle and distal convoluted tubule.

The fetus normally produces a small amount of hypotonic urine and urinates it into the amniotic fluid. Subsequently, the fetus swallows the amniotic fluid. Renal agenesis results in no urine formation and therefore a reduction in volume of amniotic fluid (**oligohydramnios**). Anencephalic fetuses have no swallowing function but do produce urine, leading to the excessive volume of amniotic fluid (**polyhydramnios**). Urine production is normal in bladder exstrophy which does not become apparent as a clinical problem until after birth. Blockage of the gastrointestinal tract would also lead to polyhydramnios.

Answers and Tutorial on Items 3-5

The answers are: **3-D; 4-D; 5-A**. The most appropriate next test would be a **karyotype analysis** followed by measurements of serum steroids. You would discover that the patient had a 46, XY normal male karyotype and normal testosterone levels. Further tests would reveal a **deficiency in testosterone receptor**. This patient has **testicular feminization syndrome**. There is an increased risk of seminoma in undescended testes and orchiectomy would be appropriate for the left testicle in the left labium majorum and the right testicle in the inguinal canal or body cavity. While genetically male, this patient would have a female gender identity but would be sterile because of a lack of ovaries and hyalinization of seminiferous epithelium in undescended testes. Because of the presence of a Y chromosome, H-Y antigen and **testis determining factor** would be present. Paramesonephric duct derivatives (uterine tubes, uterus and upper portion of vagina) would be absent due to müllerian inhibiting substance produced by the testes.

Answers and Tutorial on Items 6-10

The answers are: **6-A; 7-C; 8-C; 9-C; 10-B.** Figure 3.1 is the karyotype of a female child with primary **nondisjunctional trisomy 13** (Patau's syndrome). This congenital anomaly occurs in approximately 1/20,000 live-born children. The appropriate shorthand notation designating this kind of aneuploidy is 47, XX, +13. During synapsis of the first meiotic metaphase, homologous chromosomes pair. If this pairing leads to failure of separation of chromosomes, gametes are produced with either an extra copy of some particular chromosome or lacking that copy of the chromosome. A human female is born with all of her oocytes arrested in the first meiotic metaphase. Meiosis I is not completed in the human female until just before ovulation. Consequently, synapsis can last for many years. Increasing maternal age leads to higher incidence of non-dysjunctional chromosomal anomalies including **Patau's syndrome**. When nondisjunction occurs during oogenesis, the ova contain either two copies of chromosome 13 or no copies of chromosome 13 instead of the normal single copy of chromosome 13. When an ovum containing two copies of chromosome 13 is fertilized by a haploid sperm, three copies (2 maternal and one paternal) are found in the zygote and subsequent developmental stages resulting in trisomy 13 (Patau's syndrome). The common symptoms peculiar to trisomy 13 are holoprosencephaly, microphthalmia, anophthalmia, cleft lip, cleft palate and polydactyly. Congenital heart defects are found in Patau's syndrome but are found in other conditions as well, eg, in Down and Edward's syndrome. Children with trisomy 13 usually die soon after birth.

Answers and Tutorial on Items 11-14

The answers are: **11-E; 12-C; 13-A; 14-D**. The leading cause of death among premature infants is **respiratory distress syndrome**. A fetus 30 weeks from the last menstrual period is 28 weeks into a gestation. At 28 weeks gestational age, **type II pneumocytes** first differentiate and begin to secrete surfactant. The most abundant phospholipid in surfactant is **lecithin**. The sphingomyelin levels in amniotic fluid are relatively constant throughout gestation but the lecithin levels begin to rise slowly at 28 weeks. Once many type II cells differentiate, they secrete substantial quantities of surfactant which enters the amniotic fluid due to fetal respiratory movements. Due to increasing surfactant secretion, the lecithin/sphingomyelin ratio increases. Type II cell differentiation is a steroid dependent process. Treatment of women with certain steroid drugs will stimulate precocious differentiation of type II cells and thus reduce the risk of respiratory distress syndrome in premature infants.

Answers and Tutorial on Items 15-17

The answers are: **15-E; 16-E; 17-A**. Premature rupture of fetal membranes often leads to **chorioamnionitis** with elevated temperature and elevated white blood cell count. The normal white blood cell count is approximately 5,000/mm^3. Under normal circumstances, the fetus develops in a sterile environment and is therefore not exposed to bacterial antigens. Consequently, fetal lymph nodes lack **germinal centers**. At birth, the fetus is suddenly exposed to an entire new population of bacterial antigens. This potential problem is dealt with in three ways. First, during gestation, the fetus is passively immunized against bacterial antigens by transplacental transport of maternal IgGs. Higher molecular weight IgM is not transported across the placenta. Second, if the child is breast fed, colostrum contains high concentrations of secretory IgAs that bind to enteric bacteria and prevent their adhesion to the gastrointestinal epithelium. Third, once the fetus becomes exposed to bacterial antigens, his or her own lymph nodes (if antigens are lymph-born) and spleen (if the antigens are blood-born) become activated. Germinal centers represent areas where B lymphocytes, in conjunction with helper T cells and antigen-presenting macrophages are becoming activated. This activation involves decreasing nuclear condensation and increasing cytoplasm to produce the intracellular machinery for IgG synthesis. Once stimulated, B cells differentiate into immunoglobulin secreting plasma cells. Germinal centers also contain large numbers of macrophages.

Answer and Tutorial on Item 18

The answer is: **18-D**. **Rh isoimmunization** occurs in fetuses with Rh^- mothers and Rh^+ fathers. The Rh antigen is controlled by a dominant gene and therefore the fetus of an Rh^- mother and Rh^+ father would be Rh^+. Rh isoimmunization is more severe with each pregnancy because the maternal immune system has a memory for Rh isoimmunization. Normally, the placental trophoblast serves as a barrier between fetal and maternal blood, although microvascular accidents allowing mixture of fetal and maternal blood are inevitable. When fetal RBCs leak into the maternal blood supply, they are recognized as foreign antigens by the maternal immune system. Maternal IgGs are produced against the fetal RBCs and these are transported functionally intact across the placenta into the fetal circulatory system. Here, these IgGs bind to fetal RBCs and cause their destruction in the fetal liver and spleen. The resulting anemia stimulates fetal erythropoiesis in the bone marrow, liver and spleen. Consequently, enlargement of the liver and spleen occurs. Excessive destruction of fetal RBCs results in accumulation of bile pigments and thus **jaundice**.

Answers and Tutorial on Items 19-20

The answers are: **19-C; 20-A**. There is a high probability that the mother is an alcoholic. Her obesity, hepatomegaly and spider angiomas are highly suggestive of alcoholism. Her denial of alcohol consumption during pregnancy is suspicious. Alcoholism is especially common among American Indians. The child shows many of the features of **fetal alcohol syndrome** (FAS) including short stature, facial abnormalities and mild mental retardation. Alcohol and acetaldehyde are known teratogens. They cross the placenta rapidly and persist in the fetus long after being cleared from the maternal system. The fetal hepatic detoxification functions for alcohol are poorly developed. Experimental studies in mammalian embryos suggest that one of the primary causative events in FAS teratogenesis is inhibition of cell migration. Neural crest cells migrate into the pharyngeal apparatus where they participate in morphogenesis of facial bones. The mid-facial hypoplasia characteristic of FAS children is most likely due to defects in neural crest cell migration.

Answers and Tutorial on Items 21-22

The answers are: **21-C; 22-C**. This patient is suffering from **Hirschsprung's disease** or colonic aganglionosis. Biopsy of the distal colon would reveal that the parasympathetic ganglia and other neuronal elements of the myenteric plexus are absent from the narrowed portion of the colon. Ganglia are present in the distended portion of the colon. The neurons of the myenteric plexus are derived from the **neural crest** and the congenital anomaly is due to abnormal neural crest cell migration to the colon. Neural crest cells also contribute to dorsal root ganglia; form the adrenal medulla; form Schwann cells, myelinating cells in the peripheral nervous system; form meninges; form melanocytes and form odontoblasts, the dentin-secreting cells of tooth germs.

Answers and Tutorial on Items 23-24

The answers are: **23-D; 24-A**. Maternal oxygenated blood is supplied to the placenta from branches of the **uterine arteries**. These vessels empty into the **intervillous space** where they carry O_2 to and remove CO_2 from capillaries in chorionic villi. The deoxygenated maternal blood returns to the uterine veins and eventually the maternal pulmonary circulation, where CO_2 is expelled and fresh O_2 is dissolved in maternal blood for return to the uterine artery. Deoxygenated fetal blood enters the placenta through the umbilical arteries. These blood vessels send branches into the chorionic villi where there is a complex anastomosing network of capillaries. In these villi, fetal blood becomes oxygenated and then drains back into the umbilical vein. The umbilical vein carrying oxygenated fetal blood empties into the fetal inferior vena cava, shunts by the liver through the ductus venosus and enters the right atrium. Before birth, this blood is then mostly shunted through the foramen ovale into the left atrium and then into the fetal systemic circulation. Some of this oxygenated blood mixes with deoxygenated blood returning to the right atrium from the superior vena cava and then enters the right ventricle where it is pumped into the pulmonary artery. Most of the blood leaving the right ventricle is shunted away from the lungs into the systemic circulation at the arch of the aorta by way of the **ductus arteriosus**.

Answers and Tutorial on Items 25-29

The answers are: **25-D; 26-B; 27-B; 28-E; 29-A**. **Figure 3.2** is the karyotype of a female child with primary nondisjunctional **trisomy 18** (Edwards' syndrome). This congenital anomaly occurs in approximately 1/8,000 live-born children. The appropriate shorthand notation designating this kind of aneuploidy is 47, XX, +18. During synapsis of the first meiotic metaphase, homologous chromosomes pair. If this pairing leads to failure of separation of chromosomes, gametes are produced with either an extra copy of some particular chromosome or lacking that copy of the chromosome. A human female is born with all of her oocytes arrested in the first meiotic metaphase. Meiosis I is not completed in the human female until just before ovulation. Consequently, synapsis can last for many years. Increasing maternal age leads to higher incidence of non-disjunctional chromosomal anomalies including **Edwards' syndrome**. When non-disjunction occurs during oogenesis, the ova contain either two copies of chromosome 18 or no copies of chromosome 18 instead of the normal single copy of chromosome 18. When an ovum containing two copies of chromosome 18 is fertilized by a haploid sperm, three copies (two maternal and one paternal) are found in the zygote and subsequent developmental stages resulting in trisomy 18 (Edwards syndrome). The common symptoms peculiar to trisomy 18 are microcephaly, prominent occiput, low-set pointed ears, micrognathia, overlapping fingers and rounded feet with a large calcaneus. Cardiovascular and renal defects are also commonly found in Edwards' syndrome but are found in other conditions as well, eg, cardiovascular defects are also common in Down syndrome. Children with trisomy 18 usually die soon after birth.

Answers and Tutorial on Items 30-34

The answers are: **30-B; 31-C; 32-A; 33-C; 34-C**. **Figure 3.3** is an example of a **normal female karyotype**. Fetal tissue samples must be gathered for karyotype analysis. In prenatal diagnosis, fetal cells can be gathered by amniocentesis or chorionic villus sampling. Following collection of fetal cells, they can be grown in tissue culture. Treatment of cultures of cells with the drug **colchicine** results in the arrest of cell division at metaphase. Chromosomes on the metaphase plate can then be spread, stained, photographed and mounted in a karyotype. This karyotype is a normal female karyotype described by the shorthand notation 46, XX. This is a **euploid** karyotype. Aneuploid karyotypes have numerical anomalies so that there are more or less than 46 chromosomes. Trisomy and monosomy are examples of **aneuploid** karyotypes. Klinefelter syndrome (47, XXY) is an example of sex chromosome aneuploidy. Trisomy 21 (Down syndrome), 47, XX, +21 in a female is an example of an autosomal aneuploidy. Testicular feminization syndrome is due to a lack of the testosterone receptor and would be associated with a normal male karyotype (46, XY). Turner's syndrome is due to a lack of a second X chromosome (45, X). Sickle cell anemia is due to a point mutation in the hemoglobin gene and would be associated with either a normal male or normal female karyotype.

Answer and Tutorial on Item 35

The answer is: **35-E**. This child has the **tetralogy of Fallot**. The mild cyanosis and dyspnea are caused by the poor vascular perfusion of the lungs due to the pulmonary artery stenosis and ventricular septal defect with large right to left shunt. Abnormally high pressure in the right ventricle due to the overriding aorta causes **right ventricular hypertrophy** and is largely responsible for the radiological findings. The systolic murmur is due to turbulence of blood flow through the right ventricular outflow tract. The primitive heart, prior to ventricular septation, has a single large ventricle which leads into a large ventricular outflow tract called the conus cordis. The conus cordis leads into the truncus arteriosus which in turn supplies blood to the aortic sac and aortic arches. The tetralogy of Fallot is the most frequently seen abnormality caused by unequal division of the conus cordis and truncus arteriosus. This defect is caused by an anterior displacement of the truncoconal septum, a flap of tissue that forms in the conus cordis and truncus arteriosus to divided the ventricular outflow tracts. Prior to birth, the **ductus arteriosus**, a derivative of the left distal 6th aortic arch, provides a shunt between the pulmonary and the systemic circulation. Soon after birth, the ductus arteriosus closes and degenerates, leaving behind a ligamentum arteriosum. In many cases of tetralogy of Fallot, there is also a persistent ductus arteriosus.

Answers and Tutorial on Items 36-37

The answers are: **36-C; 37-D**. During formation of the **mature antral follicle**, the first meiotic division is completed just before ovulation, leading to the formation of the **secondary oocyte** and the **first polar body**. It is thought that fertilization normally needs to occur within about 1 day of ovulation. When spermatozoa reach the immediate environment of the primary oocyte (and associated corona radiata and zona pellucida), the **acrosome reaction** occurs, leading to the release of hydrolytic enzymes used to degrade the extracellular matrix between granulosa cells of the **corona radiata** and for lysis of the zona pellucida. When the tip of the acrosome contacts the primary oocyte, **cortical granules** are discharged and they cause changes in the oocyte membrane rendering it unfertilizable by additional spermatozoa (**block to polyspermy**). At **fertilization**, the second meiotic division occurs, leading to formation of the **ovum** and the **second polar body**. A third polar body sometimes forms as a result of completion of meiosis II in the first polar body. Fertilization also initiates development and results in the **haploid male pronucleus** entering the cytoplasm of the ovum, where it fuses with the **haploid female pronucleus**, leading to formation of the **diploid zygote nucleus**.

Answers and Tutorial on Items 38-40

The answers are: **38-A; 39-C; 40-E**. During **implantation**, the blastocyst, which was formerly floating freely in the lumen of the female reproductive tract, attaches to and invades the **endometrium**. Implantation occurs normally in the **posterior wall** of the uterine body.

The outer epithelial **trophoblast** of the blastocyst adheres specifically to endometrial epithelial cells and then differentiates into two layers, the **cytotrophoblast** and the **syncytiotrophoblast**. The cytotrophoblast proliferates and daughter cells fuse to form the syncytiotrophoblast which degrades and invades first the endometrial epithelium and then the endometrial stroma. The syncytiotrophoblast also secretes an important glycoprotein hormone called human chorionic gonadotropin (**hCG**). This hormone stimulates the **corpus luteum** to secrete **progesterone** and thus maintains the progestational state. Without a corpus luteum during the first trimester, the pregnancy would fail.

In humans, implantation is **interstitial**, ie, the developing conceptus becomes completely engulfed by maternal tissue. The syncytiotrophoblast invades maternal tissue by degrading it and eventually degrades maternal blood vessels as well. The surface of the syncytiotrophoblast increases dramatically, first by the formation of lacunae and later, in collaboration with the cytotrophoblast, fetal connective tissue, and fetal blood vessels, contributes to **placental villi**. The syncytiotrophoblast is the boundary between the fetal tissue and is bathed directly in maternal blood. Its invasiveness is limited by the formation of **decidual cells**. These differentiate from endometrial stroma and form a shell around the implantation site, limiting the invasiveness of the conceptus.

Answers and Tutorial on Items 41-44

The answers are: **41-B; 42-A; 43-C; 44-D**. During early development, the **embryoblast** (inner cell mass) becomes divided into two layers, the **epiblast** and the **hypoblast**. During gastrulation, three primary germ layers, **ectoderm**, **mesoderm**, and **endoderm** are formed. During neurulation, the ectoderm forms a neural plate in the dorsal midline and this plate rolls up into a neural tube during neurulation. Just prior to the fusion of the dorsal neural folds, certain neuroectodermal cells leave the neuroepithelium and migrate to scattered and sometimes distant sites. This population of cells is known as the **neural crest**. The non-neural ectoderm will be called surface ectoderm.

The **ectoderm** forms the neuroectoderm and the surface ectoderm. The **neuroectoderm** forms the **neural tube** and **neural crest**. The neural tube forms the brain and spinal cord. **Surface ectoderm** forms the outer surface epithelium of skin (epidermis) and its appendages, ie, hair and hair follicles, sweat and sebaceous glands, and the epithelial exocrine glandular portion of the mammary glands. Surface ectoderm also forms the corneal epithelium, the lining of the oral cavity anterior to the stomodeum (and thus enamel of teeth and parts of some salivary glands), and the lining of the anal canal posterior to the proctodeum.

Neural crest forms the neurons and glial cells in dorsal root ganglia, the myenteric plexus, and some other parasympathetic ganglia and sympathetic ganglia. In addition it forms the dentin secreting odontoblasts of teeth, melanocytes, Schwann cells (PNS myelinating cells), the adrenal medulla, and pia-arachnoid meninges. The neural crest makes an important contribution to head mesenchyme and thus contributes to pharyngeal arch cartilage, bone, connective tissue, and the pupillary muscles and ciliary muscles in the eye. It also forms calcitonin-secreting parafollicular cells in the thyroid, parts of the cardiac outflow tracts (eg, the truncoconal septum), and some enteroendocrine cells.

Mesoderm forms the entire cardiovascular system and its contents, blood. Most connective tissues (general and special) are also mesodermal derivatives. Therefore, except for those formed by neural crest, all other bones, cartilages, ligaments, tendons, fascia, aponeuroses, The vast bulk of the skeletal and smooth muscle in the body is formed by mesoderm (except for the pupillary muscles which are derived from the neural crest). Most of the urogenital system also arises from mesoderm.

Endoderm forms the epithelial lining of the gastrointestinal tract and its diverticula including the salivary glands, lungs, thyroid gland (follicular epithelial cells only), liver, pancreas, and gall bladder and their ducts. The transitional epithelium lining the urinary bladder is also endodermally derived.

Answers and Tutorial on Items 45-46

The answers are: **45-I; 46-K**. The growth of the amnion is an important feature in the establishment of the basic vertebrate body plan in humans. The **head fold of the amnion** (A) sculpts the head and tucks the **stomodeum** (G) and cardiac anlage from a dorsal cranial position to a ventral (rotated) position caudal to the forebrain. Similarly, the **tail fold of the amnion** (B) tucks the **proctodeum** (H) (precursor of the hymen) under the tail. The lateral folds of the amnion push the lateral plate mesoderm down around the **yolk sac**, sculpting the tubular gut. The growth of the amnion also pinches off the yolk sac (I) and forms the connecting stalk into an umbilical cord, leaving a small remnant of the yolk sac projecting from the umbilical cord. The yolk sac remains connected to the midgut by a **vitelline duct** (J). Persistent vitelline duct remnants can lead to formation of **Meckel's diverticulum**. This anomaly is seen in about 1% of adults, most commonly as a small diverticulum in the ileum and more commonly in men than in women. It often contains ectopic gastric tissue and can lead to ileal ulceration.

Intraembryonic mesoderm is divided in segmentally arranged **somites** (F) which are connected to segmentally arranged masses of **intermediate mesoderm** (E). The intermediate mesoderm then leads into **lateral plate mesoderm**. Somites become divided into **sclerotomes** (precursors of vertebral bodies and the annulus fibrosus) and **dermomyotomes** (precursors of segmental dermis and skeletal muscle). Intermediate mesoderm forms most of the urogenital system. The intraembryonic coelom forms by coalescence of small clefts in the lateral plate and finally splits it into an outer (superficial) **somatopleuric (somatic) mesoderm** (C) and an inner (deep) **splanchnopleuric (splanchnic) mesoderm** (D). The somatic mesoderm forms body wall structures, while the splanchnic mesoderm forms smooth muscle and connective tissue surrounding visceral organs, eg, enteric smooth muscle and cardiac muscle.

The **septum transversum** (K) is a mass of mesoderm that lies caudal to the heart primordium but cranial to the vitelline duct. It makes a major contribution to the formation of the diaphragm. The liver diverticulum grows into the septum transversum, eventually forming liver parenchymal cells. The mesenchymal tissue in the septum transversum forms blood vessels and connective tissue in the liver.

Answers and Tutorial on Items 47-48

The answers are: **47-C; 48-B**. The **cerebrum** in **Figure 3.4** is formed by the telencephalic hemispheres which are in turn derived from the prosencephalon (forebrain). The **cerebellum** (B) forms in the rhombic lip of the metencephalon which is in turn derived from the rhombencephalon (hindbrain). It has cortical grey matter like the cerebrum but contains Purkinje cells (neurons) and Golgi neurons peculiar to the cerebellum. The **medulla oblongata** (C) forms from the myelencephalon which in turn develops from the caudal portion of the rhombencephalon. The **corpus callosum** is D. The **pons** (E) forms from the metencephalon of the rhombencephalon.

Answers and Tutorial on Items 49-52

The answers are: **49-C; 50-C; 51-A; 52-B**. In many children with **lumbosacral myelomeningocele**, a kind of **spina bifida cystica**, there are associated defects in the brain stem and cerebellum known as the **Arnold-Chiari malformation**. The etiology of this and other neural tube defects is poorly understood but it appears that there are both genetic and environmental factors at work here, ie, its etiology is **multifactorial**. In the example shown in **Figure 3.5**, there is elongation of the brain stem and herniation of the lower part of the cerebellum through the foramen magnum. **Hydrocephalus** is frequently associated with the Arnold-Chiari malformation and is most likely secondary to it. One plausible sequence of events follows. Compression of the cerebellum can lead to obstruction of the foramen of Magendie. This leads to intraventricular accumulation of cerebrospinal fluid and thus, frequently, to hydrocephalus. The Arnold-Chiari malformation is a relatively common CNS abnormality (about 1/1000 births).

Answers and Tutorial on Items 53-54

The answers are: **53-E; 54-A**. The ultrasonogram in **Figure 3.6** shows an example of a fetus with an **encephalocele**. This is a type of **neural tube defect**. Neural tube defects show a complex multifactorial etiology with both genetic and environmental factors contributing to an increased incidence. In this case, the base of the occipital bone is poorly formed. During early development, the neural tube induces formation of the bony structures protecting the central nervous system such as the neural arches and the vault of the skull. In many types of neural tube defects, there is both abnormal formation of nervous tissue leading to neurological deficits and abnormal formation of the overlying bony structures normally protecting the nervous system. In encephalocele, meninges protrude into the space created by abnormal formation of the base of the occipital bone. Fetal blood and cerebrospinal fluid contains **α-fetoprotein**. In many neural tube defects, this α-fetoprotein leaks into the amniotic fluid (where it can be measured as an indication of neural tube defects) and may cross into the maternal circulation and subsequently be detected by an assay of maternal serum α-fetoprotein.

Neural tube defects range in severity. In **spina bifida occulta**, there is only an absence of the bony neural arch of vertebral bodies and a small likelihood of neurological deficits. In **rachischisis**, there is a complete failure of closure of the neural tube, so that the brain and spinal cord does not form. **Anencephalic fetuses** have a failure of closure of the neural tube beginning in the cranial region. Thus, the spinal cord is intact but the brain is malformed.

Answers and Tutorial on Items 55-60

The answers are: **55-G; 56-B; 57-A; 58-C; 59-D; 60-G**. The **pituitary gland** is derived from two different embryonic anlage. The adenohypophysis (source of major endocrine secretions of pituitary, eg, TSH, ACTH, Growth Hormone, FSH and LH) is derived from an evagination of the roof of the mouth (ectoderm) called **Rathke's pouch**. Rathke's pouch derivatives include the pars distalis, pars tuberalis, and pars intermedia of the adenohypophysis. The neurohypophysis (place where releasing hormones are released) is derived from an evagination of the floor of the brain (ectoderm) called the **infundibulum**.

The **thyroid gland** (B) arises from a diverticulum of the foregut (endoderm) at the root of the developing tongue. The anlage of the thyroid descends through the neck region as the proximal root of a **thyroglossal duct**, a structure which usually degenerates but may persist, forming ectopic thyroid tissue anywhere along the route of descent. The main thyroid follicular epithelial cells, which secrete thyroxine, are endodermally derived. The calcitonin-secreting parafollicular **C cells** of the thyroid originate in the **neural crest** (neuroectoderm).

The **pancreas** (C), both exocrine acinar tissue and endocrine islet tissue, arises from dorsal and ventral pancreatic rudiments which form as diverticula at the duodenal (inferior) portion of the foregut (endoderm). During gut rotation, the dorsal and ventral pancreatic rudiments fuse to form a single gland. Earlier theories of neural crest origin for islet tissue appear to be unsupported by experimental evidence.

The **testes** (D) and **ovaries** (E) have important endocrine roles. The chief endocrine tissue of the testis is a diffuse collection of interstitial **Leydig cells**. These arise from genital ridge mesenchyme and secrete testosterone. The chief endocrine tissue of the ovary is more complex. The **granulosa cells** of follicles and the thecal cells surrounding follicles both have an important endocrine role. The **thecal cells**, like Leydig cells, arise from genital ridge mesenchyme. The granulosa cells, like their homolog in men, the Sertoli cells, arise from coelomic epithelium. The gametogenic cell lines (oogonia and their products in women, spermatogonia and their products in men) are derived from **primordial germ cells**, a diploid cell line arising in the yolk sac and migrating to the gonadal precursor early in development.

The **adrenal glands** (F) have a population of medullary cells that originate in neural crest (neuroectoderm) and cortical cells that are arise from the coelomic epithelium and migrate into the adrenal anlage.

The **parathyroid glands** (G) usually are found as a superior pair (derived from fourth pharyngeal pouch epithelium) and an inferior pair (derived from third pharyngeal pouch epithelium). Due to their extensive developmental migrations, the position and even number of parathyroid glands can be variable.

The **pineal gland** (H) is entirely derived from the central nervous system. It arises as an evagination of the roof plate of the brain in the region of the epithalamus.

ANSWER AND TUTORIAL ON ITEM 61

The answer is: **61-B**. While many different clinical entities may show developmental anomalies in the eyes and ears, ocular development is most profoundly disrupted in Trisomy 13 where microphthalmia is common. In **Trisomy 21**, speckling of the iris and oblique palpebral fissures are common but relatively minor manifestations of the disease.

Many different clinical entities affect the development of the auditory system. In **Trisomy 18**, the auricle is dysmorphic in a characteristic way. In mandibulofacial dysostosis, the development of the first pharyngeal arch is altered. Thus, the auricles, external auditory meatus, and middle ear ossicle can be abnormal, leading to conduction hearing loss. Rubella infections often target developing neuroepithelium and commonly leading to ocular and auditory abnormalities. **Potter's syndrome** is associated with oligohydramnios and the auricle is commonly abnormal.

ANSWER AND TUTORIAL ON ITEM 62

The answer is: **62-D**. **Hematopoiesis** begins very early in development. Primitive red blood cells are first detectable in the embryo as early the end of the second week of development, and soon after this, there are numerous interconnected vessels formed in the **yolk sac**, connecting stalk, and chorionic villi. These vessels contain primitive (nucleated) red blood cells. By the middle of the fourth week, an unseptated but beating heart tube is propelling nucleated red blood cells around the embryonic body, through the connecting stalk into the chorionic villi.

Relatively minor erythropoiesis and still less myelopoiesis occurs in the **spleen** during the third to fifth months. The spleen has a relatively minor hematopoietic role. Beginning in the sixth week, the **liver** is the major hematopoietic organ in the body. Finally, in the second month, the **bone marrow** gradually becomes dominant. Bone marrow, first in the clavicles, and then in other bones as they develop, takes on an increasingly important hematopoietic role as the hematopoietic role of the liver declines. Postnatally, hematopoiesis is restricted to the red bone marrow but the potential for **extramedullary hematopoiesis** remains in the liver and even the spleen. In cases of severe hemolytic anemia or with failure of bone marrow, red and yellow marrow, liver and spleen, can become reactivated and begin to produce blood cells. **Erythropoietic stem cells** are found in the yolk sac, spleen, liver and bone marrow but not the thymus. Lymphopoiesis and cytotoxic T lymphocyte differentiation occurs in the thymus but the undifferentiated T lymphoblasts arise in yolk sac and liver and migrate chemotactically to the thymus (under the influence of thymotactin) where they are programmed to differentiate into fully functional T lymphocytes.

ANSWER AND TUTORIAL ON ITEM 63

The answer is: **63-E**. If there is no prenatal intrauterine infection, the fetus normally develops in a sterile environment and is therefore not exposed to bacterial antigens. The mother mounts an immune response to bacterial antigens that she has been exposed to (and to which the new born infant is likely to be exposed). Maternal IgGs are then transported across the placenta, leading to **passive immunization** of the fetus. These maternally derived IgGs are slowly degraded after birth and are replaced by new IgGs produced by the infant's own immune system, secondary to exposure to environmental antigens.

Human breast milk is also an important potential source of immune protection for an infant. Breast milk is rich is several nonspecific antibacterial substances. It also has an abundant supply of immunoglobulins, including **secretory IgA**. The H and L chains of this IgA are synthesized in plasma cells in the connective tissue of the mammary gland. IgA molecules are then joined by a **J-polypeptide** and bound to epithelial cells in acini. There, a secretory component is added. The **secretory component** covers the protease-sensitive regions of the IgA molecules. These **proteolysis-resistant molecules** are then ingested by the infant, where they provide significant protection from enteric infections. Secretory IgAs are also abundant in other bodily fluids including sweat, tears, saliva, and vaginal secretions.

ANSWERS AND TUTORIAL ON ITEMS 64-66

The answers are: **64-B; 65-D; 66-B**. This patient is afflicted by **DiGeorge's syndrome**, an immunodeficiency syndrome caused by **thymic hypoplasia**. The incidence of DiGeorge's syndrome is approximately 1 in 20,000 with a M:F ratio of 1:1. Deletions in the short arm of chromosome 22 have been detected in a vast majority of cases. The severity of this syndrome is highly variable, depending upon the degree of organ hypoplasia. The immunologic problems in these infants (eg, recurrent infections by opportunistic organisms) are due to thymic aplasia or hypoplasia leading to complete or partial absence of cell-mediated immune responsiveness. The hypocalcemia is due to variable **parathyroid hypoplasia**. Patients with DiGeorge's syndrome are also commonly afflicted with atrial or ventricular septal defects and craniofacial anomalies as well. In DiGeorge syndrome, the thymic and parathyroid hypoplasia is due to failed development of the **3rd and 4th pharyngeal pouches**. Abnormal neural crest cell migration may account for the characteristic facies and cardiovascular defects associated with DiGeorge's syndrome.

ANSWERS AND TUTORIAL ON ITEMS 67-69

The answers are: **67-C; 68-B; 69-B**. **Rh isoimmunization** is common is fetuses of **Rh^- mothers** and Rh^+ fathers. The Rh antigen is controlled by a dominant gene and therefore the fetus of this couple would be Rh^+. Rh isoimmunization becomes more severe with each pregnancy because the maternal immune system has a memory for Rh antigen. Normally, the placental trophoblast provides a functional barrier between fetal and maternal blood, although **microvascular accidents** are all but inevitable. When fetal Rh^+ RBCs enter the circulation of an Rh^- mother, they are recognized as foreign by the mother and a strong immune response is mounted. The resulting maternal IgGs are transported across the placenta where they coat fetal RBCs and result in their rapid destruction in the liver and spleen. The resulting anemia triggers continued splenic and hepatic (extramedullary) and bone marrow erythropoiesis and results in **hepatosplenomegaly**. Excessive destruction of fetal RBCs leads to accumulation of heme breakdown products such as bilirubin and **jaundice**. Neonatal jaundice can be severe enough to result in brain damage. Administration of **Rhogam** postnatally clears the anti-Rh antibodies from the maternal circulation, ameliorating Rh isoimmunization in subsequent pregnancies.

Answer and Tutorial on Item 70

The answer is: **70-A**. Most cases of **cleft lip/palate** are considered to be of **mulifactorial inheritance** and are caused by the failure of fusion of the mesenchyme on each side of the cleft. Surgical repair of clefts of the palate is often delayed until cranial growth is reduced, the abnormal communication between the oral and nasal cavities often being closed initially by a prosthesis. On the other hand, clefts of the lip are repaired as soon as possible after birth. Clefts of the lip/palate are the most common malformation in man and are classified according to their relation to the incisive foramen; those posterior to the foramen are midline while those anterior are oblique. Most children with this anomaly have normal intelligence. Cleft lip occurs more often in men while cleft palate with or without cleft lip occurs more often in women.

The intermaxillary segment is formed by the lower part of the medial nasal prominences and gives rise to the median part of the upper lip, the incisive tooth buds and a small part of the palate anterior to the incisive foramen. In the embryo this region forms the primary palate. The lateral palatine processes or shelves begin to fuse with each other and the nasal septum during the latter part of the second month but fusion is not complete until near the end of the third month.

Answers and Tutorial on Items 71-72

The answers are: **71-D; 72-D**. Individuals with **mandibulofacial dysostosis** (**Treacher Collins syndrome**, first arch syndrome) have a normal life span and normal mental capacity. All of the other choices are correct. This condition is a manifestation of **first arch dysgenesis** accompanied by maxillary and mandibular hypoplasia and malocclusion from irregular tooth eruption. The syndrome is thought to be caused by insufficient production of neural crest cells.

Answer and Tutorial on Item 73

The answer is: **73-C**. The **thyroid gland** is the first endocrine gland to appear during embryonic life. It begins as an endodermal thickening in the floor of the primordial (primitive) pharynx that soon forms a down growth called the thyroid diverticulum. At 11 weeks, colloid begins to collect in clusters of cells forming a cavity surrounded by a single layer of cells. At this time, iodine is concentrated in the thyroid and thyroid hormone can be demonstrated. Ectopic thyroid tissue may form from remnants of the thyroglossal duct and may be found anywhere between the tongue and neck superior to the definitive thyroid gland.

Thyroglossal duct cysts may form anywhere along the course of the thyroglossal duct. The cysts may form in the tongue or in the median plane of the anterior neck, usually just inferior to the hyoid bone. The cysts are usually painless, progressively enlarging and are easily moveable.

Answer and Tutorial on Item 74

The answer is: **74-D**. The **otic vesicle** is the primordium of the membranous labyrinth of which the **cochlear duct** is a part. The cochlear duct develops from the ventral portion of the otic vesicle. Since it contains the receptors for hearing its failure to develop would result in deafness.

The **endolymphatic duct** is part of the membranous labyrinth and develops from the dorsal utricular portion of the otic vesicle.

The **malleus** (which attaches to the medial surface of the tympanic membrane) and incus are formed by the 1st pharnygeal arch mesenchyme. The stapes (which attaches to the oval window on the membranous labyrinth) is derived from 2nd pharyngeal arch mesenchyma.

The **auditory tube** develops from the 1st pharyngeal pouch. It extends laterally to become continuous with the tympanic cavity this is also a derivative of the first pouch. The ear ossicles and chorda tympani nerve located in the middle ear cavity have a surface covering of endodermally derived epithelium.

The tensor tympani muscle attaches to the malleus ear ossicle. Both of these structures are derived from the first pharyngeal arch. The stapedius muscle is derived from the second pharyngeal arch and is innervated by the facial nerve that is the nerve of the second arch.

Most types of congenital deafness are caused by genetic factors but maternal infection by the **rubella virus** during the first trimester may interfere with inner ear development resulting in congenital deafness.

Answer and Tutorial on Item 75

The answer is: **75-D**. The **umbilical cord** inserts on the **chorionic plate** of the placenta. The basal (decidual) plate of the placenta is apposed to the uterine wall. The umbilical cord is the connection between the fetal body and the placenta, is derived from the connecting stalk and, is coated by amnion. Two **umbilical arteries** are afferent to the placenta and there is a single efferent **umbilical vein**. Deoxygenated blood is carried from the fetus to the placenta by the umbilical arteries. Following gas exchange in the placenta, oxygenated fetal blood returns from the placenta to the fetus in the single umbilical vein.

The umbilical cord is about 40 cm long at term and can have numerous loops and is usually twisted. Compression of the umbilical vessels would compromise respiratory function for the fetus. The umbilical blood vessels are surrounded by a mucous connective tissue called **Wharton's jelly**. This peculiar connective tissue has an unusually large amount of amorphous ground substance rich in sulfated proteoglycans which keep it hydrated. The walls of the umbilical vessels are also quite thick due to an abundance of smooth muscle cells. These features help prevent compression of umbilical vessels.

Answers and Tutorial on Items 76-78.

The answers are: **76-A; 77-C; 78-E**. **Human chorionic gonadotrophin** is a glycoprotein secretion product of the syncytiotrophoblast. It is similar to luteinizing hormone and is required for maintenance of the corpus luteum of pregnancy. **Human somatomammotropin** (human placental lactogen) is similar to growth hormone and alters maternal carbohydrate metabolism to make glucose and fatty acids available to the fetus. It has little demonstrable effect on the development of the mammary glands in humans. The syncytiotrophoblast has little smooth endoplasmic reticulum but nevertheless produces and secretes **progesterone and estriol**, an estrogen. Progesterone is synthesized from maternal cholesterol which is taken up from maternal blood low-density lipoprotein (LDL) by a specific receptor on the syncytiotrophoblast. Progesterone is thought to inhibit contraction of uterine smooth muscle. The placenta also secretes **prostaglandins** which stimulate uterine smooth muscle contraction. The increase in prostaglandin-secreting activity of the placenta at term is probably the trigger that initiates labor.

Answers and Tutorial on Items 79-80

The answers are: **79-B; 80-B**. **Figure 3.10** is an example of the karyotype associated with **Klinefelter's syndrome**. This was the first human sex chromosome aneuploidy that was described and is clearly the result of nondisjunction of sex chromosomes. These individuals appear physically normal at puberty. They are usually tall and thin. At puberty, signs of hypogonadism become apparent with small testes and underdeveloped secondary sexual characteristics. Histologically, the frequently undescended testes may exhibit hyalinization of the seminiferous epithelium due to prolonged exposure to core body temperature. The seminiferous epithelium requires the slightly lower temperature present in the scrotum for normal spermatogenesis. Increased incidence of seminomas is often associated with Klinefelter's syndrome. Gynecomastia is also observed occasionally. The overall incidence is about 1/1000 male live-births. Many of these patients are dyslexic.

Answers and Tutorial on Items 81-82

The answers are: **81-J; 82-G**. **Thalidomide** (A) was widely used in Germany and other countries as an anticonvulsant between 1957 and 1963. It was subsequently shown to be a potent teratogen, causing an epidemic of previously rare limb defects such as phocomelia and amelia. When use of this drug was discontinued, the incidence of these limb defects once again declined to a very low level.

Alcohol (B) is a potent teratogen. Ingestion of large quantities of alcohol, especially during the early stages of development, can lead to abnormal induction of the forebrain and a severe developmental defect known as holoprosencephaly. In addition, a less severe fetal alcohol syndrome has been identified. Afflicted children exhibit growth restriction, midfacial hypoplasia, elongated philtrum and reduced upper lip, mental retardation, hyperactivity, and speech delay. Women who are pregnant or potentially pregnant should avoid all alcohol consumption.

Cocaine (C) has been shown to be teratogenic in animal studies. Studies from pregnant humans are more complex, due to the difficulty of isolating cocaine abuse as a single etiologic factor. Cocaine-abusing pregnant women frequently have other substance-abuse problems or health problems that place their fetuses at risk. Some studies suggest that there may be an increased incidence of craniofacial, CNS, cardiovascular, and genitourinary anomalies. Cocaine use can lead to vasoconstriction in placental blood vessels, increasing risk for placental abruption.

Heroin (D) has not been firmly established as a teratogenic drug. Pregnant heroin addicts often expose their fetuses to other known teratogens. Since heroin readily crosses the placenta, newborn infants of heroin-addicted mothers will also be addicted and will exhibit opiate-withdrawal symptoms.

Rubella virus (E) is the classic example of a teratogenic infectious agent. In mothers infected with rubella virus during the first 3 months of gestation, approximately 20% of their fetuses become infected. Rubella virus crosses the placenta and infects the fetus, causing deafness, congenital cataract, and heart defects.

Herpes simplex virus (F) is not a potent teratogen, although some studies suggest that it may cause a variety of CNS abnormalities. In pregnant women actively shedding herpes simplex virus from vulvar lesions, the greatest risk is transmission of the disease to the newborn during vaginal delivery. Herpes simplex infections in newborns are often fatal, due to significant immaturity of the T cell system. Cesarean delivery is indicated for such mothers.

Toxoplasma gondii (G) is an intracellular parasitic protozoan that is known to be teratogenic. Maternal infection occurs by ingesting poorly cooked infected meat or exposure to animal feces. Toxoplasma crosses the placenta, infecting the fetus and causing chorioretinitis, microcephaly or hydrocephaly, and calcifications around the brain ventricles (often visible on ultrasound). Mental retardation and microphthalmia are also found in fetal toxoplasmosis.

Accidental exposure of pregnant women to poisoned fish in Japan and fungicide-contaminated grain in Iran established that **organic mercurial compounds** (H) are potent teratogens, causing abnormal development of the cerebrum and cerebellum as well as developmental defects in the peripheral nervous system.

Synthetic progestins (I) are not potent teratogens, but there is some evidence that suggests that progestins can cause masculinization of the external genitalia of female fetuses.

High doses of **ionizing radiation** (J) were once used on pregnant women. Radiation treatments for cervical cancer during pregnancy resulted in a high incidence of CNS abnormalities in fetuses. Similarly, among those surviving pregnant Japanese women exposed to atomic bomb blasts during World War II, there was a high incidence of spontaneous abortion and mental retardation in those children that were delivered alive. Even the small doses of radiation received with diagnostic x-rays or radioisotopes should be minimized in pregnant women. **Table 3.1** provides a convenient summary of other potentially teratogenic prescription medications.

Table 3.1 Clinical Features of Some Important Teratogenic Prescription Drugs

Drug	Possible Teratogenic Effects
Diethylstilbestrol	Causes Vaginal and cervical CA in women exposed in uter
Tetracycline	Tooth defects
Streptomycin	Deafness
Warfarin	Cartilage and CNS defects
Trimethadione	Growth retardation, facial clefts, cardiovascular, genitourinary, and limb defects
Phenytoin	Growth retardation, CNS defects, mental retardation
Valproic acid	Craniofacial, cardiac, and musculoskeletal defects
Aminopterin, also methotrexate	CNS and skeletal defects
Tumor inhibiting drugs	Potent teratogens
ACE Inhibitors	Oligohydramnios and renal abnormalities
Retinoic acid	Facial clefts, micrognathia, heart and neural tube defects
Benzodiazepine	Fetal dependence, craniofacial defects
Lithium	Cardiovascular defects

Answer and Tutorial on Item 83

The answer is: **83-B**. A child afflicted with a severe case of **fetal alcohol syndrome** (FAS) is shown in **Figure 3.11**. This child exhibits a specific pattern of craniofacial defects. The craniofacial features of FAS include short rather than long palpebral fissures although the palpebral fissures of the child shown in Figure 3.13 are not affected. However, this child's face does exhibit maxillary hypoplasia, thin upper lips, epicanthal folds, and a short nose. Abnormal palmar skin lines and mental retardation were also present. Other associated defects are microcephaly, prenatal and postnatal growth deficiency, and heart and joint anomalies.

The incidence of FAS is estimated to be 2 per 1000 live births and is considered to be the most common cause of **mental retardation**. Moderate maternal alcohol consumption may produce fetal alcohol effects (FAE) and damages the development of brain functions resulting in infants with behavioral and learning disabilities. Binge drinking will produce FAE.

Research on laboratory animals suggests that the root cause of FAS is abnormal migration of the neural crest cells that populate the pharyngeal apparatus. In addition, the CNS effects of FAS may also be due to disruptions in cell migration. During development of the cerebrum and cerebellum, there is a great deal of migration of neuroblasts. Disruption of this process may result in mental retardation and other behavioral effects such as attention deficit disorder and hyperactivity, commonly observed in children with FAS

Answer and Tutorial on Item 84

The answer is: **84-B**. The **first trimester** is the most sensitive period because it is the time when organogenesis occurs and when cell division and differentiation are at their peak. During this period **teratogens** can cause major malformations. They do not cause defects during the 2 weeks after fertilization but teratogens that interfere with cleavage of the zygote and implantation of the blastocyst cause death and spontaneous abortion of the conceptus.

Intercourse during early pregnancy is not considered a cause of spontaneous abortion.

Lead, polychlorinated biphenyls, methyl mercury, and lithium carbonate caffeine are know to be teratogenic in man. Caffeine is the most widely consumed stimulant and is present in many beverages. Heavy consumption during pregnancy may be unsafe and should be avoided.

The earlier in pregnancy the maternal **rubella infection** occurs, the greater the chances that the embryo will be malformed.

While genetic factors are the most important cause of congenital anomalies, of the choices listed, the genetic makeup of the father is the least influential in the growth of the fetus in utero.

Answers and Tutorial on Items 85-87

The answers are: **85-G; 86-C; 87-E**. **Prune-belly** is due to a congenital absence of the abdominal wall musculature which is derived from the dermomyotomes in the lumbar region. It is 20 times more common in men than women and is often associated with urogenital anomalies. It may be caused by abnormal distention of the abdomen which secondarily prevents development of abdominal musculature.

Meckel's diverticulum is an ileal diverticulum which is a remnant of the vitelline duct (ie, none of the above). Normally, this embryonic connection between the mid-gut and the yolk sac is obliterated.

Renal agenesis is due to failed reciprocal inductive interactions between the ureteric bud and the metanephric blastema, both intermediate mesoderm derivatives. Horseshoe kidney occurs when the caudal poles of the metanephroi fuse. Cranial ascent of the fused metanephroi is blocked by the inferior mesenteric artery.

The **nucleus pulposus**, that toothpaste-like cushion surrounded by the annulus fibrosus in the intervertebral discs, is derived from the notochord. Indeed, it is the only known persistent notochordal derivative in the adult. The notochord in the center of developing vertebral bodies disappears with ossification. When the intervertebral disc is traumatically torn, often at the L4,5 level, weight on the lumbar vertebral bodies expresses the semi-liquid nucleus pulposus onto the sciatic nerve roots, causing pain and possibly loss of sensory and motor function.

Vertebral bodies can be entirely missing or may be misshapen. They are intersegmentally derived from **sclerotomes**.

Answers and Tutorial on Items 88-89

The answers are: **88-B; 89-D**. **Achondroplasia** is the most common chondrodystrophy (incidence 1 in 20,000 live births). It is caused by an **autosomal dominant mutation**. Recent evidence shows that many of these mutations occur in the gene that encodes **fibroblast growth factor-3 receptor**. Most cases arise as spontaneous new mutations with parents unaffected by achondroplasia. The heterozygous form is compatible with a long life and normal intelligence. The homozygous form is usually lethal early in life. If heterozygous parents were to have a child, it would have a 25% chance of being unaffected by achondroplasia. The remaining offspring would be 50% heterozygous affected and 25% homozygous (lethal).

Recent studies have shown that most cases of achondroplasia are due to a mutation in the gene encoding fibroblast growth factor-3 receptor. Absence of this receptor results in epiphyseal plates that do not show normal proliferative activity and thus many of the bones formed by endochondral ossification (eg, limb bones and base of skull) are abnormally short. The nasal bridge depression is due to abnormal development of the base of the skull. Adults with achondroplasia have normal mentation and are fertile. Pregnant achondroplastics are routinely delivered by cesarean section due to **cephalopelvic disproportion**.

Answers and Tutorial on Items 90-91

The answers are: **90-B; 91-B**. **Osteogenesis imperfecta** (OI) is a complex group of diseases all associated with increased fragility of bones due to mutations in the genes for the polypeptides comprising **Type I collagen**, the predominant collagen of bone. This child was afflicted by a severe variety, **OI Type II**. This form, unlike the less severe OI Type I, is almost always fatal soon after birth. The most acute problems associated with OI Type II are breathing difficulties secondary to severe reduction in the thorax and possible damage to the brain from reduced ossification of the vault of the skull.

This rare disease, whose incidence is variously stated as about 1 in 20,000 to 1 in 60,000 infants (depending on the authority cited), is caused by **autosomal dominant mutations** (most often spontaneous new mutations) altering the structure of Type I collagen. There is often severe reduction in secretion of Type I collagen. The tensile strength of bone is partially due to the presence of numerous Type I collagen fibrils. Thus, with severe decreases in Type I collagen in the extracellular matrix of bone, there is invariably a concomitant increase in bone fragility.

Answers and Tutorial on Items 92-93

The answers are: **92-B; 93-D**. Bones are dynamic organs with extensive developmental potential during childhood. Even after puberty, when growth in length of bones is no longer possible because of ossification of the **epiphyseal plate**, bones continue to have a latent capacity for reformation during fracture repair. In addition, the calcified matrix of bony tissue is constantly turning over as part of the calcium regulatory system in the body.

The growth in length of long bones during childhood is primarily due to proliferation, hypertrophy, and calcification of cartilage in the epiphyseal plate. This mechanism is accelerated during the pubertal growth spurt and then ceases after puberty due to the complete ossification of the epiphyseal plate.

In the normal steady state bone resorption by osteocytes and osteoclasts (to release calcium into the blood) is nicely balanced by bone deposition by osteoblasts (to sequester calcium from the blood). There is constant balanced deposition and resorption of bone. When a bone is fractured, osteoblasts are stimulated to secrete osteoid at the fracture site. This osteoid then calcifies to form a new **bony callus** which repairs the fracture. With advancing age, especially in post-menopausal women, bone deposition is outstripped by bone resorption, leading to **osteoporosis**.

Answer and Tutorial on Item 94

The answer is: **94-D**. The **internal limiting membrane** is located at the lumen of the neural tube but it is not really a membrane. Instead, it consists of apical tight junctions between neuroepithelial cells. The **external limiting membrane** is located at the periphery of the neural tube and is the basement membrane for the neuroepithelium. The neuroepithelium is a pseudostratified epithelium and this characteristic is due to **interkinetic nuclear migration**.

The **glia limitans** forms at the external limiting membrane as astrocyte foot processes become pushed up against the external limiting membrane from within the neuroepithelium. Astrocytes (a kind of glial cell) are definitely part of the glia limitans. It does indeed form the outer boundary of the neural tube derivatives.

Neuroblasts form many different types of neurons in the nervous system, including the cones and rods in the neural retina. Glioblasts form glial cells such as oligodendroglial cells and astrocytes. Schwann cells are neural crest derivatives responsible for PNS myelination. The neuroblasts are capable of extensive mitotic divisions after they are born. For example, in the cerebral and cerebellar cortex, an entire population of neuroblasts divides extensively to form the peripheral grey matter of the brain.

Glioblasts form several different kinds of glial cells including astrocytes and oligodendroglial cells. The latter cells are responsible for CNS myelination. The microglia are part of the mononuclear phagocyte system and arise from monocytes rather than the neuroepithelium, the source of all glioblasts.

Myelination is the result of the activity of Schwann cells (neural crest derivatives) in the PNS and oligodendroglial cells (glioblast derivatives) in the CNS . The mesaxon of the myelinating cells grows extensively in a spiral fashion around processes (axons and dendrites) to be myelinated. Myelination occurs extensively before and after birth and is more prominent in white matter than in grey matter.

ANSWERS AND TUTORIAL ON ITEMS 95-96

The answers are: **95-A; 96-B**. The **alar plate** and **alar laminae** are dorsal structures in the neural tube. They contain the cell bodies of developing sensory neurons in the spinal cord and developing neurons that form the tectal nuclei in the mesencephalon. The motor neurons develop in the basal plates. The neurons in dorsal root ganglia are neural crest derivatives.

The **basal plate** and **basal laminae** are ventral structures in the neural tube. They contain the cell bodies for developing motor neurons in the spinal cord and developing neurons that form the tegmental nuclei in the mesencephalon. They also form general visceral efferent nuclei in the rhombencephalon. The special visceral afferent nuclei in the rhombencephalon form from the alar laminae.

Notes

CHAPTER 4

Physiology and Endocrinology

DIRECTIONS (Items 1-122): For each of the numbered items that proceed, you must select the single best answer from among the lettered options listed.

Some of the numbered items will pose a question or incomplete sentence that is followed by a list of 4-5 lettered options. In all cases, select the ONE lettered option that best answers the question or completes the sentence given.

Some of the numbered items are preceded by 5-24 lettered options. In these sets, the lettered options will be preceded by a single instruction asking you to match one of the lettered options to each numbered item most closely associated with it. In all matching sets, you may use any of the lettered options once, more than once or not at all, but you should still only select ONE lettered option per numbered item.

If you wish to simulate actual USMLE testing conditions, you should aim to complete all the items in this chapter in TWO hours.

Do NOT look at the answers and tutorials until you have completed all of the items in this chapter.

Good luck!

Item 1

1. The Na^+-K^+ pump has which most crucial function for all cells?

   (A) maintains a low extracellular Na^+ concentration
   (B) maintains a high extracellular K^+ concentration
   (C) ATP hydrolysis
   (D) maintenance of cell volume
   (E) maintenance of cell surface charge

Item 2

2. The second messenger for vascular smooth muscle relaxation triggered by atrial natriuretic factor is

   (A) cAMP
   (B) cGMP
   (C) calmodulin
   (D) inositol triphosphate
   (E) arachidonic acid

Item 3

Figure 4.1 below represents synapses between two presynaptic axon terminals (A and D) and a postsynaptic dendritic process (B) in the central nervous system. The terminal at C represents an axon terminal synapsing with terminal A (an axo-axonic synapse).

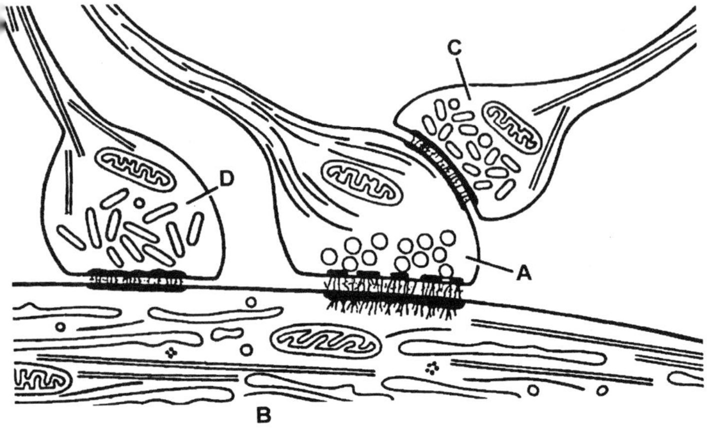

Figure 4.1

3. The neurotransmitter released by cell A causes an opening only in the K^+ channels in cell B. The effect of this would be

   (A) depolarization of the postsynaptic membrane and stimulation of an action potential
   (B) an increase in the excitability of the excitatory nerve endings
   (C) a partial depolarization of the excitatory nerve endings
   (D) opening of Na^+ channels
   (E) hyperpolarization of the postsynaptic membrane and inhibition of the action potential

Item 4

4. You can test the integrity of the vestibular system of a patient by irrigating the external auditory canal with cold or warm water. If warm water is placed into the right external auditory canal,

   (A) the slow component of nystagmus occurs to the right and the fast component to the left
   (B) no nystagmus would be seen
   (C) the slow component of nystagmus occurs to the left and the fast component to the right
   (D) both the slow and fast component of nystagmus occur to the right
   (E) both the slow and fast component of nystagmus occur to the left

Item 5

5. Your patient, known to be suffering from epilepsy, hyperventilates which causes an increase in arterial pH. The effect of this on central nervous system neural function would likely be

   (A) cerebral convulsions due to increased excitability of neurons
   (B) comatose state
   (C) decreased neuronal excitability
   (D) neuronal cell death
   (E) cerebral ischemia

Item 6

6. A patient presents with an intention tremor, scanning speech, "past-pointing," and a "drunken" gait. This patient might be expected to have a lesion involving the

   (A) cerebellum
   (B) vestibulocochlear nerve
   (C) precentral gyrus
   (D) caudate nucleus
   (E) red nucleus

Items 7-10

Figure 4.2 represents the range of frequency waves seen in the electroencephalogram of an individual under different conditions.

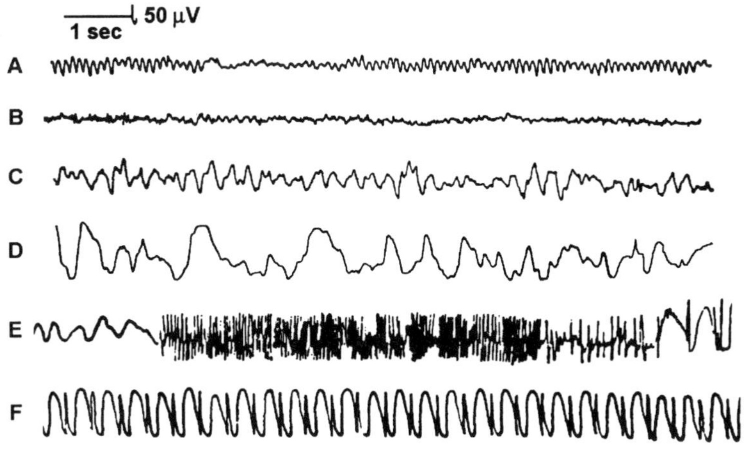

Figure 4.2

7. Which of the wave types in the above diagram is found in almost all normal adult persons when they are awake and in a quiet, resting state?

   (A) A
   (B) B
   (C) C
   (D) D
   (E) E

8. Which of the waves in the above diagram would be found during deep sleep in a normal adult?

   (A) A
   (B) B
   (C) C
   (D) D
   (E) E

9. An electroencephologram is recorded from normal resting adult with her eyes closed. The patient is then asked to open the eyes for a few seconds and they close them again. During this interval, the wave pattern of the EEG would likely be

   (A) Alpha waves changing to beta waves when the eyes open, then back to alpha waves when the eyes close again.
   (B) Beta waves changing to alpha waves when the eyes open, then back to beta waves when the eyes close again.
   (C) Delta waves changing to beta waves when the eyes open, then to alpha waves when the eyes close again.
   (D) Theta waves changing to beta waves when the eyes open, then back to theta waves when the eyes close again.
   (E) Beta waves changing to theta waves when the eyes open, then back to beta waves when the eyes close again.

10. Which of the waves in the above diagram are typical in a person during a grand mal epileptic attack?

(A) A
(B) B
(C) C
(D) D
(E) E

Item 11

11. Gamma motoneurons of the spinal cord

(A) only innervate antagonistic muscles
(B) innervate skeletal muscle fibers and cause their contraction
(C) generate activity in Ib afferent fibers
(D) prevent skeletal muscle contraction
(E) innervate intrafusal muscle fibers

Items 12-18

Figure 4.3 is a diagram of the retina with numerous lettered structures. Match the lettered structure with the most appropriate physiologic description in the items below.

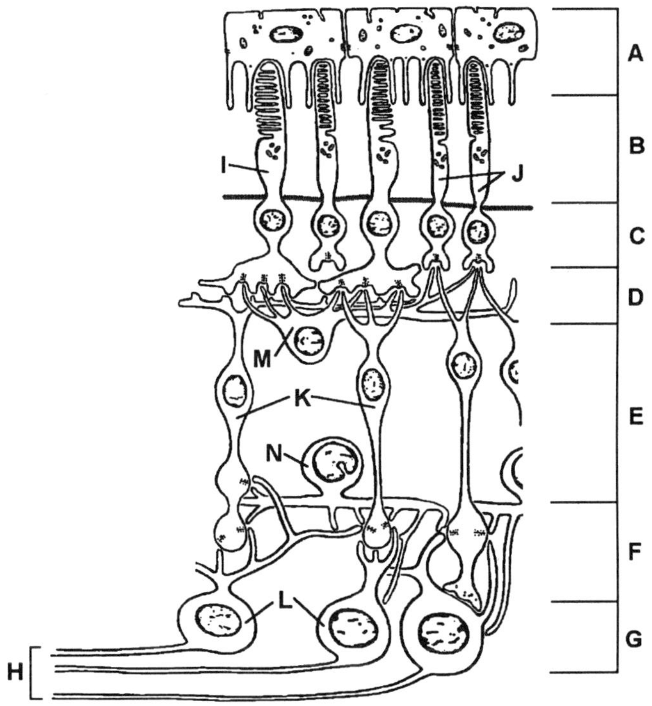

Figure 4.3

12. Layer E contains the nuclei of all of the following cells of the retina EXCEPT

    (A) ganglion cells
    (B) Müller cells
    (C) bipolar cells
    (D) amacrine cells
    (E) horizontal cells

13. The absorption of stray light and phagocytosis of disks that have been sloughed from the receptor cells occurs in which layer?

    (A) A
    (B) D
    (C) H
    (D) E and F
    (E) G and H

14. Cells responsible for scotopic vision are

(A) cell I
(B) cell J
(C) cell K
(D) cell L
(E) cell M

15. Cells most concentrated at the fovea are

(A) cell I
(B) cell J
(C) cell K
(D) cell L
(E) cell M

16. Cells responsible for color vision are

(A) cell I
(B) cell J
(C) cell K
(D) cell L
(E) cell M

17. One of the reactions in the retinal rods directly caused by absorption of light energy is

(A) dissociation of scotopsin and vitamin A
(B) decomposition of scotopsin
(C) transformation of 11-*cis* retinal to all-*trans* retinal
(D) combination of 11-*cis* retinal with opsin
(E) transformation of vitamin A to 11-*cis* retinal

18. When light strikes a retinal receptor

(A) the receptor will depolarize
(B) the receptor will hyperpolarize
(C) no change will occur in receptor membrane potential
(D) increased transmitter is released from the receptor cell
(E) bipolar cells are hyperpolarized

Items 19-25

Figure 4.4 shows an action potential recorded from a large myelinated nerve fiber. Match the lettered portion of the action potential curve with the most appropriate description of the physiologic state of the membrane.

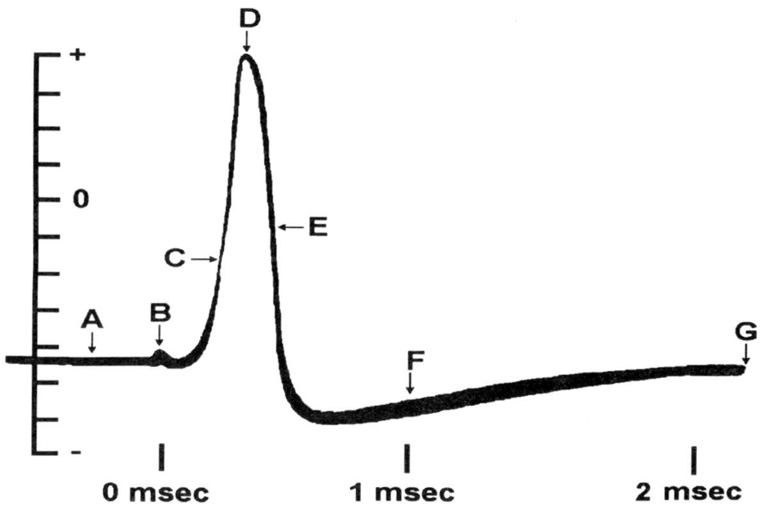

Figure 4.4

19. At this point, the membrane resting potential has been reestablished after depolarization.

20. At this point, prior to application of a depolarizing stimulus, the extracellular Na^+ is at its highest value.

21. At this point, Na^+ conductance is highest.

22. At this point, K^+ conductance is rising slowly.

23. This is a stimulus artifact.

24. At this point, Na^+ conductance is falling rapidly and K^+ conductance has peaked.

25. Reducing the external [Na^+] to 100 mEq/L would have which effect on the action potential?

    (A) 40% increase in spike height
    (B) 10% increase in spike height
    (C) no change in spike height
    (D) decrease in spike height and shift curve to right
    (E) decrease in spike height and shift curve to left

Items 26-31

Match the ocular terms below with the correct item.

(A) Myopia
(B) Hyperopia
(C) Presbyopia
(D) Emmetropia
(E) Astigmatism
(F) Accommodation
(G) Convergence
(H) Conjugate gaze
(I) Refractive power
(J) Far point
(K) Near point

26. The focal point of an eye with __________ is behind the retina.

27. The focal point of an eye with __________ is in front of the retina.

28. Movement of the two eyes together such that an image falls on the fovea of both eyes is called ____________.

29. Vision in an eye with __________ can be corrected by use of a biconvex lens.

30. Cylindrical lenses can be worn to correct __________.

31. Loss of accommodative power associated with aging is known as __________.

Items 32-34

The mother of a $3\frac{1}{2}$-year-old boy brings her child to the family doctor concerned because the child was slow to begin walking, has difficulty standing, seems clumsy, and fatigues easily. Her greatest concern is that he seems to be falling behind his peers in development of motor skills. She recalls that her maternal uncle had similar problems and died in his late teens. Physical examination revealed an unusual gate, protruding abdomen, and significant muscle weakness. Laboratory tests of the child revealed creatinuria and elevated serum levels of creatine phosphokinase (CPK). Muscle biopsy revealed elevated CPK and significant degeneration in skeletal muscle.

32. The child probably suffers from which disease?

    (A) nemaline myopathy
    (B) pyruvate decarboxylase deficiency
    (C) mitochondrial myopathy
    (D) myasthenia gravis
    (E) duchenne's muscular dystrophy

33. Skeletal muscle CPK is elevated because of

    (A) mitochondrial degeneration
    (B) degeneration of neuromuscular junctions
    (C) myosin auto-antibody accumulation
    (D) muscle fiber degeneration
    (E) lack of thin filaments

34. A principal factor in the occurrence of this disease is

    (A) lack of the protein dystrophin
    (B) inability of actin filaments to bind to the Z-line
    (C) overproduction of a myosin isoform with reduced ATPase activity
    (D) absence of gap junctions between muscle fibers
    (E) tropomyosin is not produced, hence thick filaments are unstable

Item 35

35. Increase in muscle mass due to strenuous physical activity is due primarily to

    (A) an increase in blood supply
    (B) an increase in number of neuromuscular junctions
    (C) hypertrophy of individual fibers
    (D) activation of satellite cells
    (E) an increase in testosterone receptors

Item 36

36. The chief cause of rigor mortis is

    (A) decline in ATP production
    (B) decrease in muscle temperature
    (C) decrease in muscle Ca^{2+}
    (D) release of lysosomal enzymes
    (E) death of neuromuscular junctions

Items 37-41

Figure 4.5 is a length-tension curve for normal skeletal muscle. Match the labeled portions of the curve with the appropriate description of the state of the myofibrils in the answers.

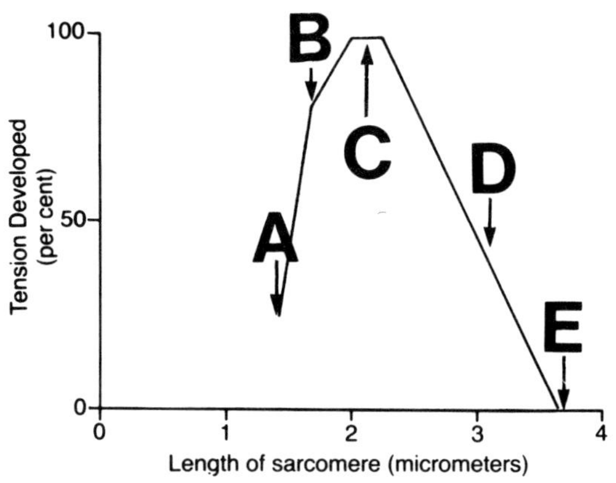

Figure 4.5

37. The thin filaments are no longer overlapping the thick filaments.

38. The sarcomere length equals the length of the thick filaments.

39. There is partial overlap between thin filaments and cross bridge rich portion of thick filaments here.

40. An increase in extent of thin filament-cross bridge interaction at this point would result in an increase in tension generated.

41. The thin filaments are overlapping here so that the Z-Z distance is minimal.

Items 42-46

Match the muscle protein in the list of answers below with the most appropriate statement concerning this protein's physiologic role in muscle contraction in the items below. Answers may be used once, more than once, or not at all.

(A) F-actin
(B) G-actin
(C) α-actinin
(D) Myosin II
(E) Myosin rod
(F) Troponin T
(G) Troponin C
(H) Troponin I
(I) Tropomyosin
(J) Titin
(K) Nebulin
(L) Cap Z
(M) Myosin heads (SF 1)

42. Forms the swinging cross bridges in sarcomeres.

43. Regulatory muscle protein which lies in the groove of the F-actin helices.

44. Homologous to calmodulin.

45. Binds actin filaments to Z-disc.

46. Most abundant subunit protein in actin filaments.

Item 47

47. Which protein is abnormal in patients with hereditary spherocytosis?

(A) Tubulin
(B) Fibronectin
(C) Collagen
(D) Integrin
(E) Spectrin

Items 48-50

Examine **Figure 4.6** below, a photomicrograph, and then choose the best response for each item. The granules in these cells are metachromatic when stained with basic dyes such as hematoxylin.

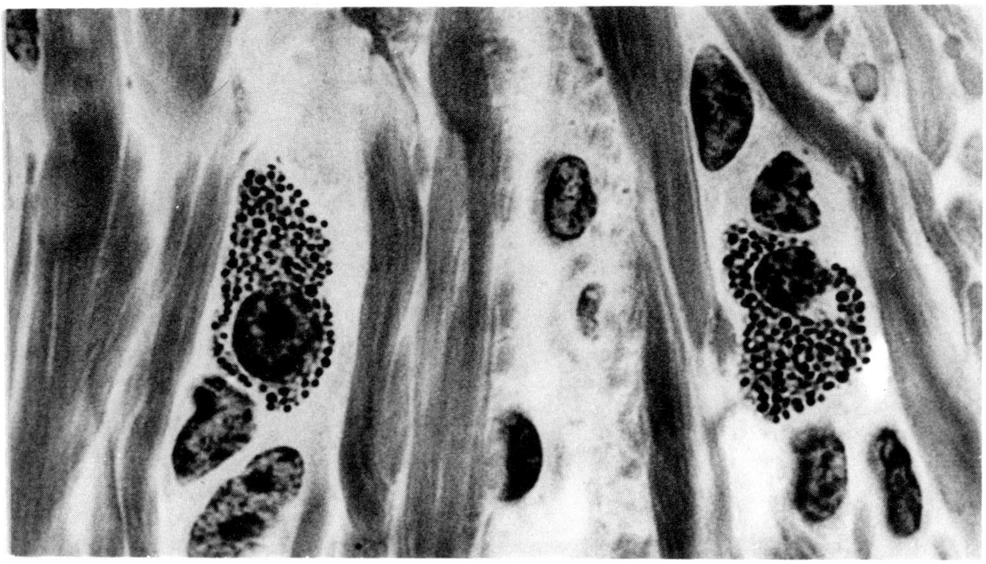

Figure 4.6

48. The metachromasia of the granules is due to

    (A) histamine
    (B) heparin
    (C) chondroitin sulfate
    (D) lysosomal hydrolases
    (E) hyaluronic acid

49. This cell is a

    (A) B lymphocyte
    (B) T lymphocyte
    (C) basophil
    (D) macrophage
    (E) mast cell

50. Degranulation would result in which primary physiologic response?

    (A) Increased capillary leakiness
    (B) Phagocytosis by macrophages
    (C) Chemotaxis of basophils
    (D) Triggering of complement cascade
    (E) Immunoglobulin synthesis

Items 51-58

Match the cell in the answers below with the most appropriate description of its physiologic role in the items below. Answers may be used once, more than once, or not at all.

(A) Erythrocyte
(B) Neutrophil
(C) Basophil
(D) Eosinophil
(E) B lymphocyte
(F) Helper T lymphocyte
(G) Suppressor T lymphocyte
(H) Cytotoxic T lymphocyte
(I) Monocyte
(J) Platelet
(K) Plasma cell
(L) Mast cell
(M) Megakaryocytes

51. This cell has an abundance of integrin on its surface. This receptor allows it to participate in clotting.

52. This cell is part of the mononuclear phagocyte system where it moves freely from blood to loose connective tissue domains.

53. This cell is specialized for phagocytosis of opsonized bacteria.

54. This cell is essentially devoid of intracellular organelles during its life span in the circulation.

55 This cell becomes clonally expanded and differentiates into an immunoglobulin-secreting plasma cell after proper antigenic stimulation.

56. This cell is the most abundant granulocyte in normal blood.

57. This cell is programmed to attack malignant cells.

58. This cell combats parasitic infestation.

Items 59-68

Match the blood compound in the answers with the most appropriate description of its physiologic role described in the items below. Answers may be used once, more than once, or not at all.

(A) Albumin
(B) Complement
(C) Transferrin
(D) Apolipoprotein
(E) Fibrinogen
(F) Hemoglobin
(G) Bilirubin
(H) Haptoglobin

59. Provides the colloidal osmotic pressure that regulates H_2O movement through capillaries

60. Carries iron in the blood

61. Group of proteins that mediated immune response after proteolysis

62. Transports triglycerides

63. Severe reduction in concentration leads to edema

64. Decreased concentration in peritoneal cavity produces ascites

65. Transports phospholipids

66. Transports cholesterol

67. Breakdown product of hemoglobin

68. Scavenges hemoglobin

Items 69-74

Figure 4.7 below represents the pressure changes that occur during the cardiac cycle.

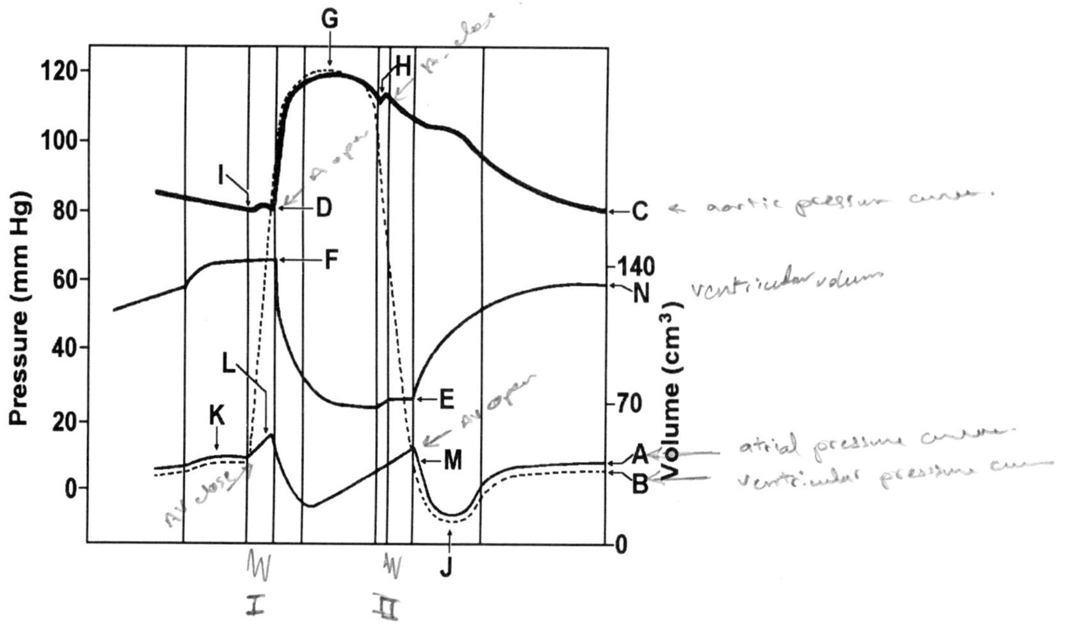

Figure 4.7

69. Which labeled point represents the closure of the AV valve?

70. The dicrotic notch is indicated by which labeled point?

71. Which labeled point represents the beginning of ventricular systole?

72. Which labeled point represents the aortic pressure curve?

73. At which labeled point would the second heart sound occur?

74. The wave labeled L is a result of

(A) decreased ventricular pressure due to closure of the aortic semilunar valve
(B) increased atrial pressure due to bulging of the mitral valve into the left atrium
(C) increased atrial pressure due to opening of the AV valves
(D) increased pressure in the pulmonary trunk due to opening of the pulmonary semilunar valve
(E) increased aortic pressure due to opening of the aortic semilunar valve

Items 75-76

75. If the end-diastolic ventricular volumes are increased (within physiologic limits)

(A) the stroke volume would be increased
(B) cardiac output would be decreased
(C) venous pressure would be decreased
(D) the force of cardiac contraction would be decreased
(E) the output of the left ventricle would exceed the output of the right ventricle

76. An increase in arterial blood pressure during systole would cause

(A) a reduction in stroke volume
(B) an increase in the velocity of blood ejection from the ventricles
(C) an increase in stroke volume
(D) a reduction of ventricular afterload
(E) a decrease in arterial pressure during diastole

Item 77

77. The type of sympathetic receptor found in myocardium is

(A) α_1-adrenergic
(B) β_1-adrenergic
(C) β_2-adrenergic
(D) gamma aminobutyric acid (GABA)
(E) dopamine

Items 78-80

A 3-year-old child is brought to a pediatrician by a concerned father who reports that his child is easily fatigued after play, becoming exhausted and breathing heavily. The pediatrician finds significant cyanosis in the child and a systolic murmur. Further tests lead to the diagnosis of tetralogy of Fallot.

78. The chief cause of the cyanosis and dyspnea is

(A) atrial septal defect
(B) ventricular septal defect
(C) right ventricular hypertrophy
(D) bypass of the pulmonary circulation
(E) patent ductus arteriosus

79. Catheterization of the right ventricle would show

(A) increased diastolic pressure
(B) increased systolic pressure
(C) decreased diastolic pressure
(D) decreased systolic pressure
(E) normal diastolic and systolic pressures

80. Tetralogy of Fallot can be corrected by

(A) family therapy
(B) medical management with a -adrenergic blocking agent
(C) surgical repair
(D) antibiotic therapy
(E) oxygen therapy

Item 81

81. Decreasing an airway diameter by half would lead to which degree of change in airway resistance?

(A) 50% decrease
(B) 50% increase
(C) 100% decrease
(D) 100% increase
(E) greater than 100% increase

Items 82-87

Figure 4.8 shows a spirometer tracing for a normal adult male during normal breathing and during forced inspiration and expiration. Match the labeled portion of the diagram with its correct designation in the items below.

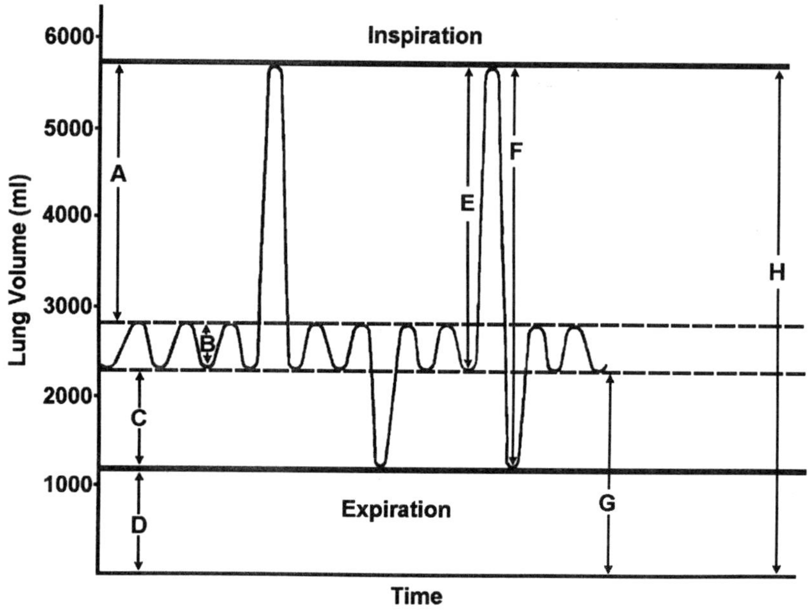

Figure 4.8

82. This is the total vital capacity of the lungs.

83. This is the tidal volume of the lungs.

84. This is the inspiratory reserve volume of the lungs.

85. This is the volume that remains after forceful expiration.

86. This is the functional residual capacity.

87. Which number is most correct for the minute respiratory volume of a normal adult female at rest in mL/minute?

(A) 2,000
(B) 3,000
(C) 4,000
(D) 5,000
(E) 6,000

Items 88-94

For each numbered statement of function in the items, match the lettered hormone whose activity most closely corresponds. Answers may be used once, more than once, or not at all.

(A) Serotonin
(B) Gastrin
(C) Cholecystokinin
(D) Secretin
(E) Neurotensin
(F) Somatostatin
(G) Motilin
(H) Insulin
(I) Glucagon
(J) Bombesin (GRP)
(K) Vasoactive Intestinal Peptide
(L) Melatonin
(M) Substance P

88. It stimulates parietal cells in the stomach to secrete hydrochloric acid and increases the constriction of the lower esophageal sphincter.

89. This product of endocrine cells found in the duodenum causes smooth muscle in the wall of the gallbladder to contract.

90. A derivative of tryptophane, this compound functions as a local activator of smooth muscle in the mucosa of various parts of the gastrointestinal tube.

91. In addition to stimulating the release of enzymes from the pancreas, this hormone has mild inhibitory effects on motility of several regions of the gastrointestinal tube.

92. This product of endocrine cells in the small intestine causes cells lining pancreatic ducts to release large quantities of water and bicarbonate.

93. The vagus nerve regulates secretion of this by virtue of the fact that vagal stimulus causes both increased release of bombesin and decreased release of somatostatin.

94. This polypeptide is produced in the duodenum and stimulates strong gastric smooth muscle contraction.

Items 95-101

Match the enzyme in the lettered answers below with the most accurate description of its physiologic role in digestion in the numbered items below. Answers may be used once, more than once, or not at all.

(A) Ptyalin
(B) Pepsinogen
(C) Enterokinase
(D) Catalase
(E) Chymotrypsinogen
(F) Deoxyribonuclease
(G) Ribonuclease
(H) Carboxypeptidase
(I) Na^+-K^+-ATPase
(J) Lipase

95. Produced by duodenal enterocytes, this cleaves trypsinogen to form trypsin.

96. Its activity is strongly dependent on emulsification of fats by components of bile.

97. This enzyme functions to allow the concentration of bile by the gallbladder and of saliva by ducts in the salivary glands.

98. An amylase found in saliva, this enzyme functions to begin the degradation of starches while food is in the oral cavity.

99. Although this protease precursor can be cleaved by several proteases, its activation is primarily due to the action of trypsin.

100. This is the precursor of an enzyme whose activity is maximal in an acid milieu.

101. This removes amino acids from the -COOH terminal of peptides and proteins.

Item 102

102. When the arterial blood pressure of an individual changes from 100 mm Hg to 150 mm Hg, the glomerular filtration rate (GFR)

   (A) remains unchanged
   (B) increases by 10%
   (C) increases by 50%
   (D) decreases by 25%
   (E) decreases by 50%

Item 103-104

103. Of the total body H_2O, the largest fraction is found in the

   (A) bone and connective tissue
   (B) plasma
   (C) interstitial fluid
   (D) intracellular fluid
   (E) transcellular fluid

104. Plasma represents what percentage of the total extracellular fluid mass of the normal human body?

   (A) 5%
   (B) 10%
   (C) 15%
   (D) 20%
   (E) 25%

Items 105-111

A 28-year-old female complains of hirsutism, acne (although she never had it as a teenager), weight gain, and amenorrhea. Your examination reveals hypertension and adipose tissue deposits in the face, neck, and abdomen, but not in the upper and lower extremities. The woman is found to have a large adrenal cortical carcinoma.

105. The most likely diagnosis of her disease is

   (A) pheochromocytoma
   (B) diabetes insipidus
   (C) congenital adrenal hyperplasia
   (D) Goodpasture's syndrome
   (E) Cushing's syndrome

106. The hirsutism seen in this patient is caused by high levels of which adrenal cortical steroid?

   (A) testosterone
   (B) estradiol
   (C) cortisol
   (D) aldosterone
   (E) corticosterone

107. The hypertension seen in this patient is caused by high levels of which adrenal cortical steroid?

   (A) testosterone
   (B) estradiol
   (C) cortisol
   (D) aldosterone
   (E) corticosterone

108. The blood of this patient would show significantly elevated levels of all of the following hormones EXCEPT

(A) cortisol
(B) corticosterone
(C) aldosterone
(D) testosterone
(E) ACTH

109. Of the following laboratory findings, which is LEAST LIKELY in this patient?

(A) elevated Na^+
(B) elevated K^+
(C) elevated androstenedione
(D) elevated testosterone
(E) elevated DHEAS

110. Which statement most accurately describes the physiologic basis for her hypernatremia?

(A) increased ADH secretion decreases renal tubule excretion of Na^+
(B) increased testosterone secretion increases renal tubule excretion of Na^+
(C) increased aldosterone secretion increases renal tubule Na^+ retention
(D) renin secretion declines due to feedback inhibition by aldosterone
(E) testosterone excess inhibits ADH secretion

111. Which statement most accurately describes the physiologic basis for her hypertension?

(A) angiotensinogen levels increase because of ACTH secretion
(B) aldosterone causes an increase in blood volume
(C) aldosterone stimulates renal K^+ excretion
(D) aldosterone inhibits renin secretion from the juxtablomerular apparatus
(E) angiotensin II levels decline

Items 112-113

A 25-year-old male was involved in a street fight. He received a severe laceration across his larynx. During his hospitalization for recovery from emergency surgery, he experienced tetany and seizures. His serum Ca^{2+} values were significantly lowered.

112. The decreased serum Ca^{2+} would most likely to be due to a decline in secretion of which hormone?

(A) thyroxine
(B) TSH
(C) calcitonin
(D) parathyroid hormone
(E) ACTH

113. Which statement most accurately describes the fundamental physiologic mechanism of action of this hormone?

(A) increases Ca^{2+} influx
(B) decreases Ca^{2+} efflux
(C) increases calcitriol synthesis
(D) decreases calcitriol synthesis
(E) mediated by the cAMP second messenger

Item 114

114. A 52-year-old man went to his doctor complaining of intermittent but severe headache, sweating, angina, anxiety and fatigue. Urinalysis revealed high levels of epinephrine, norepinephrine and their metabolites. MRI revealed a 3-cm mass in the adrenal medulla. The most likely diagnosis of this disease is

(A) Cushing's disease
(B) Zollinger-Ellison syndrome
(C) pheochromocytoma
(D) adenocarcinoma of pituitary
(E) Hashimoto's thyroiditis

Items 115-122

In the following group of hormones involved in female reproductive physiology, match the hormone in the answers with the most appropriate description of its physiologic role in the items below.

(A) FSH
(B) LH
(C) Chorionic gonadotropin
(D) Chorionic somatomammotropin
(E) Progesterone
(F) β-estradiol
(G) Inhibin
(H) Prolactin
(I) Oxytocin
(J) Gonadotrophin releasing hormone

115. When secreted from the pars nervosa, this polypeptide hormone stimulates contraction of smooth muscle in the uterus and myoepithelial cells in the mammary gland ducts.

116. This hormone is secreted by cells in the adenohypophysis. Its titer rises during pregnancy and it is required for milk secretion.

117. This hormone is secreted by the placenta. It is required for growth and development of the ducts of the mammary glands. It is also secreted by the ovary where it stimulates endometrial glandular growth prior to ovulation.

118. The release of this hormone from the pituitary gland is inhibited by dopamine. It shows marked increase in secretion during and after periods of nursing.

119. This is a glycoprotein hormone secreted by the placenta. Its chief function is to stimulate continued growth of the corpus luteum during pregnancy.

120. Small quantities of this hormone are secreted by the luteal cells of the corpus luteum. It inhibits secretion of FSH from the anterior pituitary.

121. A surge in secretion of this hormone is required for a mature ovary follicle to progress to rupture.

122. This hormone is secreted by the hypothalamus in a pulsatile fashion. It is a decapeptide.

STOP.

YOU HAVE COMPLETED THIS SECTION.

Notes

Physiology and Endocrinology

Answers and Tutorials

Answer and Tutorial on Item 1

The answer is: **1-D**. There are three basic mechanisms for transport of solutes across semi-permeable cell membranes: (1) **simple diffusion**, (2) **facilitated diffusion**, and (3) **active transport**. Simple diffusion can occur either by solutes passing through membranes, eg, lipid soluble steroids; or, by solutes passing through aqueous pores in membranes. Facilitated diffusion requires a carrier protein. Glucose, other sugars, and many amino acids cross cell membranes by facilitated diffusion. Active transport involves movement of substances up an electrochemical gradient. Na^+, K^+, H^+, and Ca^{2+} are all moved by active transport. It is mediated by integral membrane transport proteins called "pumps" and requires the hydrolysis of ATP to drive it.

The **Na^+-K^+ pump** is an important integral membrane carrier protein which spans the plasma membrane. It is found in all cell membranes in human cells. It consists of two different protein subunits. The larger subunit has a MW = 100,000 with three Na^+ binding sites and an ATP binding site on its intracellular side and 2 K^+ binding sites on its extracellular side. When Na^+ and ATP bind on the inside, the ATPase becomes activated and the protein becomes phosphorylated. This causes a conformational change in the carrier protein which expels Na^+ on the extracellular side of the membrane. In this conformation, the Na^+-K^+-ATPase binds extracellular K^+. The binding of K^+ dephosphorylates the ATPase, returning it to its original conformation and expelling K^+ at the intracellular side of the membrane. The function of the smaller subunit (MW = 55,000) is unclear at present.

The most essential role of this ion pump is to maintain the **volume of cells**. The cytosol contains many negatively charged proteins and small molecular weight solutes. These bind cations. If the ion pumps were not active in expelling more cations than they took into cells, then water would diffuse into cells, eventually causing them to swell to bursting. The Na^+-K^+ pump also establishes gradients of Na^+ and K^+ across the plasma membrane since it expels three Na^+ ions for every two K^+ taken in. Since these ion gradients contribute to the resting membrane potential, the Na^+-K^+ pump is electrogenic.

Under normal circumstances, the intracellular Ca^{2+} concentration is extremely low. The extracellular Ca^{2+} concentration is relatively high. This gradient is maintained by a Ca^{2+} pump which is quite similar to the Na^+-K^+ pump in that it has a carrier protein with ion binding sites and an ATPase activity. The **carrier proteins** in mitochondria and the endoplasmic reticulum are distinct from those in the plasma membrane. In resting muscle cells, the cytosol (location of the myofibrils) has a 10-7 M [Ca^{2+}]. In contrast, there is a large store of Ca^{2+} in the sarcoplasmic reticulum. When a nerve action potential reaches the motor end plate of a muscle cell, it causes a depolarization of the sarcolemma which in turn causes an increase in the Ca^{2+} permeability of the sarcoplasmic reticulum. This results in a rush of Ca^{2+} ions into the region of the myofibrils, increasing [Ca^{2+}] to 10-5 M, a crucial event for initiating the sliding of thick and thin filaments relative to one another. These sliding filaments ultimately result in forceful contraction of the entire cell.

Epithelial sheets in many locations in the human body are capable of polarized transport of ions between different compartments. Examples of these transporting epithelia are found in the gastrointestinal tract, kidney tubules, exocrine glands, the ciliary body and the choroid plexus. This polarized transport, for example as seen with Na^+ transport out of the proximal convoluted tubules (PCTs) in the kidney, involves active transport of Na^+ out of cells on the lateral and basal surfaces. The apical surface of PCT epithelial cells is freely permeable to Na^+ and water by diffusion. Thus, when Na^+ is actively pumped out of cells at the lateral and basal surfaces, water exits these cells by osmosis at the same locations. Individual epithelial cells are joined apically by an extensive network of tight junctions that are impermeable to Na^+ ions, to prevent leakage of extracellular Na^+ into the lumen.

Answer and Tutorial on Item 2

The answer is: **2-B**. Hormones bind specifically to receptors, located either in the cell membrane or in the cytoplasm. Receptors have high affinity for their respective hormones. Hormones circulate at exceedingly low concentrations in the interstitial fluids, eg, in the range 10^{-15}-10^{-9} molar. Receptors have a recognition domain that binds the hormone and a transduction domain that couples hormone binding and alteration of cellular function.

Group I hormones are lipophilic, and, except for T3 and T4, are derived from cholesterol. These hormones are associated with carrier (transport) proteins in blood. This association circumvents problems with solubility and also prolongs the hormone half-life in plasma ($t_{1/2}$ = days). Free hormone diffuses across the plasma membrane readily and rapidly associates with receptors in the nucleus or cytosol to form a ligand-receptor complex which serves as the intracellular messenger. The hormone-receptor complex now undergoes an activation reaction, rendering it able to bind to the hormone response element of DNA. When the activated ligand-receptor complex binds to the hormone response element of DNA, selective transcription occurs, resulting in the synthesis of mRNAs. This leads immediately to the production of new proteins and a change in metabolic activity in target cells. Group I ligands include androgens, calcitriol, estrogens, glucocorticoids, mineralocorticoids, progestins, and thyroid hormones.

Group II hormones are hydrophilic polypeptides or catecholamines that have a short plasma half-life ($t_{1/2}$ = minutes) because they are not bound to transport proteins. Their receptors are located in the plasma membrane and lead to the formation of second messengers such as cyclic AMP (cAMP), the widespread cyclic nucleotide derived from ATP by the enzyme adenylate cyclase.

The **adenylate cyclase system** is extraordinarily complex. Interaction between ligand and receptor can lead either to the activation or inactivation of adenylate cyclase. For example, ACTH, ADH, FSH, glucagon, PTH, and TSH among others are all hormones that stimulate adenylate cyclase. Here we will call them H_s and they bind to receptor, R_s. In contrast, acetylcholine, angiotensin II, and somatostatin among others are all hormones that inhibit adenylate cyclase. Here we will call them H_i and they bind to receptor, R_i. This process is mediated by GTP-dependent regulatory proteins, called G_s and G_i. These **G proteins** are each composed of three subunits, α, β, and γ. The β and γ subunits are similar in G_s and G_i but the α subunits are distinct (α_s and α_i). This trimer, in the presence of GTP, is converted to a GTP-α_s or GTP-α_i complex and a β-γ complex. The GTP-α_s complex stimulates the catalytic portion of adenylate cyclase, leading to formation of cAMP from ATP. The GTP-α_i complex inhibits the catalytic portion of adenylate cyclase, preventing formation of cAMP from ATP.

In higher organisms, cAMP binds to protein kinase which consists of an inactive heterotetramer with two regulatory subunits and two catalytic subunits. Cyclic AMP binds to the regulatory subunits and dissociates them from the catalytic subunits, rendering them enzymatically active. The catalytic subunits in turn catalyze the transfer of γ phosphate from ATP to serine or threonine residues generating many different phosphoproteins including calcium/calmodulin-dependent kinase, myosin light chain kinase, phosphorylase kinase, and pyruvate dehydrogenase kinase. These phosphoproteins are then thought to have diverse physiologic effects. Regulation can occur at several levels including degradation of cAMP by phosphodiesterase and/or dephosphorylation by phosphoprotein phosphatases.

Cyclic GMP, which is synthesized from GTP under the influence of guanylate cyclase, can serve as a second messenger for atrial natriuretic factor (ANF). ANF binds to the membrane guanylate cyclase and causes dramatic increases in cGMP levels which in turn leads to diuresis, vasodilation, and inhibition of aldosterone secretion.

Answer and Tutorial on Item 3

The answer is: **3-E. Synaptic transmission** is a one-way conductance between cells which involves release of neurotransmitter synthesized in the presynaptic terminal and interaction of this neurotransmitter with a specific receptor in the postsynaptic cell membrane. Depolarization of the presynaptic cell results in an influx of Ca^{2+} into the presynaptic terminal from the extracellular fluid. This influx of Ca^{2+} is required for the release of neurotransmitter by exocytosis.

Brief repetitive stimulation results in accumulation of Ca^{2+} within the presynaptic cell, so that subsequent stimulation at a lower voltage permits efficient excitation-secretion coupling. This post-tetanic potentiation persists until Ca^{2+} stores are depleted. It is not dependent on catabolism or synthesis of neurotransmitter and is independent of transport of axoplasmic protein and the postsynaptic receptor. The physiologic significance of this phenomenon is unclear, but post-tetanic potentiation may function in short-term storage of information.

The **transmitter** released by the presynaptic neuron alters the conductance at the postsynaptic plasma membrane to one or more ions by binding to receptors on the plasma membrane of the postsynaptic cell. It is the specificity of these receptors that determines whether the net effect is inhibitory or excitatory. A specific transmitter may have either effect depending on the site of action. Thus, **acetylcholine** is excitatory at the neuromuscular junction but is inhibitory when released by the vagus nerve at cardiac muscle junctions.

The action of acetylcholine (ACh) is terminated by acetylcholinesterase (AChE), which hydrolyzes ACh to acetate and choline. The choline is pumped into the nerve terminal and used in the resynthesis of new ACh. The other transmitters listed are inactivated by re-uptake into the nerve terminal. A variety of drugs act by preventing re-uptake of the neurotransmitter into the nerve terminal or, in the case of ACh, by blocking the action of AChE.

When the effect of a neurotransmitter is to open only K^+ channels in the postsynaptic membrane, the postsynaptic cell becomes hyperpolarized (the resting membrane potential becomes more negative). This is called an **inhibitory postsynaptic potential** (IPSP). The postsynaptic cell sums the incoming excitatory postsynaptic potentials (EPSPs) and the inhibitory postsynaptic potentials (IPSPs). If the sum of inputs depolarizes the cell to threshold, then an action potential is triggered. If the sum of inputs is below threshold, then no action potential is fired. The action potential itself is not altered in magnitude. It is an "all or none" phenomenon.

In presynaptic inhibition (illustrated by the axo-axonic synapse terminal in **Figure 4.1**), δ aminobutyric acid (GABA) is released which opens Cl^- channels on the postsynaptic terminal A. The increase in Cl^- conductance produces a rather long-lived depolarization of the excitatory (postsynaptic) nerve terminal bringing it close to threshold. This partially depolarized excitatory terminal will then release less transmitter in response to an action potential (since less Ca^{2+} enters the nerve terminal) resulting in a smaller EPSP.

Neurons are highly responsive to changes in pH of the surrounding interstitial fluids. A rise in arterial pH from the 7.4 (normal) to 7.8 to 8.0, often causes cerebral convulsions because of increased excitability of the neurons. This can be demonstrated by having a person who is predisposed to epileptic convulsions hyperventilate. This elevates the pH of the blood (alkalosis) momentarily, but even this short interval can often precipitate an epileptic attack. On the other hand, acidosis greatly depresses neuronal activity; a fall in pH from 7.4 to below 7.0 usually causes a comatose state. For instance, in very severe diabetic or uremic acidosis, coma always develops.

Brain
Neuronal activity ↑ Alkalosis → excitability
↓ Acidosis → Comatose

Answer and Tutorial on Item 4

The answer is: **4-C**. The **vestibular apparatus** consists of two sac-like organs (**saccule** and **utricle**) with neuroepithelium called the **macula** and three **semicircular canals** with neuroepithelium called the **crista**. Both the maculae and the cristae (and the **organ of Corti** for that matter) have mechanoreceptors in them called hair cells. There are minor structural variations in hair cells in different neuroepithelia of the vestibular apparatus but, regardless of location, they share certain common physiologic features. Hair cells have a single nonmotile cilium called the kinocilium and an array of tall modified microvilli called stereocilia. Stereocilia are deformed by motion. This deformation then triggers changes in membrane permeability leading to generation of action potentials in hair cells.

The **semicircular canals** are responsible for detecting angular accelerations of the head. The utricle and saccule are responsible for detecting linear acceleration, linear deceleration, and the static position of the head. The hair cells of the semicircular canals are part of the neuroepithelium (the crista) within the ampulla (the expanded end of the semicircular canal). The kinocilium and stereocilia of the hair cells are embedded in a gelatinous structure called the cupula, which projects into the ampullary space. The hair cells of the utricle and saccule are part of the macula (utriculi and sacculi). The apical projections are embedded in a gelatinous otolithic membrane rich in small calcium carbonate crystals called otoliths.

Bipolar neurons within the vestibular ganglion make synaptic connection with the hair cells in both maculae and all three cristae. Central processes of these bipolar neurons, in turn, connect to the vestibular nuclei of the brainstem via cranial nerve VIII, the vestibulocochlear nerve.

The **hair cells** of the horizontal canals are oriented with the kinocilium located closest to the utricle. Head movements that bend the stereocilia toward the utricle cause the hair cells to depolarize, while movements that bend the stereocilia away from the utricle cause hyperpolarization. For example, when the head is rotated toward the left, the endolymph in the left horizontal semicircular canal pushes the cupula and stereocilia toward the utricle. This occurs because the fluid lags behind the head movement and causes the cupula to move toward the right. Movement of the cupula to the right pushes the stereocilia toward the kinocilium causing a depolarization. At the same time, the hair cells within the right horizontal canal are pushed away from the utricle and hyperpolarize. When the head stops rotating, the fluid continues to move, pushing the cupula in the opposite direction. This causes the hair cells in the left horizontal canal to hyperpolarize and those in the right horizontal canal to depolarize. The information generated by the activity of the semicircular canals is used by the CNS to interpret the speed and direction of head movements and to make the appropriate adjustments in posture and eye position.

With rotation of the head to the left, the eyes move toward the right in order to prevent an image from moving off the fovea of the retina. When the eyes have rotated as far as they can, they are rapidly returned to the center of the orbit. If rotation of the head continues, the eyes once again move in the direction opposite the head rotation. These movements of the eyes are called **nystagmus**. The direction of nystagmus is designated according to the direction of the fast component, although this is opposite to the movement induced by stimulation from the semicircular canal. The fact that vestibular stimulation evokes nystagmus provides a basis for clinical tests of vestibular function.

Stimulation of the vestibular apparatus, whether by motion of the body or by artificial means, produces definite conscious effects which take the form of a false sense of motion. **Vertigo** is a sensation of whirling where the individual may have a feeling that his body is rotating, or it may seem that external objects are spinning around. **Ménière's** disease is characterized by sudden attacks of severe vertigo, usually associated with unilateral deafness and tinnitus, and with nausea, vomiting, and prostration. Examination during an attack shows that the patient has fine rotatory nystagmus, which is maximal on gaze opposite to the affected side. Generally, there are no ocular palsies, cranial-nerve signs, or long-tract signs. Patients characteristically complain of a sense of fullness in the affected ear and audiograms will show a high-tone hearing loss with recruitment but not tone decay. Edema with increased pressure of fluid in the labyrinth is thought to be responsible for this condition.

Caloric or thermal tests of nystagmus permit the vestibular system of each side to be tested separately. The subject is usually seated with the head tilted backward about 60° to bring the horizontal semicircular canal into a vertical plane. The external auditory canal is irrigated with cold or warm water. Warm water raises the temperature of the endolymph in the semicircular canal, causing fluid movement. Stimulation of hair cells by the current flowing past the ampulla produces nystagmus. With warm water in the right ear, the current going up produces a flow equivalent to flow to the left in the horizontal position. Thus the nystagmus has its slow component to the left and its fast component to the right. If cold water is used, the current is reversed and nystagmus is in the opposite direction.

Answer and Tutorial on Item 5

The answer is: **5-A**. **Synaptic transmission** is a one-way conductance between cells which involves release of neurotransmitter synthesized in the presynaptic terminal and interaction of this neurotransmitter with a specific receptor in the postsynaptic cell membrane. Depolarization of the presynaptic cell results in an influx of Ca^{2+} into the presynaptic terminal from the extracellular fluid. This influx of Ca^{2+} is required for the release of neurotransmitter by exocytosis.

Brief repetitive stimulation results in accumulation of Ca^{2+} within the presynaptic cell, so that subsequent stimulation at a lower voltage permits efficient excitation-secretion coupling. This post-tetanic potentiation persists until Ca^{2+} stores are depleted. It is not dependent on catabolism or synthesis of neurotransmitter and is independent of transport of axoplasmic protein and the postsynaptic receptor. The physiologic significance of this phenomenon is unclear, but post-tetanic potentiation may function in short-term storage of information.

The transmitter released by the presynaptic neuron alters the **conductance** at the postsynaptic plasma membrane to one or more ions by binding to receptors on the plasma membrane of the postsynaptic cell. It is the specificity of these receptors that determines whether the net effect is inhibitory or excitatory. A specific transmitter may have either effect depending on the site of action. Thus, acetylcholine is excitatory at the neuromuscular junction but is inhibitory when released by the vagus nerve at cardiac muscle junctions.

The action of **acetylcholine** (ACh) is terminated by acetylcholinesterase (AChE), which hydrolyzes ACh to acetate and choline. The choline is pumped into the nerve terminal and used in the resynthesis of new ACh. The other transmitters listed are inactivated by re-uptake into the nerve terminal. A variety of drugs act by preventing re-uptake of the neurotransmitter into the nerve terminal or, in the case of ACh, by blocking the action of AChE.

When the effect of a neurotransmitter is to open only K^+ channels in the postsynaptic membrane, the postsynaptic cell becomes hyperpolarized (the resting membrane potential becomes more negative). This is called an **inhibitory postsynaptic potential** (IPSP). The postsynaptic cell sums the incoming **excitatory postsynaptic potentials** (EPSPs) and the inhibitory postsynaptic potentials (IPSPs). If the sum of inputs depolarizes the cell to threshold, then an action potential is triggered. If the sum of inputs is below threshold, then no action potential is fired. The action potential itself is not altered in magnitude. It is an "all or none" phenomenon.

In **presynaptic inhibition** (illustrated by the axo-axonic synapse terminal in **Figure 4.1**), **gamma aminobutyric acid** (GABA) is released which opens Cl^- channels on the postsynaptic terminal A. The increase in Cl^- conductance produces a rather long-lived depolarization of the excitatory (postsynaptic) nerve terminal bringing it close to threshold. This partially depolarized excitatory terminal will then release less transmitter in response to an action potential (since less Ca^{2+} enters the nerve terminal) resulting in a smaller EPSP.

Neurons are highly responsive to changes in pH of the surrounding interstitial fluids. A rise in arterial pH from the 7.4 (normal) to 7.8 to 8.0, often causes cerebral convulsions because of increased excitability of the neurons. This can be demonstrated by having a person who is predisposed to epileptic convulsions hyperventilate. This elevates the pH of the blood (alkalosis) momentarily, but even this short interval can often precipitate an epileptic attack. On the other hand, acidosis greatly depresses neuronal activity; a fall in pH from 7.4 to below 7.0 usually causes a comatose state. For instance, in very severe diabetic or uremic acidosis, coma always develops.

Answer and Tutorial on Item 6

The answer is: **6-A**. The cerebellar cortex consists of three layers: **molecular**, **Purkinje**, and **granular**. The outermost molecular layer contains two types of neuron, the stellate and basket cells that form connections within the cerebellum. The Purkinje cell layer contains the large, flask-shaped Purkinje cells whose axons form the only efferent projection from the cerebellum. The Purkinje cell axons synapse in the deep cerebellar nuclei or the vestibular nuclei. The granule cells of the innermost granular layer give rise to the parallel fibers that project to the molecular layer.

Afferents to the cerebellum terminate either in the granule cell layer as mossy fibers or upon the dendrites of Purkinje cells as the climbing fibers. Mossy fiber afferents are derived from areas such as the spinal cord, pontine nuclei, vestibular nuclei and deep cerebellar nuclei. Climbing fibers are thought to derive exclusively from the inferior olivary nucleus. Both mossy fiber and climbing fiber inputs are excitatory. The Purkinje cells, the only route for all information exiting from the cerebellar cortex, are inhibitory to the deep cerebellar and vestibular nuclei.

The cerebellum participates with other central nervous system structures in the execution of a wide variety of movements. It is needed to maintain the proper posture and balance for walking and running; to execute sequential movements for eating, dressing, and writing; to participate in rapidly alternating repetitive movements and in smooth pursuit movements; and to control certain properties of movements, including trajectory, velocity, and acceleration.

The cerebellum is responsible for muscle synergy throughout the body. It coordinates the action of muscle groups and times their contractions so that movements are performed smoothly and accurately. Voluntary movements can proceed without assistance from the cerebellum, but such movements are clumsy and disorganized. Lack of motor skill as a result of cerebellar dysfunction is called asynergia or cerebellar ataxia.

The clinical signs of **cerebellar dysfunction** can be separated into those resulting from disease of the midline zone and those resulting from disease of the hemispheres. The midline zone of the cerebellum consists of the vermis, the flocculonodular lobe and the fastigial nuclei. Disease of these regions produces disorders of stance and gait. The stance is usually broad-based with the feet wide apart. There may be a severe truncal tremor. A number of disturbances of ocular function result from cerebellar disease, the most prominent of which is nystagmus. Nystagmus consists of rhythmical oscillatory movements of one or both eyes occurring with the eyes gazing straight ahead or with ocular deviation.

Ataxia, scanning speech, dysmetria, and an intention tremor all are classic findings in a patient with a lesion involving the cerebellum. Ataxia results chiefly from the combined effects of dysmetria and decomposition of movement. There are errors in the sequence and speed of the components of each movement. An ataxia of gait results in a veering of the path from side to side with difficulty walking in a straight line (drunken gait).

Decomposition of movement occurs when an action which normally requires the cooperative movement of several joints is not properly coordinated, but the action is broken down into its component parts. **Dysmetria** is a disturbance of the trajectory or placement of a body part during active movements. The limb may fall short of its goal in hypometria, or it may extend beyond its goal in hypermetria (past-pointing). In cerebellar disease, speech may be slow, slurred, and labored (**dysarthria**), but comprehension remains intact and grammar does not suffer. Scanning speech is due to asynergy of the muscles used in speaking. In scanning speech, the spacing of sounds is irregular with pauses in the wrong places. Persons with cerebellar disease also exhibit **dysdiadochokinesia**, which is a loss of ability to stop one movement and follow it immediately by the directly opposite action. This is apparent on attempting to make rapid alternating movements of pronation and supination of the hands, or by tapping quickly with the fingers. The tremor of cerebellar dysfunction is usually an **intention tremor**. It is evident during purposeful movements, but absent or diminished with rest.

Answers and Tutorial on Items 7-10

The answers are: **7-A; 8-D; 9-A; 10-E**. **Figure 4.2** shows electrical recordings from the surface of the brain or from the outer surface of the head, demonstrating continuous electrical activity in the brain. The undulations in the recorded electrical potentials as shown in **Figure 4.2** are called brain waves and the entire record is called an **electroencephalogram** (EEG). The discharge of a single neuron or single nerve fiber in the brain can never be recorded from the surface of the head. Instead, many thousands or even millions of neurons or fibers must fire synchronously to allow the potentials to summate enough to be recorded through the skull.

The types of waves that can occur in normal persons can be classified as alpha, beta, theta and delta waves. **Alpha waves** (A) are rhythmic waves occurring at a frequency of between 8 and 13 per second and are found in the EEGs of almost all normal adult persons when they are awake in a quiet, resting state of mental activity. These waves occur most intensely in the occipital region but can also be recorded from the parietal and frontal regions of the scalp. During deep sleep, the alpha waves disappear entirely. When the awake person's attention is directed to some specific type of mental activity, the alpha waves are replaced by asynchronous, higher-frequency but lower-voltage beta waves.

Beta waves (B) occur at frequencies of more than 14 cycles per second and as high as 25. These are most frequently recorded from the parietal and frontal regions of the scalp during activation of the central nervous system or during tension. The alpha rhythm is replaced by an asynchronous discharge of beta waves on opening the eyes.

Theta waves (C) have frequencies of between 4 and 7 cycles per second. These occur mainly in the parietal and temporal regions in children, but they also occur during emotional stress in some adults, particularly during disappointment and frustration. Theta waves also occur in many brain disorders.

Delta waves (D) include all the waves of the EEG below 3.5 cycles per second and sometimes as low as one cycle every 2-3 seconds. These occur in very deep sleep, in infancy, and in serious organic brain disease.

Epilepsy is characterized by uncontrolled excessive activity of either a part or all of the central nervous system. **Grand mal epilepsy** (E) is characterized by extreme neuronal discharges in all areas of the neural cortex, deep parts of the cerebrum, brainstem and thalamus. The EEG is characterized by a high-voltage (100 μV), synchronous discharges over the entire cortex. In patients with **petite mal epilepsy** (F) the EEG shows a classic three cycles per second spike and wave form.

Answer and Tutorial on Item 11

The answers is: **11-E**. **Muscle spindles** are proprioceptors that relay information on length and tension of muscles to the nervous system. They are encapsulated structures 3-4 mm in length, consisting of a connective tissue sheath that encloses several intrafusal muscle fibers. The end of the spindle is attached to skeletal muscle fibers (extrafusal fibers). The spindles are dispersed throughout the muscle in parallel to the extrafusal fibers. The spindle will stretch as the muscle relaxes (lengthens) and shortens as the muscle contracts. There are two types of intrafusal fibers, nuclear bag fibers, and nuclear chain fibers. Nuclear bag intrafusal fibers have cell nuclei clustered into a bag-like structure in the central region of the fiber. The nuclear chain fibers contain a single row of nuclei in the central region of the fiber. Both types of fiber are innervated by the gamma motor neurons and both are supplied with sensory nerve endings. The very large **group Ia afferent fibers** innervate both types of muscle spindle fiber and are referred to as primary afferents (annulospiral endings). In addition, the nuclear chain fibers, and to a lesser extent, the nuclear bag fibers are also supplied by group II afferents (secondary endings or flower spray endings).

A normal, live muscle which appears to be fully relaxed still possesses a small amount of tension. If it is palpated in a resting state, the muscle will be found to have a quality of resilience rather than complete flabbiness. When it is passively stretched by moving one of the joints, a certain amount of resistance will be encountered in the muscle which is not related to any conscious effort on the part of the patient. These characteristics—subdued activity at rest, and involuntary reaction opposing mechanical stretch—are the chief clinical manifestations of **muscle tone** (tonus).

A muscle loses its tonus at once if the ventral roots containing its motor nerve fibers are cut or if the ventral horn motoneurons (alpha motor neurons), which give origin to the ventral root fibers, are destroyed. Tonus is likewise abolished by cutting the dorsal nerve roots that contain sensory fibers from the muscle. Damage to the corticospinal tracts would result in an increase in muscle tone.

The **gamma motoneurons** are the small neurons of the ventral horn of the spinal cord that innervate the intrafusal fibers of the muscle spindles. When a skeletal muscle contracts, the intrafusal muscle fiber becomes slack and the Ia afferents stop firing. By stimulating the intrafusal muscle fibers during a contraction, the gamma motoneurons prevent the intrafusal muscle fibers from becoming slack and thus maintain Ia afferent activity during the contraction.

The **myotatic**—or stretch—**reflex**, is a spinal cord reflex that prevents further stretch of muscle by stimulating contraction of muscle fibers. It is important in preventing oscillation and jerking movements. The function of the intrafusal fibers within skeletal muscle is to inform the nervous system of the length and rate of change in length of the extrafusal muscle fibers. The reflex is normally subject to both facilitation and inhibition by higher centers.

The **stretch (myotatic) reflex** can be tested by tapping the patellar tendon. This stretches the quadriceps femoris muscle; and, since the muscle spindles are in parallel with the extrafusal fibers of the quadriceps, they will also be stretched. This stretching will stimulate the sensory endings in the spindle, in particular the primary afferents (Ia). The latter neurons monosynaptically stimulate the alpha motor neurons that supply the quadriceps and polysynaptically inhibit the antagonistic muscles. Consequently, the quadriceps will suddenly contract causing extension of the leg.

A second type of proprioceptor input comes from the **Golgi tendon organs** which transmit information regarding the force generated at the musculotendinous junction. Golgi tendon organs are encapsulated structures located in the tendons near the muscle insertion. Within the capsule, sensory nerve endings (**Ib afferents**) terminate in small bundles of collagenous fibers of tendons. The Golgi tendon organs are primarily tension recorders in series with the muscle fiber and respond to the velocity of contraction and to steady-state contraction of the muscle. They polysynaptically inhibit the agonistic muscles and facilitate the antagonistic muscles. This is responsible for the clasp-knife phenomenon in upper motor neuron lesions in which there is a sudden release of a spastic

Answers and Tutorial on Items 12-18

The answers are: **12-A; 13-A; 14-B; 15-A; 16-A; 17-C; 18-B**. **Figure 4.3** shows the retina which is comprised of three basic cell types (neurons, pigmented epithelial cells, and neuronal support cells) divided into 10 histologically defined layers. The outer most layer (A), the **pigmented epithelium** absorbs stray light and phagocytoses disks that have been sloughed from the outer segments of receptor cells. The next layer (B) contains the **photoreceptive portions of rods and cones**, two distinct types of photoreceptor cells. Their nuclei are found in the **outer nuclear layer** (C).

The membrane of the outer segment of rods and cones invaginates to form stacks of photopigment-rich disks. In rods, the disks pinch off and become independent of the cell membrane as they undergo constant renewal. Disks are formed initially at the basal pole of the outer segment and migrate through the outer segment until they reach the apical pole. Here, the disintegrating disks are phagocytosed by the pigmented cells. The inner segments contain numerous mitochondria as well as the nucleus of the rod or cone.

The **cones** (I) are the only cells involved with color vision. Cones function at high light intensities and, therefore, are responsible for day (photopic) vision. Cones are not as sensitive as rods to low levels of illumination. Highly modified cones are packed closely together in the fovea centralis, the portion of the retina with maximal visual acuity. Rods function at low light intensities and are responsible for night (scotopic) vision. **Rods** (J) are absent in the fovea. They are confined to the peripheral retina where visual acuity is minimal.

Müller cells are glial elements that have cell bodies in the inner nuclear layer (E). Müller cell processes span most of the thickness of the retina. Their basal surfaces rest on the inner limiting membrane (basement membrane for the neural retina) and their apical surface make tight junctions with the rods and cones, forming the outer limiting membrane. Müller cell processes also fill the spaces between photoreceptor cells and are supportive.

The interneurons consist of three cell types: bipolar cells, horizontal cells, and amacrine cells. Their cell bodies are located in the **inner nuclear layer** (E). Bipolar cells synapse with the photoreceptor terminals of rods or cones in the **outer plexiform layer** (D) and with **ganglion cells** (L) located in the **inner plexiform layer** (F). The dendrites of ganglion cells receive their input from the bipolar cells. Ganglion cells have their cell bodies in the **ganglion cell layer** (G). The axons of ganglion cells course along the retina and form the optic nerve layer (H) which proceeds to the optic disk to form the optic nerve. The processes of horizontal cells (N) are confined to the outer plexiform layer. They form a triad synapse at the junction of the photoreceptor terminals and the bipolar cells. The **amacrine cells** (M) form complex synapses in the **inner plexiform layer** (F) at the junction of the bipolar cells and the dendrites of the ganglion cells.

These different neuronal cell types function within the retina as follows: (1) the photoreceptors of the rods and cones are stimulated by light; (2) the horizontal cells transmit signals horizontally in the outer plexiform layer from the rods and cones to the bipolar cell dendrites; (3) the bipolar cells transmit signals from the rods, cones, and horizontal cells to the inner plexiform layer, where they synapse with either amacrine cells or ganglion cells; (4) the amacrine cells transmit signals in two directions, either directly from bipolar cells to ganglion cells or horizontally within the inner plexiform layer between the axons of bipolar cells, the dendrites of ganglion cells and/or other amacrine cells; (5) the ganglion cells transmit output signals from the retina through the optic nerve to the brain.

The light-sensitive chemical in the retinal rods is called **rhodopsin** (or visual purple). It is a combination of the protein scotopsin and the carotinoid pigment retinal (also called retinene). The retinal is in the configuration called **11-*cis* retinal**. Light immediately changes the *cis* structure of 11-*cis* retinal to **all-*trans* retinal**. The physical structure of the all-*trans* retinal no longer combines in a stable fashion with scotopsin and the two dissociate. The all-*trans* retinal is then converted to all-*trans* retinol (**vitamin A**). During this process, the color of the photopigment changes from purple to pink, consequently, this process is called bleaching. The all-*trans* retinol is then enzymatically isomerized to 11-*cis* retinol and then enzymatically oxidized to 11-*cis* retinal. The 11-*cis* retinal then spontaneously combines with opsin, reforming rhodopsin. A deficiency of vitamin A prevents the regeneration of rhodopsin. For this reason, lack of vitamin A leads to night blindness.

The receptor cells of the retina have a resting membrane potential of about -40 mV due to a high Na^+ conductance. The high Na^+ conductance is maintained by the presence of cGMP. When light strikes a receptor, photoisomerization of 11-*cis* retinal is accompanied by the activation of a G protein called transducin, which causes cGMP levels to decrease. The reduction of cGMP levels causes the Na^+ channels to close which in turn causes the receptor to hyperpolarize. The result of this hyperpolarization is a reduction in release of receptor cell transmitter, the bipolar cells depolarize and the ganglion cell is stimulated. The hyperpolarization of retinal receptors is different from other receptors which are depolarized when activated by a stimulus.

Transmission of most signals occurs in the retina by electrotonic conduction and not by action potentials. The only retinal neurons that transmit visual signals by action potentials are the ganglion cells. Electrotonic conduction means direct flow of electrical current in the neuronal cytoplasm from the point of excitation to the output synapses. The importance of electrotonic conduction is that it allows graded conduction of signal strength. Thus, for the rods and cones, the hyperpolarizing output signal is directly related to the intensity of illumination; the signal is not all-or-none, as would be the case for action potential conduction.

Each ganglion cell receives synaptic input from many bipolar cells, which, in turn, receive input from a large number of receptor cells. All of the receptor cells that connect directly to a ganglion cell through bipolar cells form the receptive field center for that ganglion cell. The ganglion cell is also influenced by receptors that connect to the bipolar cells through horizontal cells. The output of horizontal cells is always inhibitory. Receptor cells lying within an annulus surrounding the receptive field of the ganglion cell form the receptive field surround. When light strikes the receptors in the receptive field center of a ganglion cell, the ganglion cells in the receptive field surround are inhibited through the horizontal-to-bipolar-to-ganglion cell pathway.

Answers and Tutorial on Items 19-25

The answers are: **19-G; 20-A; 21-C; 22-D; 23-B; 24-E; 25-D.** **Figure 4.4** shows an **action potential** recorded with an intracellular electrode impaling a large myelinated nerve fiber and a second electrode placed in extracellular fluid. The charge separation generated by differences in ion concentration creates an electrical potential difference called the membrane potential. The membrane potential at equilibrium, **resting potential** (A), is caused by a high extracellular [Na^+] (142 mEq/L) and a corresponding low intracellular [Na^+] (14 mEq/L); and, by a low extracellular [K^+] (4 mEq/L) and a corresponding high intracellular [K^+] (140 mEq/L). These concentration differences are generated by the activity of Na^+-K^+-ATPase and result in a resting potential (A) of approximately -90 mV. At resting potential, the Na^+ conductance is extremely low. In contrast, the K^+ conductance is much higher. That is, the plasma membrane is more leaky to K^+ than to Na^+.

The resting potential can be perturbed by current that is either depolarizing or hyperpolarizing depending upon the direction of flow. Depolarization occurs when the membrane potential is decreased (eg, -90 mV to -70 mV), and hyperpolarization occurs when the membrane potential is increased (eg, -90 mV to -110 mV).

The larger the current applied, the larger the perturbation of the membrane potential. Above a certain threshold strength, a depolarizing current will trigger an action potential. The action potential differs from local depolarization in that the polarity of the membrane potential actually reverses (eg, the interior of the cell is now positive with respect to the exterior) and the action potential propagates along the fiber without decreasing in magnitude.

Once the membrane is depolarized to threshold, Na+ rushes into the cell, leading to **rapid depolarization** (C). The Na+ conductance increases rapidly, reaching a peak value which corresponds roughly to the **peak in the action potential** (D) and then falls rapidly to the resting potential. A stimulus can result in a **stimulus artifact** (B) due to a brief opening of the voltage-gated Na^+ channels.

In addition to increases in Na^+ conductance, the action potential is caused in part by changes in K^+ conductance. The K^+ conductance increases more slowly and reaches a maximum midway in the **repolarization phase** (E) and then returns to basal levels slowly. The K^+ conductance starts at a higher level then Na^+ conductance and reaches a lower magnitude. The rapid return of the membrane potential is due to the decline in Na^+ conductance and the increase in K^+ conductance, as seen in **Figure 4.9**.

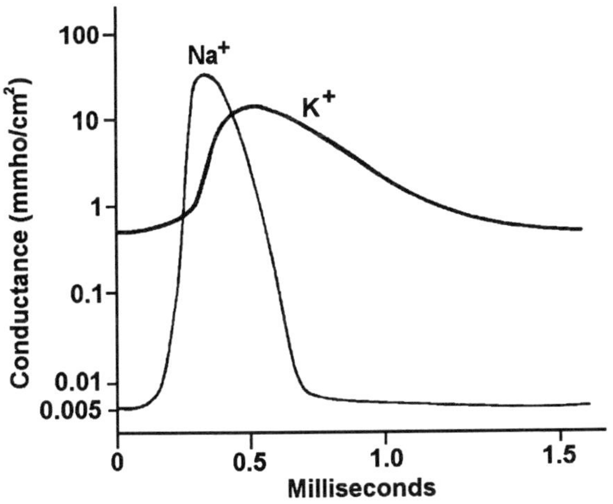

Figure 4.9

These differences in the time course of ion conductances lead first to a **sudden depolarization** (C) as Na^+ rushes in followed by an inactivation of the Na^+ channels; and, then a repolarization (E) as K^+ exits the cell. At (D) there is a **positive overshoot** of membrane potential. This is basically due to the fact that the Na^+ channels open much more rapidly than the K^+ channels. At (F), the membrane potential is actually more negative than at rest. This **afterpotential** is caused by the relatively greater delay in closure of K^+ channels compared to Na^+ channels, so the exterior of the cell becomes more positive and the interior becomes more negative. Eventually, both channels return to the **resting state** and the resting potential returns to -90 mV (G). Lowering of extracellular [Na^+] to 100 mEq/L would lower the height of the spike and would shift the curve to the right.

Answers and Tutorial on Items 26-31

The answers are: **26-B; 27-A; 28-H; 29-A; 30-E; 31-C**. In **emmetropia** (D), the eye is normal. Parallel light rays from distant objects are in sharp focus on the retina when the ciliary muscle is completely relaxed. This means that the emmetropic eye can see all distant objects clearly, with its ciliary muscle relaxed, but to focus objects at close range it must contract its ciliary muscle and thereby provide various degrees of accommodation.

Myopia (nearsightedness) (A) results from an axial length of the eye that is too long for the refractive power of the eye. In this case, the focal point is in front of the retina; thus, distant objects cannot be focused on the retina. An object can be seen clearly if it is moved closer to the eye so that the image forms on the retina. In severe myopia, the far point may be only 10-15 cm from the eye. As the object is moved closer to the eye, the lens accommodates for near vision. Myopes have near points very close to the eye. Thus, they are able to do fine work without magnifying glasses. A diverging lens can be placed in front of a myopic eye, reducing its refractive power. When wearing such a lens, the myope can see distant objects clearly.

Hyperopia (farsightedness) (B) results from an axial length of the eye that is too short for the refractive power of the eye. In this case, distant objects cannot be focused clearly because the focal point is in back of the retina. In overcoming this abnormality, the ciliary muscle may contract to increase the curvature of the lens. Therefore, the far-sighted person use accommodation to focus distant objects on the retina. Since some amount of accommodation is used to see distant objects, there is not so much available for near vision. Thus the near point in hyperopes is further from the retina than normal. A converging lens can be placed in front of a hyperopic eye to increase its refractive power. When wearing a diverging lens, a hyperope can see distant objects clearly without accommodation.

The **near point** (K) is the nearest point at which an object can be seen clearly. A typical young adult can increase refractive power by 12 D (diopters) where a diopter is equal to 1 over the focal length of the lens. At a maximum lens power of 70.8 D, the near point is about 8.3 cm from the eye. The **far point** (J) is the distance from the eye that an object must be placed so that it can be clearly seen without accommodation. For a normal person, this is 6 m.

Presbyopia (C) is loss of accommodative power associated with aging. As an individual ages, the elastic recoil of the lens decreases, and it is unable to bulge as much when the ciliary muscle contracts. Because the accommodative power is lost in presbyopia, the near point moves farther from the eye. A converging lens is used to substitute for the lost accommodative power. The use of these lenses in reading glasses makes near vision possible.

Astigmatism (E) is due to an uneven cornea. Normally, the cornea has a spherical surface; in astigmatism, it has more of an oblong (egg-shaped) surface. As a result, the power of the lens is different in different axes. Images formed with an astigmatic lens are distorted. For example, a point is seen as a line, and a line appears to have a halo on either side of it. Cylindrical lenses can be worn by an astigmatic individual. These lenses add refractive power in only one axis and thus allow the lens system to behave as a spherical surface. The **refractive power** (I) of a lens is the degree to which the lens bends light rays and is measured in diopters.

Accommodation is the reflex mechanism by which the eye forms a clear image of near objects. Accommodation consists of three components: (1) contraction of the ciliary muscle which releases tension on the zonular fibers of the lens and thus allows the lens to "round up"; (2) **convergence** (G), where the gaze of the two eyes shifts toward the center of the head to keep both eyes focused on the object; and (3) pupillary constriction which reduces the area through which light can enter the eye and thereby reduces spherical aberration. This increases the depth of focus (the degree to which the image can form in front of or behind the retina and still appear to be in focus).

Conjugate gaze (H) is a reflex eye movement controlled by the vestibular system and its connections to the nuclei of cranial nerves III, IV and VI. In response to movement of the head, the eyes move reflexly in an attempt to maintain the image on the fovea of both eyes.

Answers and Tutorial on Items 32-34

The answers are: **32-E; 33-D; 34-A**. This child is suffering from **Duchenne's muscular dystrophy** (DMD). This genetically linked condition is maternally transmitted, only to male children. It usually manifests in the first decade of life as difficulty in standing and walking. Muscle weakness initially appears in muscles of the hip girdle and upper legs. Later, the condition involves muscles of the arms and respiratory system, with death usually occurring before age 20. Biopsies show muscle fibers of highly variable size, as well as degenerating fibers and fibers being broken down and phagocytosed. Patients fail to produce the protein **dystrophin**. This is a member of the spectrin superfamily, with a MW = 427,000. Dystrophin is found underneath the sarcolemma in normal muscle, especially where membrane folds are formed, eg, at myotendinous and neuromuscular junctions. It also interacts with actin filaments, stabilizing their side-side association as well as binding to the amino-terminus. Muscles from DMD patients are fragile and rupture easily. They also show reduced levels of enzymes normally found in the sarcoplasm with concomitant increases in serum levels of creatine phosphokinase, lactate dehydrogenase, and glucose phosphoisomerase. Urinary levels of creatine are usually elevated. It is believed that one of the normal functions of dystrophin is to stabilize the sarcolemma against the physical stresses caused by frequent folding during cycles of contraction and relaxation.

Answer and Tutorial on Item 35

The answer is: **35-C**. **Fast twitch fibers** are specialized for rapid forceful contractions but are easily fatigued. Muscles rich in fast twitch fibers (eg, gastrocnemius) can grow considerably as a result of repeated usage during athletic training. Their most significant response to increased work loads is hypertrophy of individual fibers. In addition, there is a considerable increase in blood supply to such muscles.

Slow twitch muscles are specialized for repeated contraction over extended periods. Muscles rich in slow twitch fibers (eg, soleus) hypertrophy much less extensively than fast twitch fibers. As a result of training, slow twitch fibers increase functional capacity by changing their ability to utilize O

(eg, increased myoglobin content, increased mitochondria, increased oxidative mitochondrial enzymes, and increased capillary beds to deliver more O_2).

Answer and Tutorial on Item 36

The answer is: **36-A**. Certain muscles in the body are specialized for brief bursts of rapid and powerful contraction. For example, the quadriceps femoris and gastrocnemius are especially well developed in sprinters. These muscles are rich in **fast twitch (white) fibers**. These fibers have a larger diameter, more extensive sarcoplasmic reticulum, more folds in their neuromuscular junctions, more glycolytic enzymes, less myoglobin, and fewer mitochondria. As a result, they are capable of performing rapidly and powerfully, but they fatigue easily as a result of accumulation of lactate during anaerobic metabolism.

Other muscles are specialized for prolonged contraction. These muscles have a relative abundance of **slow twitch (red) fibers**. These fibers have a smaller diameter, less extensive sarcoplasmic reticulum, less complexly folded neuromuscular junctions, fewer glycolytic enzymes, more myoglobin, and more mitochondria. As a result, they are capable of performing consistently. They fatigue less easily because their richer supply of mitochondria allows them to produce ATP aerobically.

When a person dies, initially, their muscles become rigid (**rigor mortis**). Death results in a cessation of respiration. Consequently, ATP is no longer formed. The binding of SF 1 of myosin to actin is irreversible when there is no ATP present. During normal contraction, ATP binding to SF 1 releases the myosin cross bridge from the actin. Without ATP, cross bridges remain firmly bound. Later, the lysosomal enzymes present in muscle tissue are released, causing a degradation of the muscle proteins leading to a loss of rigor mortis.

Answers and Tutorial on Items 37-41

The answers are: **37-E; 38-A; 39-D; 40-D; 41-A**. **Figure 4.5** shows a **length tension curve** for normal skeletal muscle. Variations in the amount of tension potentially generated by contraction are directly related to the extent of overlap between the thin filaments and the thick filaments. What is critical is the number of cross bridges the thick filaments can make in contact with the thin filaments. At **maximal length** (E), the Z-discs are pulled so far apart that there is no overlap between thick and thin filaments. Since there is not contact between cross bridges and thin filaments, no tension can be generated at this length. As the Z-discs move closer together, **decreasing sarcomere length** (D), there is partial overlap between thick and thin filaments, allowing generation of modest tension. When there is complete **overlap between thick and thin filaments** (C and B), the maximal tension can be generated. However, as the Z-discs move even **closer** (A), the thin filaments collapse, decreasing the tension generated by contraction.

Answers and Tutorial on Items 42-46

The answers are: **42-M; 43-I; 44-G; 45-C; 46-B**. The **thin filaments** of skeletal and cardiac muscle (microfilaments in other motile cells) consist of two helically wound fibrous strands of F-actin (A) composed of many subunits of globular **G-actin** (B) strung together like a string of pearls. Tropomyosin (I) is an elongated regulatory muscle protein that fits in the groove of the F-actin helices, spanning 7 G-actin subunits. A three subunit troponin complex sits at the head of the tropomyosin molecule. **Troponin** consists of troponin T (F) which links the other troponins to tropomyosin; troponin C (G) which binds Ca^{2+}; and troponin I which inhibits interaction between actin and myosin head groups.

Thin filaments insert into the Z-disc of **sarcomeres**. The disc consists mainly of **α-actinin** (C), a protein with considerable homology to dystrophin and spectrin, other proteins that are involved in binding actin rich proteins to the cell membrane. Cap Z (L) is another protein that binds to the + end of actin filaments and secures them in the Z-disc.

The **thick filaments** of skeletal and cardiac muscle contain many closely packed **myosin II** (D) molecules. Myosin II consists of a long fibrous component with two helically arranged segments each capped by a globular head. Treatment of myosin II with papain yields a long myosin rod (E) and two **myosin heads** (M) (SF 1 fragments). The myosin heads are the cross bridges that bind tightly to actin during muscle contraction. Thick filaments are anchored to the Z-discs by a large fibrous protein called **titin** (J). **Nebulin** (K) is another large fibrous protein that may regulate the sarcomere structure. It binds to the Z-disc and is closely associated with thin filaments. Perhaps it functions to regulate the size of the thin filaments.

The **swinging cross bridges** are polarized to form arrowhead-like complexes on the thick filaments. The direction of the arrowheads points to the middle of the sarcomere away from the Z-discs. When these cross bridges become attached to the thin filaments and move toward the center of the sarcomere, the Z-discs move together, shortening the entire sarcomere.

Answer and Tutorial on Item 47

The answer is: **47-E**. **Pernicious anemia** is primarily due to gastric abnormalities leading to a decrease in production of **gastric intrinsic factor** (GIF), a secretion product of parietal cells in gastric glands. GIF is required for vitamin B_{12} absorption. Vitamin B_{12} and folic acid are both required for DNA synthesis and therefore normal erythropoiesis. When they are absent or deficient in the diet, eg, in intestinal malabsorption → sprue, in alcoholics, in gastrectomy patients, or in malnourished people, the hematocrit falls.

Sickle cell anemia is a variety of hemolytic anemia prevalent in African-Americans. It is caused by a single amino acid substitution in the chain of hemoglobin, resulting in the formation of hemoglobin S. This mutant form of hemoglobin readily crystallizes in RBCs, giving them an abnormal sickle shape and rendering them more susceptible to destruction in the spleen.

Polycythemia vera is caused by hyperplasia of bone marrow. Huge excesses of RBCs are produced so that the hematocrit rises to as high as 70. It is distinct from the increases in hematocrit due to living at high elevation (an example of secondary polycythemia due to hypoxia).

Erythroblastosis fetalis is an example of a disease of unborn fetuses caused by maternal-fetal RBC surface antigen incompatibility. It is often seen in Rh positive fetuses carried by Rh negative mothers. Fetal RBCs cross the placenta and enter the maternal circulation. The maternal immune system produces antibodies against the fetal RBCs. These antibodies cross the placenta and bind to the surface of fetal RBCs. The fetal spleen and liver become enlarged as they destroy fetal RBCs and remain hematopoietically active in an attempt to compensate for the hemolytic anemia. Excessive destruction of fetal RBCs releases hemoglobin which can also lead to jaundice in the fetus.

In **hereditary spherocytosis**, RBCs are abnormally small and spherical rather than the normal biconcave discs. As a result, RBCs are more fragile and less deformable, rendering them more susceptible to removal by the spleen. This condition is caused by a mutation in spectrin, an important cytoskeletal protein of RBCs, essential for maintaining their normal shape.

Answers and Tutorial on Items 48-50

The answers are: **48-B; 49-E; 50-A**. **Figure 4.6** is a photomicrograph of two **mast cells** in the lamina propria (mucosal connective tissue) of the trachea. Notice the round nucleus with peripheral blocks of heterochromatin and the prominent cytoplasmic granules. These granules are **metachromatic** when stained with basic dyes such as hematoxylin because they are rich in the sulfated glycosaminoglycan heparin, a potent anticoagulant. Mast cell granules also contain histamine and eosinophil chemotactic factors. Mast cells also release leukotriene C (slow reactive substance of anaphylaxis).

Mast cells have **IgE** bound to their cell surface via receptors. When a person is sensitized to antigens such as those found in pollen or bee venom, IgEs are produced and bind to the mast cell surface. Second exposure to the antigen causes degranulation of mast cells which results primarily in induction of leakiness in capillaries (induced by histamine) followed by edema, inflammation, and, in severe cases, anaphylactic shock.

Mast cells bear some similarities to **basophils** but are distinct cell types. The mast cell has a round, unlobulated nucleus. In contrast, the basophil (a member of the granulocyte series), has a multilobed nucleus. In addition, their granules differ chemically.

Answers and Tutorial on Items 51-58

The answers are: **51-J; 52-I; 53-B; 54-A; 55-E; 56-B; 57-H; 58-D**. The **erythrocyte** (A) is the most abundant cell in whole blood. It is a biconcave disc 7 μm in diameter. It consists essentially of a plasma membrane surrounding cytoplasm with highly concentrated hemoglobin. Once in the circulation, it has no intracellular organelles. The life span of the RBC is normally 120 days. Its main function is to transport O_2 and CO_2 between the lungs and the rest of the body.

There are three kinds of granulocytes in normal peripheral blood. These include the most numerous **neutrophils** (40-75% of circulating leucocytes) (B), the least numerous **basophils** (less than 1% of circulating leucocytes) (C), and the **eosinophils** (1-6% of circulating leucocytes) (D). Neutrophils are chemotactically attracted to sites of inflammation particularly those caused by bacteria. Here, they engulf invading microorganisms by phagocytosis and destroy them using their lysosomes. Basophils release the anticoagulant heparin and histamine when their surface IgEs are challenged by an immunizing antigen such as that found in bee venom. While functionally related to **mast cells** (L), basophils are morphologically distinct. These two cells probably represent distinct cell types with similar functions. Eosinophils are cells specialized for killing the larvae of parasites. They are summoned to the sites of parasitic infestation by eosinophil chemotactic factor which is released from the granules of mast cells and basophils.

There are two major classes of agranulocytes in normal peripheral blood. These are **monocytes** (I) (2-10% of circulating leucocytes) and lymphocytes (20-45% of circulating leucocytes). Monocytes are highly mobile phagocytic cells. They are part of a complex system of bone marrow-derived phagocytic cells in the body called the mononuclear phagocyte system (MPS). In addition to blood monocytes, the MPS includes macrophages (abundant in the skin, lungs, and immune organs), microglial cells in the CNS, Kupffer cells in the liver, and osteoclasts.

Lymphocytes play a key role in all immune responses. In contrast to neutrophils and macrophages, they are activated by specific agents (antigens). Although morphologically similar, the lymphocytes are a heterogeneous collection of functionally distinct cells classified as B and T lymphocytes. **B lymphocytes** (E) are important for humoral immunity. When stimulated by antigen presented by macrophages, they differentiate into immunoglobulin-secreting **plasma cells** (K). T lymphocytes govern cell-mediated immune responses and include three subtypes: helper T lymphocytes, suppressor T lymphocytes, and cytotoxic T lymphocytes. **Helper T lymphocytes** (F) up-regulate the immune response by secreting mitogenic lymphokines such as the interleukins. **Suppressor T lymphocytes** (G) down-regulate the immune response. **Cytotoxic (killer) T lymphocytes** (H) bind to foreign cell surface antigens and kill them by punching holes in their plasma membranes by insertion of perforins.

Platelets (J) are circulating fragments derived from **megakaryocytes** (M) found in the bone marrow. They have a cell surface receptor called integrin which recognizes and binds to fibronectin-fibrin in blot clotting.

Never let monkeys eat Bananas
Neutrophils, lymphocyte, monocytes, eosinophils, Basophils

serum + fibrinogen = plasma

Answers and Tutorial on Items 59-68

The answers are: **59-A; 60-C; 61-B; 62-D; 63-A; 64-A; 65-D; 66-D; 67-G; 68-H**. **Blood** is a tissue consisting of various types of cells suspended in plasma. It functions as a vehicle for transport of gases, nutrients, metabolic waste products, hormones, and cells throughout the body. Blood treated with anticoagulants can be separated into plasma and blood cells by centrifugation. If blood is allowed to clot and then centrifuged, the cell-depleted fluid devoid of fibrinogen is called serum. In the normal adult, the normal volume of plasma is about 3.5L. It contains many substances such as electrolytes to maintain osmolality and pH of the blood, as well as proteins that function as carrier molecules or mediators of immune response.

Albumin (A) is the most abundant protein in plasma. It is synthesized in the liver. Because of its size (MW = 65,000), albumin does not permeate closed capillary endothelium and thus provides a colloidal osmotic pressure that regulates diffusion of H_2O from interstitial tissues into the vasculature. When the concentration of albumin is severely decreased, H_2O leaves the capillaries and accumulates in the interstitial tissue compartment. This fluid accumulation in the interstitial spaces is called edema. If it accumulates in the peritoneal cavity, it is called ascites.

In addition to albumin, other proteins are present in plasma. They can be classified as carrier proteins or proteins involved in immune responses. Specific carrier proteins include: **transferrin** (C) that transports iron; **apolipoprotein** (D) that transport triglycerides, cholesterol, and phospholipids; and **haptoglobin** (H) that scavenges **hemoglobin** (F) from lysed RBCs for delivery to the liver. The proteins involved in immune functions include **immunoglobulins** (E) and **complement** (B). Immunoglobulins are secreted into the blood stream by plasma cells which are derived from stimulated lymphocytes. Complement is a system of proteins that mediate three effects. First, some components of complement may act as opsonins. Second, others are chemotaxins that attract neutrophils. Third, these proteins mediate direct osmotic lysis of pathogenic cells. **Bilirubin** (G) is a hemoglobin breakdown product that is normally eliminated in bile.

Answers and Tutorial on Items 69-74

The answers are: **69-D; 70-H; 71-I; 72-C; 73-H; 74-B**. The heart receives venous blood from the body and lungs and propels that blood into the pulmonary and systemic circulations. This process is called the cardiac cycle and it involves two events: (1) **diastole**, relaxation of the muscular walls of the heart chambers, followed by (2) **systole**, a contraction of the walls of the heart. The relationships between the pressure changes that occur and mechanical events in the heart are represented by **Figure 4.7**. Curve A represents the **atrial pressure curve**; B is the **ventricular pressure curve**; C is the **aortic pressure curve**. Point D is the point in the cycle when the **AV valves close** while point E is when the **AV valves open**. Point F is the point in the cycle when the aortic valve closes while point G is when the **aortic valve opens**. Point H is termed the **dicrotic notch**. The portion of the graph labeled I represents systole while the portion labeled J represents **diastole**. Points K, L and M are points on the atrial pressure curve.

The two atria contract almost simultaneously and the resulting increase in atrial pressure (A) is termed the a wave (K). The ventricular pressure at the end of atrial contraction is the ventricular end-diastolic pressure, which, for the left ventricle is normally less than 12 mm Hg.

Just after the onset of the **QRS complex**, the pressure in the ventricles increases due to the onset of ventricular contraction (systole). Rising ventricular pressure now exceeds atrial pressure closing the AV valves. Closure of the AV valves is the major factor in producing the first heart sound (S_1). The backflow of blood even causes the bicuspid valve to bulge into the atrium, producing a continued increase in atrial pressure (c wave of the atrial pressure curve—L). Pressure within the ventricle continues to increase (period of isovolumic contraction) until it exceeds the pressure in the aorta, opening of the aortic (and pulmonary) semilunar valves. Now blood rushes into the aorta and pulmonary trunk. The drop in pressure against the bicuspid valves causes a sudden drop in the atrial pressure. The pressure within the atria increases as blood from the venae cavae and pulmonary veins flows in. At the point where the AV valves open (E), atrial pressure again deceases as blood flows into the ventricles.

With the onset of the QRS complex and ventricular contraction (systole), pressure within the ventricles rises rapidly and blood pushes against the underside of the semilunar valves.

Opening of the semilunar valves (G) causes an increase in the aortic pressure but left ventricular pressure continues to rise due to the powerful contraction of the ventricular musculature. As blood leaves the ventricle, the pressure begins to decrease and the onset of diastole causes a rapid decline in ventricular pressure. When ventricular pressure falls below that of the atrium, the bicuspid valve opens and allows blood to enter the ventricle, starting another cardiac cycle. With the decrease in ventricular pressure the aortic valve closes (creating the second heart sound). Additionally, there is a minor back-flow of blood into the cusps of the aortic valve, which raises the aortic pressure momentarily. This sudden increase in pressure is referred to as the dicrotic notch.

Answers and Tutorial on Items 75-76

The answers are: **75-A; 76-A**. **Stroke volume** is the volume of blood that is ejected with each beat of the heart. Both ventricles must pump the same volume of blood during any significant time interval. Normally, the stroke volume of each ventricle averages 70 mL of blood, but the stroke volume varies with changes in ventricular contractility, arterial pressure (afterload), and end-diastolic volume. Cardiac output equals stroke volume times heart rate. The normal cardiac output of an average man is 5.5 L/minute and the average heart rate is 70 beats/minute. Thus, the stroke volume is 5.5 L/minute/70 beats/minute = 78.5 mL.

One of the major factors that controls the force of cardiac contraction is the initial length, or preload, of the muscle fibers. An increase in end-diastolic volume lengthens the cardiac fibers, which, up to an optimum, exposes more of the myosin heads (cross bridge sites) to actin. The additional cross bridges allow the heart to generate more force with each contraction. Thus, an increase in preload produces a stronger contraction and a greater volume of blood is pumped by the heart. These effects result in a higher pressure being generated by the myocardium.

Increased contractility (**positive inotropism**) results in a stronger contraction so that the ventricles are able to eject more blood from the same diastolic volume, and stroke volume increases. An increased contractility occurs with sympathetic stimulation to the heart (eg, during exercise).

Decreased contractility (**negative inotropism**) occurs in heart failure and results in a decreased stroke volume. In this condition, the ventricle increases in size because of the rise in residual ventricular volume. The increased ventricular volume raises stroke volume toward normal through the Frank-Starling mechanism. Cardiac output is maintained by increasing the heart rate.

In **severe ventricular failure**, both cardiac output and stroke volume are decreased and the ventricular diastolic pressure is high. The increased ventricular diastolic pressure causes high venous pressure, which is reflected back to the capillaries and produces leakage of fluid into the tissues (edema).

In **left heart failure**, fluid accumulates in the lungs (pulmonary edema), causing difficulty in breathing (dyspnea) and the inability to breathe when lying down (orthopnea). During right heart failure, edema occurs in the feet and ankles (dependent edema) since the high venous pressures occur in the systemic veins.

Arterial pressure during systole affects the ejection of blood from the ventricles and is termed the ventricular afterload. The higher the arterial pressure, the greater the afterload that the ventricle must overcome. An increase in arterial pressure causes a reduction in the stroke volume and a decrease in the velocity of ejection from the ventricle.

Ventricular end-diastolic volume affects the stroke volume because of the Frank-Starling relationship. The greater the ventricular end-diastolic volume, the stronger the contraction and the larger the stroke volume. The ventricular end-diastolic volume increases if the pressure in the atria or the central veins increases because the higher pressure can stretch the ventricular walls. The ventricular end-diastolic volume also increases if the distensibility of the ventricles increases or if the heart rate slows, which allows more time for the blood to enter the ventricles.

Answer and Tutorial on Item 77

The answer is: **77-B**. All preganglionic sympathetic fibers are **cholinergic**, while sympathetic postganglionic fibers may be either **adrenergic** or cholinergic. Sympathetic postganglionic cholinergic fibers innervate some exocrine glands and sweat glands and are the vasodilator fibers in skeletal muscles of certain species. The receptors of the effector cells are muscarinic.

There are two major types of adrenergic receptor of sympathetic mediators. adrenergic receptors are stimulated most strongly by **epinephrine** and **norepinephrine** and cause vasoconstriction. There are two types of **α-adrenergic receptors**: α_1 is located on the myocyte and α_2 is located on blood vessels. **β-receptors** are of two types β_1 and β_2, both of which are most strongly stimulated by isoproterenol and least stimulated by norepinephrine. **The β_1 receptors** are located in the myocardium (but not the coronary arteries), and activation of these receptors results in positive inotropic and chronotropic responses (increase rate and force of contraction). **The β_2 receptors** are located in other body tissues, and stimulation of these receptors leads to inhibition (eg, bronchodilation or vasodilation). Pharmacologic agents are available that can stimulate or block the β_1 or β_2 receptors individually.

The administration of a **β-adrenergic blocking drug** would reduce heart rate as well as cardiac contractility so that cardiac output would be significantly reduced. Vagal stimulation can cause marked cardiac slowing, but ventricular end-diastolic volume can increase, so that stroke volume increases sufficiently to compensate for the reduced heart rate. Stimulation of the sympathetic system will cause a sequence of changes including a rise in heart rate, arterial pressure and total peripheral resistance.

An **α-adrenergic agonist** increases peripheral resistance, which raises arterial blood pressure. This results in baroreceptor stimulation, causing a reflex slowing of the heart rate. An -adrenergic blocking drug has the opposite effect. Cholinergic blocking agents and β-adrenergic agonists increase heart rate. A β-adrenergic blocking agent would reduce heart rate and contractility, resulting in a decreased cardiac output and a reduced arterial pressure.

All adrenergic agonists would cause an increase in heart rate as a direct effect on the SA node, isoproterenol having the greatest effect and norepinephrine the least. A drug such as **epinephrine**, which has both α- and β-adrenergic properties and excites both receptors about equally, can increase contractility and peripheral resistance so that a large increase in arterial pressure occurs, which can then affect the baroreceptors and result in a reflex slowing of cardiac rate. **Norepinephrine** excites mainly a receptors but has a slight effect on β receptors as well.

Answers and Tutorial on Items 78-80

The answers are: **78-D; 79-B; 80-C. Tetralogy of Fallot** is caused by a congenital defect in heart development leading to four major anatomical defects; (1) pulmonary artery stenosis; (2) ventricular septal defect (VSD); (3) over-riding aorta (ie, the aorta straddles the ventricular septal defect; and (4) right ventricular hypertrophy. In many instances, the ductus arteriosus, which serves as a by-pass shunt for the pulmonary circulation in utero, remains patent. The cyanosis and dyspnea seen in these patients is due to a by-pass of the pulmonary circulation. Right ventricular hypertrophy is due to significant increases in right ventricular blood pressure that would be detected with catheterization.

Tetralogy of Fallot is most successfully treated by a complex surgical procedure that closes the VSD, opens the pulmonary artery, closes the patent ductus arteriosus if necessary, and reconstructs the outflow tracts of the ventricles assuring adequate blood supply to both the pulmonary and systemic circuits. This surgical procedure can increase the otherwise limited life expectancy of 3-4 years to nearly normal.

Answer and Tutorial on Item 81

The answer is: **81-E. Airway resistance** is responsible for most of the resistance during breathing. The airway resistance changes dramatically with changes in airway diameter. A disease state that decreases airway diameter to half its healthy equivalent would result in a dramatic increase in airway resistance, perhaps a 16-fold increase. In **chronic obstructive pulmonary disease** (COPD), the airway diameter can be reduced by bronchoconstriction and mucus accumulation. Examples of COPD include chronic bronchitis, cystic fibrosis, asthma, and emphysema. **Respiratory syncytial virus** causes acute pulmonary disease, especially in children, but is not an example of a COPD.

The **tone of smooth muscle** that surrounds the airways affects their diameter and therefore resistance. Smooth muscle reacts to both parasympathetic and sympathetic nervous activity. Stimulation of the parasympathetic fibers releases acetylcholine which causes smooth muscle contraction (thus constricting the airways); while sympathetic activation releases norepinephrine which relaxes smooth muscle causing dilation of the airway. Epinephrine and β_2 adrenergic agonists are powerful bronchodilators and are useful for treatment of asthma. In addition, there are large numbers of enteroendocrine cells in the respiratory system whose secretions alter airway diameter. Substance P is a potent bronchoconstrictor and stimulator of mucus secretion. Vasoactive intestinal peptide has the opposite effect.

Answers and Tutorial on Items 82-87

The answers are: **82-H; 83-B; 84-A; 85-D; 86-G; 87-E**. The volumes and capacities of the human lung vary in men and women, the former being about 20% greater than the latter. The numbers below are those for a normal healthy adult male of 70 kg. They also vary considerably with body size, extent of athletic training, and even altitude at which the individual lives. For example, people who live in mountainous regions have larger lungs and larger volumes and capacities than comparable people living at low altitudes. The figures listed below are for a normal adult living at low altitude. **The tidal volume** (B) is the amount of air inhaled or exhaled during each resting breath. It is about 400 mL in women and 500 mL in men. The **total inspiratory capacity** (E) of the lungs is 3500 mL and includes tidal volume of 500 mL and **inspiratory reserve volume** (A) of 3000 mL. The **expiratory reserve volume** (C) is the amount of air that can be forcibly expelled at the end of a normal expiration. It usually presents about 1000 mL. After the most forceful expiration possible, 1200 mL of air remains in the lungs as **residual volume** (D). The **vital capacity** (4600 mL) (F) is the sum of the inspiratory residual volume, the tidal volume, and the expiratory reserve volume. The **functional residual capacity** (G) is the amount of air left in the lungs after a normal expiration. It equals the sum of expiratory reserve volume and residual volume and amounts to about 2300 mL. The **total lung capacity** (H) is the sum of the vital capacity and the residual volume. It represents the total volume of the lungs at maximal inspiration. It amounts to about 5800 mL.

The minute respiratory volume is the tidal volume multiplied by the respiratory rate. In a resting adult, the normal tidal volume is 500 mL and the respiratory rate is about 12 breaths/minute. Thus, the minute respiratory volume is about 6000 mL/minute.

Answers and Tutorial on Items 88-94

The answers are: **88-B; 89-C; 90-A; 91-D; 92-C; 93-B; 94-G**. The glandular secretions of the GI tract are elicited by the actions of specific regulator substances (**secretagogues**) on the secretory cells. These secretagogues can be classified as neurocrine, endocrine, or paracrine. Neurocrine secretagogues are released from neurons that innervate the secretory target cells. Endocrine secretagogues (hormones) are blood borne substances produced by cells located at a distance from their target cell. Paracrine substances are released locally and reach their target cell by diffusion. In general, these secretagogues modulate secretory activity via one of two second messenger systems: (1) increases in adenylate cyclase/cAMP levels or (2) increases in inositol triphosphate (IP3)/intracellular Ca^{2+}. Secretagogues that act via cAMP can potentiate the effects of those that use Ca^{2+} as second messengers and vice versa.

Six classes of secretagogues modulate the secretory activity of pancreatic acinar cells. These can be grouped by the second messenger systems that mediate their effects: (1) regulators of intracellular Ca^{2+} include cholinergic agents, **cholecystokinin** (C), **bombesin** (J), and **substance P** (M); and (2) regulators of cAMP levels include **secretin** (D) and **vasoactive intestinal peptide** (VIP) (K).

Several secretagogues are released by the mucosa of the pyloric stomach and duodenum, notably **serotonin** (A), cholecystokinin, and **gastrin** (B). These stimulate smooth muscle contraction. Serotonin (A) is made by cells scattered throughout the GI mucosa. It is a derivative of the amino acid tryptophane and stimulates the contraction of mucosal smooth muscle cells in the vicinity of its site of release. **Motilin** (G) is a polypeptide, produced by mucosal cells in the duodenum, which acts as a strong stimulator of smooth muscle contraction in the wall of the stomach.

Gastrin (B) is a polypeptide hormone that has multiple effects including stimulation of gastric parietal cells to release HCl and stimulating smooth muscle of the lower esophageal sphincter to contract. The release of gastrin is itself controlled by a variety of factors including, indirectly, vagal nerve activity which increases release of the hormone bombesin (J) which in turn stimulates parietal cells and inhibits the release of **somatostatin** (F). Secretion of **cholecystokinin** (C) is stimulated both by the vagus nerve and by the presence of fatty foodstuffs entering the lumen of the small intestine. One of the main effects of cholecystokinin is to stimulate contraction of the smooth muscle in the wall of the gallbladder, causing bile to be released via the common bile duct into the lumen of the duodenum. Cholecystokinin (previously also called pancreozymin because of this effect) also causes the pancreatic ducts to release copious amounts of a watery mix containing bicarbonate, which helps to neutralize the acidity of chyme entering the duodenum from the stomach.

Three hormones, **secretin** (D), **neurotensin** (E), and vasoactive intestinal peptide (VIP) (K) are produced in the brain and in the GI tract. Secretin and VIP cause smooth muscle relaxation. In addition, secretin stimulates pancreatic acinar cells to release a mixture of hydrolytic enzymes. Neurotensin (E) is released at several places in the brain and in the small intestine but its effects on the digestive system are not well understood. Somatostatin (F) is secreted by cells in the pyloric stomach and duodenum. It inhibits gastrin release.

Insulin (H) and **glucagon** (I) are both polypeptides produced in the pancreatic islets of Langerhans. They work antagonistically to regulate the storage and release of glucose by the liver. **Melatonin** (L), produced in the pineal, is a derivative of serotonin. It has no known direct effect on the digestive system.

ANSWERS AND TUTORIAL ON ITEMS 95-101

The answers are: **95-C; 96-J; 97-I; 98-A; 99-E; 100-B; 101-H.** Many of the activities of the digestive system depend on specific enzymes, including ones that break down food and/or aid in its processing. The salivary amylase, **ptyalin** (A), begins the digestion of starches in the oral cavity, releasing sugars that help trigger the cephalic phase of gastrointestinal secretion and movement. **Pepsinogen** (B), the inactive precursor of the protease pepsin, is secreted by the chief cells of the main gastric glands. Pepsin requires a low pH (such as found in the stomach) to be active. **Enterokinase** (C) is an enzyme produced by the absorptive cells lining the small intestine (enterocytes) that cleaves trypsinogen to trypsin, thus activating it. **Catalase** (D), an enzyme found in peroxisomes, converts hydrogen peroxide to water and oxygen.

The enzymes released by pancreatic acinar cells include precursors of a number of hydrolases that are activated and function to digest foodstuffs in the lumen of the small intestine. Pancreatic enzymes include the following: **chymotrypsinogen** (E) which is activated to chymotrypsin, a protease, when cleaved by trypsin; **deoxyribonuclease** (F) and **ribonuclease** (G) which hydrolyse DNA and RNA respectively into smaller fragments that are then absorbed; carboxypeptidases (H) which cleave amino acids from the carboxy-terminus of proteins and polypeptides; and, **lipases** (J) which breakdown fatty components of food provided the fats are first emulsified (broken down into smaller particles and maintained in suspension) by components of bile.

In other organs of the GI tract, luminal contents are concentrated by the passive movement of water across the epithelium due to the active transport of ions across the basal plasma membrane of these epithelial cells. Active transport utilizes Na^+-K^+-ATPase (I) which hydrolyses ATP to transport potassium into a cell and sodium out against their respective concentration gradient. In the epithelial cells that line the lumen of the gallbladder, this water transfer concentrates bile; and, in the ducts of the salivary glands (H), concentrates saliva.

ANSWER AND TUTORIAL ON ITEMS 102

The answer is: **102-A**. Filtration of blood across the glomerular basement membrane depends on the difference between glomerular capillary hydrostatic pressure (45 mm Hg) and the sum of Bowman's capsule hydrostatic pressure (10 mm Hg) and the plasma protein osmotic pressure (28 mm Hg). Thus, the net pressure supporting glomerular filtration is 7 mm Hg. Due to the extreme porosity of the fenestrated glomerular capillaries and the gaps between the foot processes of podocytes, approximately 180 L/day of glomerular filtrate is produced. The **glomerular filtration rate** (GFR) can easily be calculated as 125 mL/minutes. This rate is relatively invariant, even with large changes in blood pressure. A substantial increase in blood pressure will result in a concomitant decrease in blood flow through the afferent arteriole due to smooth muscle contraction. Also, the macula densa in the distal convoluted tubule detects changes in rate of production of glomerular filtrate and feeds back on the afferent arteriole to autoregulate GFR.

Stimulation of sympathetic nerve fibers to the kidney causes **vasoconstriction** in the afferent arteriole, leading to a decrease in the GFR. Factors that vasoconstrict efferent arterioles will increase the GFR. Conversely, a decrease in vascular tone will result in an increase in GFR. Catecholamines are also potent vasoconstrictors of the afferent arterioles and will therefore cause a significant decrease in GFR.

Answers and Tutorial on Items 103-104

The answers are: **103-D; 104-E**. **Total body H_2O** (TBW) represents about 50% of the total body weight, with women having a lower percentage for TBW due to the fact that they have more adipose tissue. Of this TBW, about 33% is in extracellular fluid and 67% is in intracellular fluid. Thus, the intracellular fluid is the largest single component of the total body H_2O. Extracellular fluid makes up about 33% of the TBW and includes four different sub-components: plasma, interstitial fluid (the fluid between cells and lymph), the fluid in bone and connective tissue, and transcellular fluid. **Plasma** is the fluid component of blood. It represents about 25% of the extracellular fluid, with the rest being interstitial fluid, bone and connective tissue fluid, and transcellular fluid. Transcellular fluid is defined as the fluid contained within lumina lined by epithelium and includes cerebrospinal fluid, aqueous humor, endolymph, sweat, milk, serous fluids, digestive secretions, and bile.

Plasma and interstitial fluid have similar ionic composition. The most abundant cation of plasma and interstitial fluid is Na^+ with a concentration of 143 mOsm/liter in plasma and 140 mOsm/liter in interstitial fluid but only 14 mOsm/liter in intracellular fluid. The K^+ concentration of plasma and interstitial fluid is relatively low at 4.2 mOsm/liter for plasma and 4.0 mOsm/liter for interstitial fluid. Conversely, intracellular fluid has a high K^+ concentration at 140 mOsm/liter. Plasma and interstitial fluid have little Ca^{2+} while intracellular fluid has essentially none. The predominant anion of plasma and interstitial fluid is Cl^- at 108 mOsm/liter. The most obvious difference between plasma and interstitial fluid is the protein concentration, a fact that leads to a 20 mm Hg excess total osmotic pressure in plasma compared to interstitial fluid. Plasma has 1.2 mOsm/liter protein while interstitial fluid has only 0.2 mOsm/liter. The Na^+, Cl^-, glucose, and urea concentrations in plasma and interstitial fluid are essentially alike.

Answers and Tutorial on Items 105-111

The answers are: **105-E; 106-A; 107-D; 108-E; 109-B; 110-C; 111-B**. This patient suffers from **Cushing's syndrome**. There are three basic pathologic processes that lead to Cushing's syndrome: (1) pituitary tumors producing excessive ACTH; (2) hypothalamic insensitivity to cortisol; and (3) adrenal cortical tumors. This patient was discovered to have a large adrenal cortical carcinoma.

Pituitary tumors or hypothalamic disorders leading to cortisol insensitivity could both result in high levels of ACTH secretion which would in turn elevate all of the adrenal cortical steroids. In this patient, the cortical tumor results in high levels of cortisol secretion which in turn feeds back on the hypothalamus, inhibiting release of CRF and secondarily inhibiting pituitary release of ACTH. This patient would have elevated levels of all adrenal cortical steroids including testosterone, androstenedione, DHEAS, cortisol and corticosterone but little or no ACTH.

The **hirsutism** and **amenorrhea** are caused by excessive secretion of androgens including testosterone. The hypertension is caused by excessive secretion of aldosterone. Aldosterone causes an increase in renal retention of Na^+ which has an indirect effect on increasing blood volume and therefore blood pressure. Under normal physiologic circumstances, when blood pressure falls, the juxtaglomerular apparatus releases renin. This proteolytic enzyme causes the cleavage of angiotensinogen to angiotensin I which is subsequently cleaved to angiotensin II, a peptide that stimulates release of aldosterone from the adrenal cortex. Excessive aldosterone will also elevate blood Na^+ as a result of increased renal retention of Na^+ and a concomitant decreased K^+ in the blood.

Answers and Tutorial on Items 112-113

The answers are: **112-D; 113-B**. The man suffers from damage to his **parathyroid glands** due to the laceration. The chief cells of the parathyroid gland secrete **parathyroid hormone** (PTH), a 9500 MW, 84 amino acid polypeptide essential for mobilization of bound Ca^{2+} in the body.

The fundamental physiologic effect of PTH is to increase plasma Ca^{2+} and decrease plasma phosphate. These actions are mediated via the cAMP second messenger system. Soon after administration of PTH, the cAMP levels in target cells in the bone, kidney and gut increase. This increase in cAMP then causes secretion of enzymes by osteoclasts for bone resorption, resulting in elevated blood Ca^{2+} levels within minutes.

PTH effects bone metabolism by several processes. First, it stimulates Ca^{2+} mobilization by osteocytes, the mature cells of bones. This process transfers free Ca^{2+} from bone canalicular fluid to the blood. Second, it stimulates bone degradation by osteoclasts to liberate bound Ca^{2+} and phosphate. Finally, chronic PTH stimulates osteoclasts to secrete hydrochloric acid and lytic enzymes which together degrade larger areas of bone. With chronic pathologic over production of PTH, gross osteoporosis can develop.

PTH alters renal function by increasing Ca^{2+} uptake in the ascending loops of Henle, distal convoluted tubules, and the collecting tubules. In addition, PTH diminishes phosphate ion uptake in the proximal convoluted tubules, leading to a sudden increase in urinary excretion of phosphate. PTH also increases the rate of resorption of NH_4^+ and H^+.

PTH increases intestinal absorption of Ca^{2+} and phosphate indirectly by increasing renal synthesis of 1,25-dihydroxy-cholecalciferol from vitamin D. This metabolite of vitamin D is required for PTH to be effective. It may work by increasing cell membrane Ca^{2+} transport.

Answer and Tutorial on Item 114

The answer is: **114-C**. This man suffers from **pheochromocytoma**, a chromaffin cell tumor in the adrenal medulla. Hypersecretion of catecholamines results in hypertension, severe headache, sweating, heart palpitations, angina, and anxiety. If the patient were given phentolamine, an adrenergic blocker, a marked decrease in blood pressure would be noted. A β-adrenergic antagonist such as propranolol would be used to reduce tachycardia. In most patients, the tumors secrete predominantly norepinephrine.

About 80% of the catecholamines released from the adrenal medulla by sympathetic stimulation is **epinephrine**, the remaining 20% being **norepinephrine**. Epinephrine and norepinephrine exert their effects by binding to plasma membrane receptors classified as either α or β. Epinephrine has a stronger stimulatory effect on β-adrenergic receptors. Norepinephrine reacts predominantly with α-adrenergic receptors. Both catecholamines increase glucose production. They stimulate hepatic glycogenolysis by way of the Ca^{2+}-activated glycogen phosphorylase and concurrently depress glycogen synthetase activity. They also stimulate gluconeogenesis, leading to release of glucose from the liver. In addition, they increase muscle glycogenolysis which increases plasma lactate levels. Furthermore, epinephrine activates hormone-sensitive lipase, thereby increasing plasma free fatty acids. Mobilized free fatty acids are then used to generate ketone bodies used as energy substrates in muscle, liver and renal cortex. These actions help restore plasma glucose levels to be used for energy in the central nervous system.

Catecholamines exert a number of divergent systemic effects by binding to β-adrenergic receptors. For example, epinephrine has a stronger stimulatory effect on β-adrenergic receptors, and thus has a greater stimulatory effect on heart rate. Norepinephrine causes strong constriction of most blood vessels. Epinephrine has a weaker effect on the blood vessels of muscle. Epinephrine also has a much more dramatic effect on glucose metabolism than norepinephrine.

Answers and Tutorial on Items 115-122

The answers are: **115-I; 116-H; 117-F; 118-I; 119-C; 120-G; 121-B; 122-J**. **Follicle-stimulating hormone** (FSH) (A) is a 30,000 MW glycoprotein hormone secreted by gonadotropes of the adenohypophysis. In women, FSH levels rise during the preovulatory phase of follicular growth in the ovary. It is primarily responsible for the proliferation of granulosa cells in the developing ovarian follicles. Rising plasma estradiol levels and follicular inhibin suppress FSH secretion by negative feedback. In men, FSH binds to receptors on Sertoli cells and its secretion is required, along with testosterone, to maintain normal spermatogenesis. Sertoli cells also secrete **inhibin** (G), another glycoprotein hormone which has negative feedback effects on FSH secretion by the adenohypophysis [and perhaps a weaker effect on **gonadotrophin-releasing hormone** (J) (GnRH) secretion by the hypothalamus].

Luteinizing hormone (LH) (B) is a 30,000 MW glycoprotein hormone secreted by gonadotropes of the adenohypophysis. In women, it is required for growth of the preovulatory follicles. A transient spike in LH is required for the final phases of follicular maturation and rupture that occurs at ovulation. In men, LH stimulates Leydig cells to secrete testosterone. In turn, testosterone directly decreases GnRH secretion from the hypothalamus, consequently resulting in a depression of LH secretion by gonadotropes. There is also a weak direct inhibition of testosterone on LH secretion by gonadotropes.

Human chorionic gonadotropin (hCG) (C) is a 39,000 MW glycoprotein with considerable homology to LH. It is secreted by the syncytiotrophoblast of the placenta. The secretion of hCG is high enough soon after implantation that it can be used as a sensitive pregnancy test. During the first 12 weeks of gestation, hCG levels rise rapidly and then fall off to a much lower level over the next 8 weeks. It stimulates secretion of progesterone and estrogen from the corpus luteum that forms from the mature follicle after ovulation. It also stimulates testosterone secretion by the testes in a male fetus, thus leading to development of male internal and external genitalia.

Human chorionic somatomammotropin (hCS) (D) is 38,000 MW protein which serves as a growth factor. It is first detectable at about the fifth week of pregnancy. As the placenta grows, the secretion of hCS increases. Although it is lactogenic in laboratory animals, administration to human subjects appears to have little direct effect on lactation. It has some structural homology to growth hormone and appears to have weak growth hormone-like activity. It stimulates lipolysis and depresses maternal insulin sensitivity. This raises glucose for fetal growth and development.

Progesterone (E) is a sex steroid secreted by the ovary and placenta. The ovarian progesterone, secreted in large quantities after ovulation by the corpus luteum, stimulates secretion of glands in the uterus and uterine tubes. These secretions are thought to be trophic substances to support the early development of the conceptus. Progesterone also stimulates mammary gland development by causing growth of secretory units.

β-estradiol (F) and the related estrogens, estrone and estriol, are sex steroids secreted by the ovary. They stimulate glandular development in the endometrium and stimulate ciliary beating in the uterine tubes. Estrogens also cause extensive development of the endometrial stroma and extensive fat deposition and growth of the ducts of the mammary glands. Estrogens also cause rapid growth of the skeleton at puberty to result in the female dimorphisms of the skeleton, eg, broader pelvis, and deposition of fat in the thighs and buttocks.

Inhibin (G) is a glycoprotein hormone secreted by luteal cells in the corpus luteum or Sertoli cells in the testis. It has a negative inhibitory feedback effect on the pituitary gland, decreasing FSH secretion by the adenohypophysis, causing corpus luteum involution late in the menstrual cycle, and decreasing spermatogenesis.

Prolactin (H) is a single polypeptide with 198 amino acids. It is secreted by acidophilic lactotropes of the adenohypophysis. The prolactin levels rise linearly during early pregnancy, reaching an 8-10 fold increase at birth. Soon after birth, prolactin secretion gradually declines to a baseline value with intermittent bursts of secretion surrounding nursing events. Prolactin (along with estrogen and progesterone) is required for development of the secretory units of the breasts. Prolactin also is required for the secretory activity of breasts during lactation. The hypothalamus inhibits secretion of prolactin by prolactin inhibitory hormone (PIH) (dopamine) and stimulates prolactin secretion by prolactin-releasing factor (PRF). A decrease in circulating prolactin will trigger LH release and initiate cycling.

Oxytocin (I) is a nonapeptide secreted by the neurohypophysis. Oxytocin secretion during the later stages of labor stimulates massive uterine contractions. In addition, the stimulus of suckling at the nipple causes release of oxytocin from the neurohypophysis, leading quickly to myoepithelial cell contraction around milk-laden alveoli and the copious ejection of milk from the breasts.

Gonadotrophin releasing hormone (GnRH) (J) is a decapeptide secreted in a pulsatile fashion from the hypothalamus. It is carried down the hypothalamic-hypophyseal portal system to the adenohypophysis where it stimulates gonadotropes to release LH and FSH.

Notes

CHAPTER 5

Biochemistry and Molecular Biology

DIRECTIONS (Items 1-107): For each of the numbered items that proceed, you must select the single best answer from among the lettered options listed.

Some of the numbered items will pose a question or incomplete sentence that is followed by a list of 4-5 lettered options. In all cases, select the ONE lettered option that best answers the question or completes the sentence given.

Some of the numbered items are preceded by 5-24 lettered options. In these sets, the lettered options will be preceded by a single instruction asking you to match one of the lettered options to each numbered item most closely associated with it. In all matching sets, you may use any of the lettered options once, more than once or not at all, but you should still only select ONE lettered option per numbered item.

If you wish to simulate actual USMLE testing conditions, you should aim to complete all the items in this chapter in ONE hour and 50 minutes.

Do NOT look at the answers and tutorials until you have completed all of the items in this chapter.

Good luck!

Items 1-5

Examine the labeled titration curve for glutamic acid in **Figure 5.1** below and then choose the best answers for the items below the titration curve.

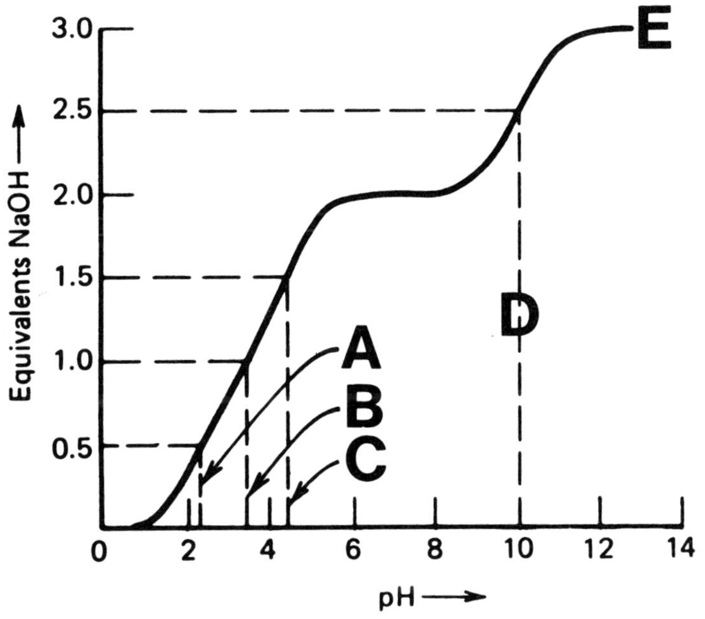

Figure 5.1

1. At which point on the curve would the amino acid be in the zwitterionic form?

2. At which point on the curve would addition of more base have no effect on the net charge of the molecule?

3. At which point on the curve would the molecule have a net charge of +1 and addition of further base would cause ionization of the α-COOH?

4. At which point on the curve would the molecule have a net charge of -1?

5. At which point on the curve would polyglutamic acid have no net electrophoretic mobility?

Items 6-8

The rate of many enzymatic reactions such as the one shown below

$$E + S \rightleftharpoons ES \rightleftharpoons E + P$$

can be described by the Michaelis-Menten equation

$$v_0 = \frac{V_m[S]}{K_m + [S]}$$

6. When Michaelis-Menten kinetics apply, the shape of the reaction velocity as a function of substrate concentration curve is

   (A) linear with negative slope
   (B) linear with positive slope
   (C) sigmoidal
   (D) parabolic
   (E) hyperbolic

7. Competitive inhibitors have which effect on the Lineweaver-Burk plot?

   (A) increasing inhibitor concentration does not change slope of curve
   (B) increasing inhibitor concentration increases K_m
   (C) increasing inhibitor concentration changes V_m
   (D) increasing inhibitor concentration decreases the slope of curve
   (E) all curves intersect that the same place on the X-axis

8. Noncompetitive inhibitors have which effect on the Lineweaver-Burk plot?

   (A) increasing inhibitor concentration does not change slope of curve
   (B) increasing inhibitor concentration increases K_m where $k_I = k_I$
   (C) increasing inhibitor concentration does not change V_m
   (D) increasing inhibitor concentration decreases the slope of curve
   (E) all curves intersect the same place to the left of the Y-axis

Items 9-14

For each description of the basic building blocks of proteins, select the most appropriate chemical compound.

(A) Glycine
(B) Arginine
(C) Proline
(D) Valine
(E) Threonine
(F) Serine
(G) Glutamic acid
(H) Desmosine
(I) Lysine
(J) Tyrosine
(K) Phenylalanine

9. This abundant neutral amino acid is a major constituent of collagen. It is the simplest amino acid with a hydrogen atom for an R group.

10. This uncommon amino acid is an important constituent of cross-links in elastin.

11. This common basic amino acid is involved in formation of Schiff bases in collagen cross-linking.

12. This common acidic amino acid is abundant in many proteins and is an important intermediate for the synthesis of the nonessential amino acids proline and arginine.

13. This aromatic amino acid is an important precursor for melanin. It can also be iodinated to form thyroxine.

14. This imino acid is abundant in collagen.

Item 15

15. The ionization of acetic acid is described by the following simple equation

$$HA \rightleftharpoons H^+ + A^-$$

When the pH of a solution of acetic acid is equal to the pK, the ratio of the anion concentration to the following un-ionized acid concentration $\frac{[A^-]}{[HA]}$ is

(A) 0
(B) 1.0
(C) 1.5
(D) 2.0
(E) 2.5

Item 16

16. The most abundant immunoglobulin in plasma is

(A) IgA
(B) IgD
(C) IgE
(D) IgG
(E) IgM

Item 17

17. Which statement best characterizes changes in serum LDH following myocardial infarction?

(A) LDH_1 becomes less than LDH_2
(B) LDH_1 becomes greater than LDH_2
(C) LDH_1 remains unchanged
(D) LDH_5 decreases
(E) LDH profiles remain unchanged

Items 18-21

A 7-year-old woman is pallid and short with fat deposits in her face. She has a markedly distended abdomen due to hepatomegaly. Laboratory tests reveal hypoglycemia after fasting, hyperlipidemia, lactic acidemia, hyperuricemia and gout-like tenderness and swelling in the joints of the extremities.

18. The most likely diagnosis of this disease is

(A) Sandhoff disease
(B) von Gierke's disease
(C) cystic fibrosis
(D) Pompe's disease
(E) Duchenne muscular dystrophy

19. The cause of the elevated lactic acid levels in blood is

(A) inefficient utilization of lactate for glucose synthesis
(B) abnormal conversion of lactate to pyruvate
(C) accelerated glycogenolysis
(D) lack of glucagon

20. Which enzyme would be lacking in this disease?

(A) lactate dehydrogenase
(B) β-glucuronidase
(C) glucose-6-phosphatase
(D) β-galactosidase
(E) α-1,4 glucosidase

21. The cause of the hyperuricemia is

(A) stimulation of the urea cycle
(B) blockage of ornithine transcarbamoylase
(C) hypersecretion of glucocorticoids
(D) hyposecretion of ACTH
(E) stimulated hepatic purine degradation

Items 22-31

Examine **Figure 5.2** below, a diagram of the tricarboxylic acid cycle, and then match the labeled step with the correct functional biochemical description of that step in the items below the diagram.

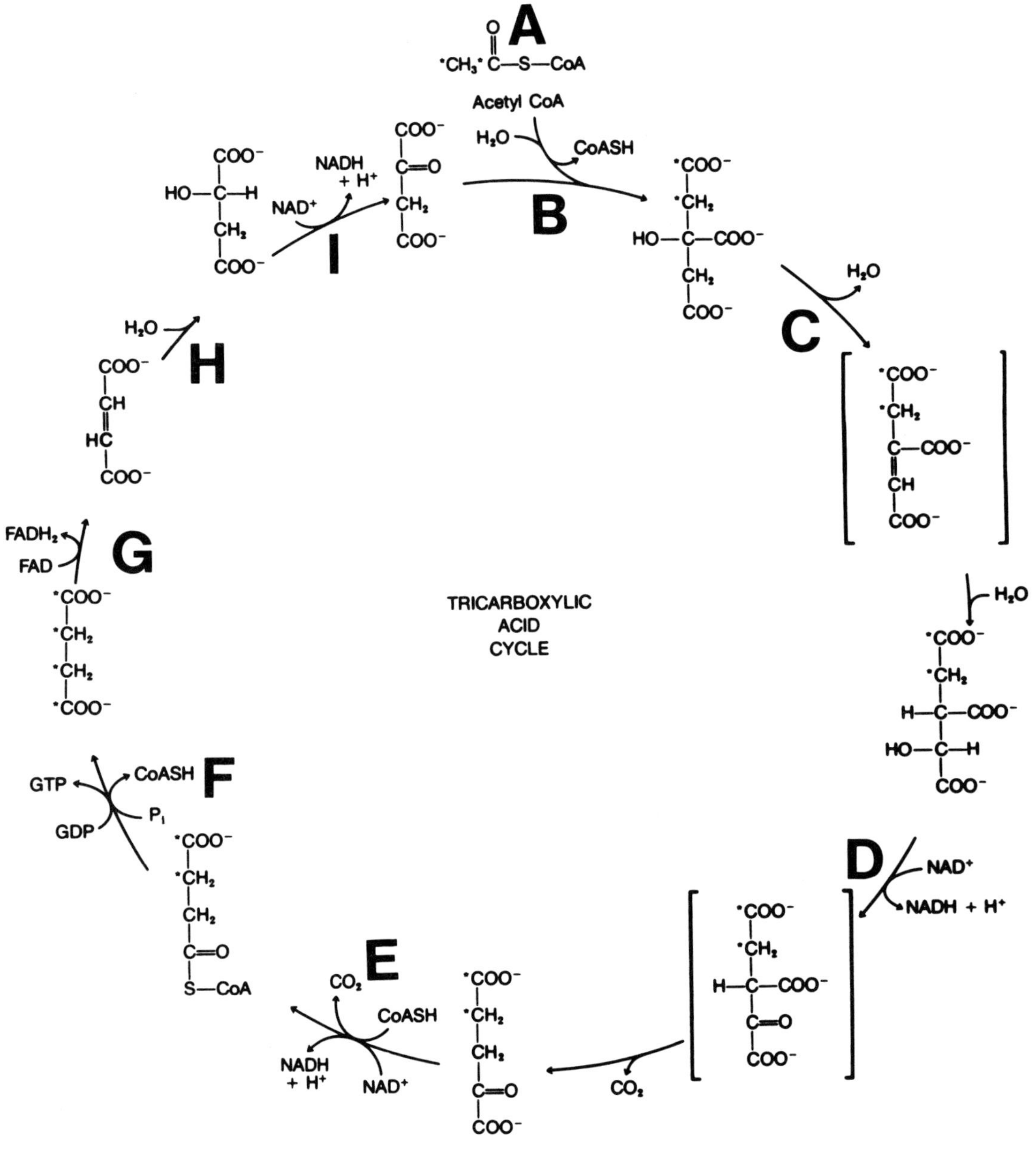

Figure 5.2

22. This step is catalyzed by citrate-condensing enzyme.

23. This step results in the production of NADH, requires Mg^{2+} and ADP as cofactors and is catalyzed by isocitrate dehydrogenase.

24. The enzyme which converts pyruvate to this compound requires CoASH, TPP, Mg^{2+}, NAD^+, FAD and $LipS_2$ as cofactors.

25. This enzyme causes the production of $FADH_2$ by the oxidation of succinate to fumarate.

26. This enzyme requires CoASH as a cofactor. It converts α-ketoglutarate to succinyl CoA.

27. This enzyme converts succinyl CoA to succinate and requires GDP as a cofactor.

28. This enzyme converts malate to oxaloacetate and requires NAD^+ as a cofactor.

29. The enzyme fumarase is used at this step to convert fumarate to malate.

30. This enzyme requires Fe^{2+} and GSH as cofactors. It converts citrate to CIS-aconitate.

31. Which set of enzymatic steps listed below contains the correct steps where reduced nucleotides are produced?

    (A) A, E, G and H
    (B) B, C, D and G
    (C) E, F, G and H
    (D) D, E, G and I
    (E) A, D, E and F

Item 32

32. Which enzyme is effected first by epinephrine binding to epinephrine receptor in a liver cell?

    (A) phosphorylase b
    (B) phosphorylase a
    (C) phosphorylase kinase
    (D) adenylate cyclase
    (E) protein kinase

Item 33

33. Which enzyme is deficient in galactosemia?

    (A) galactokinase
    (B) galactosyltransferase
    (C) epimerase
    (D) lactase
    (E) galactose-1-phosphate uridyl transferase

Items 34-37

A 1-month-old male infant became progressively weak and listless. He developed enlargement of the heart and abnormalities on the EKG with enlarged QRS complexes and a shortened PR interval. Biopsy of skeletal muscle followed by electron microscopy revealed moderately electron dense granular deposits in membrane delimited vesicles. The child died of heart failure in his 18th month.

34. The most likely diagnosis of this disease is

    (A) Sandhoff disease
    (B) von Gierke's disease
    (C) cystic fibrosis
    (D) Pompe's disease
    (E) Duchenne muscular dystrophy

35. The organelle most effected in this disease is the

    (A) nuclear envelope
    (B) plasma membrane
    (C) mitochondria
    (D) lysosome
    (E) microtubule

36. Which enzyme would be lacking in this disease?

    (A) α-1,6 glucosidase
    (B) β-glucuronidase
    (C) neuraminidase
    (D) β-galactosidase
    (E) α-1,4 glucosidase

37. The granular material seen in electron microscopic biopsies is

    (A) glycolipids
    (B) lipofuscin
    (C) amyloid deposits
    (D) glycogen
    (E) proteoglycan aggregates

Items 38-42

Match the enzyme in the glycolytic pathway with the most appropriate description of the action of this enzyme described in the items below.

(A) Hexokinase
(B) Glucose phosphate isomerase
(C) 6-phosphofructo-1-kinase
(D) Fructose-biphosphate aldolase
(E) Triose phosphate isomerase
(F) Glyceraldehyde 3-phosphate dehydrogenase
(G) Phosphoglycerate kinase
(H) Phosphoglycerate mutase
(I) Enolase
(J) Pyruvate kinase
(K) Lactate dehydrogenase

38. This enzyme of the priming stage of glycolysis converts glucose 6-phosphate to fructose 6-phosphate.

39. This enzyme of the splitting stage of glycolysis results in the formation of substrates for triose phosphate isomerase.

40. This enzyme of the oxidoreduction-phosphorylation stage of glycolysis reduces pyruvate by the consumption of NADH and H^+.

41. Starting with glucose in the glycolytic pathway, this enzyme phosphorylates a substrate and results in the consumption of the second mole of ATP/mole glucose.

42. This enzyme dehydrates 2-phosphoglycerate to produce a substrate for pyruvate kinase.

Items 43-47

The following is a list of mitochondrial enzymes. Match the most appropriate description of the enzyme in the items with the enzyme in the list below.

(A) Monoamine oxidase
(B) Phospholipase A
(C) Kynurenine hydroxylase
(D) Adenyl kinase
(E) Succinate dehydrogenase
(F) NADH dehydrogenase
(G) Cytochrome c oxidase
(H) Pyruvate dehydrogenase
(I) Isocitrate dehydrogenase
(J) Ornithine transcarbamoylase

43. This important TCA cycle enzyme is found in the mitochondrial matrix.

44. This enzyme is present in the outer mitochondrial membrane. It inactivates epinephrine.

45. This enzyme is found in the intermembrane space of mitochondria.

46. This important constituent of the electron transport chain is found in the inner mitochondrial membrane. It catalyzes the terminal step in the electron transport chain.

47. This enzyme is found in the mitochondrial matrix. It is a massive multi-subunit complex with a MW = 8×10^6.

Items 48-49

A female infant was delivered at 39 weeks of a normal pregnancy. She had severe megaloblastic anemia which was not ameliorated by vitamin B_{12} or folic acid. Her urine contained crystals of orotic acid. The diagnosis of orotic acidemia/aciduria was made.

48. Oral administration of which compound would lessen orotate excretion?

    (A) uridine
    (B) adenine
    (C) guanine
    (D) carbamoyl phosphate
    (E) PRPP

49. Which of the following enzymes is the patient most likely lacking?

    (A) hypoxanthine-guanine phosphoribosyl transferase
    (B) dihydroorotase
    (C) carbamoyl phosphate synthetase II
    (D) orotodylic pyrophosphorylase-orotodylic decarboxylase
    (E) phosphoribosyl pyrophosphate synthetase

Items 50-52

The drug 5-fluorouracil (5-FU) is a potent antimetabolite used for cancer chemotherapy.

50. Which enzyme is inhibited by this drug?

    (A) DNA polymerase
    (B) thymidine kinase
    (C) reverse transcriptase
    (D) thymidylate synthetase
    (E) HGPRT

51. Which compound would accumulate in 5-FU treated patients?

    (A) dTMP
    (B) dUMP
    (C) hypoxanthine
    (D) xanthine
    (E) ATP

52. 5-FU works as a cancer chemotherapy agent by

    (A) depolymerizing microtubules
    (B) preventing microfilament assembly
    (C) arresting mitosis at metaphase
    (D) blocking DNA synthesis
    (E) blocking DNA transcription

Items 53-54

53. Which of the following amino acids is an essential amino acid, ie, one that can not be formed from other dietary compounds?

    (A) methionine
    (B) cysteine
    (C) serine
    (D) glycine
    (E) alanine

54. Tyrosine is a nonessential amino acid. It can be synthesized directly from which essential amino acid?

    (A) alanine
    (B) phenylalanine
    (C) serine
    (D) glycine
    (E) threonine

Items 55-58

An internist examines a 50-year-old obese man who complains of aching joints. He reported awakening two nights ago with intense pain in his big toe. Physical examination reveals swelling, tenderness and an asymmetric tophus on his big toe. Blood and urine chemistry reveal strikingly elevated levels of uric acid. The diagnosis of primary gout is made by observations of crystals of sodium urate in urine and an aspirate of the arthritic joint on his big toe.

55. Which drug is most effective in preventing uric acid accumulation for treating primary gout?

    (A) cytochalasin B
    (B) colchicine
    (C) cycloheximide
    (D) allopurinol
    (E) hypoxanthine

56. This drug is an inhibitor of which enzyme?

    (A) guanase
    (B) urate dehydrogenase
    (C) xanthine oxidase
    (D) PRPP Synthetase
    (E) HGPRT

57. This drug is converted into which product?

    (A) alloxanthine
    (B) xanthine
    (C) urate
    (D) cytochalasin D
    (E) cycloheximide

58. In addition to arthritis, what other condition is most often associated with primary gout?

    (A) dementia
    (B) urolithiasis
    (C) biliary atresia
    (D) alcoholism
    (E) hypoglycemia

Item 59

59. The enzyme aspartate transaminase, also known as glutamate:oxaloacetate transaminase requires which of the following cofactors?

(A) NAD
(B) thiamine
(C) pyridoxal phosphate
(D) FAD
(E) ATP

Item 60

60. Arginase results in the formation of what compound from arginine?

(A) ornithine
(B) citrulline
(C) carbamoyl phosphate
(D) fumarate
(E) argininosuccinate

Item 61

61. The methyl group which is added to norepinephrine in the synthesis of epinephrine is derived from which compound?

(A) S-adenosyl methionine
(B) acetyl CoA
(C) tetrahydrofolic acid
(D) threonine
(E) serine

Item 62

62. Aspirin is a widely used drug. Its pleiotropic effects are due to the fact that it is

(A) a stimulator of PGE_2 synthesis
(B) a phospholipase inhibitor
(C) a stimulator of PGF_{2a} synthesis
(D) a cyclooxygenase inhibitor
(E) a stimulator of arachidonic acid synthesis

Item 63

63. The complete β-oxidation of palmitic acid would have a net yield of how many ATP molecules?

(A) 135
(B) 129
(C) 122
(D) 110
(E) 106

Item 64

64. Which tissue is primarily involved in the synthesis of the apoprotein component of VLDLs?

(A) white adipose tissue
(B) brown adipose tissue
(C) liver parenchyma
(D) small intestinal epithelium
(E) vascular endothelium

Item 65-66

65. Which of the following membranes has the highest relative lipid content?

(A) red cell membrane
(B) myelin
(C) Golgi membranes
(D) rough endoplasmic reticulum
(E) outer mitochondrial membrane

66. Which of the following membranes has the highest relative protein content?

(A) red cell membrane
(B) myelin
(C) Golgi membranes
(D) rough endoplasmic reticulum
(E) inner mitochondrial membrane

Item 67

67. Which of the following substances is LEAST LIKELY to move across the plasma membrane by mediated transport?

(A) testosterone
(B) glucose
(C) aspartate
(D) glutamate
(E) galactose

Items 68-74

Match the lipids below with the most appropriate description in the items below.

(A) Phosphatidylcholine
(B) Phosphatidylethanolamine
(C) Phosphatidylserine
(D) Phosphatidylinositol
(E) Sphingomyelin
(F) Glucocerebroside
(G) Sulfatide
(H) Ganglioside G_{M1}
(I) Ganglioside G_{M2}
(J) Ganglioside G_{M3}
(K) Cholesterol

68. This lipid accumulates in Tay-Sachs disease.

69. This lipid accumulates in Gaucher's disease.

70. This lipid accumulates in Niemann-Pick disease.

71. This lipid is a sphingolipid containing ceramide and phosphocholine.

72. This lipid is part of the protein kinase C activation chain.

73. This lipid is abundant in surfactant.

74. This lipid is important for regulating membrane fluidity.

Items 75-82

Match the water-soluble vitamins below with the most appropriate description of their biochemical role in the items below.

(A) Vitamin B_1
(B) Riboflavin
(C) Niacin
(D) Vitamin B_6
(E) Pantothenic acid
(F) Folic acid
(G) Vitamin B_{12}
(H) Ascorbic acid

75. This vitamin is a precursor of the hydrogen acceptor of isocitrate dehydrogenase in the TCA cycle.

76. This vitamin serves as an essential cofactor for collagen cross-linking.

77. This vitamin is required for the interconversion of tetrahydrofolate and N5-methyl tetrahydrofolate.

78. This vitamin is a precursor of an essential coenzyme for α-ketoglutarate dehydrogenase.

79. This vitamin is a precursor of the hydrogen acceptor of succinate dehydrogenase in the TCA cycle.

80. This vitamin is a precursor of a cofactor involved in transaminase reactions.

81. This vitamin is a precursor of a compound involved in the transfer of methyl groups during purine biosynthesis.

82. This vitamin is an important constituent of acetyl CoA.

Items 83-84

83. The best approximation to average daily basal metabolic rate in a normal human adult is

    (A) 0.1 kcal/kg
    (B) 1.0 kcal/kg
    (C) 2.0 kcal/kg
    (D) 20.0 kcal/kg
    (E) 200.0 kcal/kg

84. The most important initial source of blood glucose during fasting is

    (A) muscle glycogen
    (B) muscle protein
    (C) liver triglycerides
    (D) liver glycogen
    (E) liver protein

Items 85-87

Figure 5.3 below shows the metabolism of sex steroids. Certain key enzymatic steps are labeled with letters. Match the clinical scenario in the items most closely associated with an enzymatic deficiency. If the clinical scenario is not associated with an enzymatic defect in sex steroid biosynthesis, the answer G = none of the above should be selected.

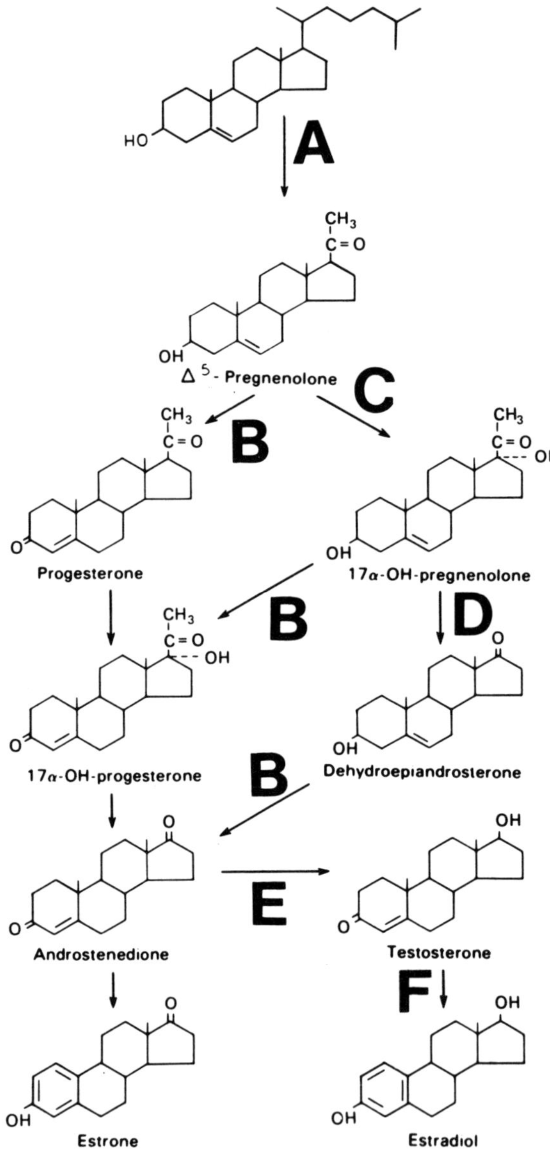

Figure 5.3

85. A patient was born with a female karyotype and female external genitalia. She remained sexually infantile, never menstruated and had hypertension associated with hypokalemia and alkalosis. The gonads appeared normal.

86. A patient was born with a male karyotype and male internal genitalia. Significant levels of androstenedione but not testosterone are detected. At puberty, gynecomastia and incomplete masculinization of secondary sexual characteristics was observed.

87. A patient was born with a female karyotype and had normal female external genitalia at birth. At the normal time of puberty, however, the patient exhibited primary amenorrhea with complete lack of development of female secondary sexual characteristics. The patient has hypertension and a normal level of corticosterone but depressed levels of cortisol, androstenedione, testosterone and estrogens.

Items 88-93

Match the elements listed below with the most appropriate description of their biochemical role in the items.

(A) Calcium
(B) Iron
(C) Iodine
(D) Fluorine
(E) Zinc
(F) Copper
(G) Chromium
(H) Selenium
(I) Manganese
(J) Molybdenum

88. This micronutrient is incorporated into the amorphous ground substance of bones and teeth. It is especially important for hardening tooth enamel.

89. This micronutrient is essential for normal functioning of myoglobin.

90. This micronutrient is an essential component of RNA and DNA polymerase.

91. This micronutrient is contained in cytochrome oxidase c and lysyl oxidase.

92. This micronutrient is required for the synthesis of thyroxine.

93. This micronutrient is a component of xanthine oxidase.

Items 94-97

Two African-American parents of a 1-year-old boy report that while their child seemed normal for the first 6 months of life, he is failing to thrive. The child has swollen joints and cutaneous ulcerations on his ankles. The child's hematocrit is 20 percent and elevated plasma hemoglobin values are present. Microscopic examination of blood smears reveals normochromic erythrocytes with an elongated, crescent shape. Other laboratory tests are used to make the diagnosis of sickle cell anemia.

94. Which of the following erythrocyte proteins is mutated in this disease?

(A) spectrin
(B) ABO antigen
(C) actin
(D) α-hemoglobin
(E) β-hemoglobin

95. This disease is associated with which amino acid substitution?

(A) alanine substituted for valine
(B) leucine substituted for arginine
(C) glycine substituted for valine
(D) valine substituted for glutamic acid
(E) serine substituted for threonine

96. Prenatal diagnosis of this disease is accomplished by

(A) analysis of restriction endonuclease fragments
(B) analysis of mutant hemoglobin
(C) detection of abnormal fetal erythrocytes
(D) karyotype analysis
(E) maternal serum α-fetoprotein screening

97. The most likely cause of erythrocyte abnormalities seen in this disease is

(A) disruption of peripheral microtubule bundles
(B) loss of spectrin-membrane interaction
(C) hemoglobin precipitation
(D) serum albumin polymorphism
(E) lack of glyceraldehyde-3-phosphate dehydrogenase

Items 98-104

Examine the diagram of a polynucleotide in **Figure 5.4** below. Then match the correct lettered structure with the description in the items below the diagram.

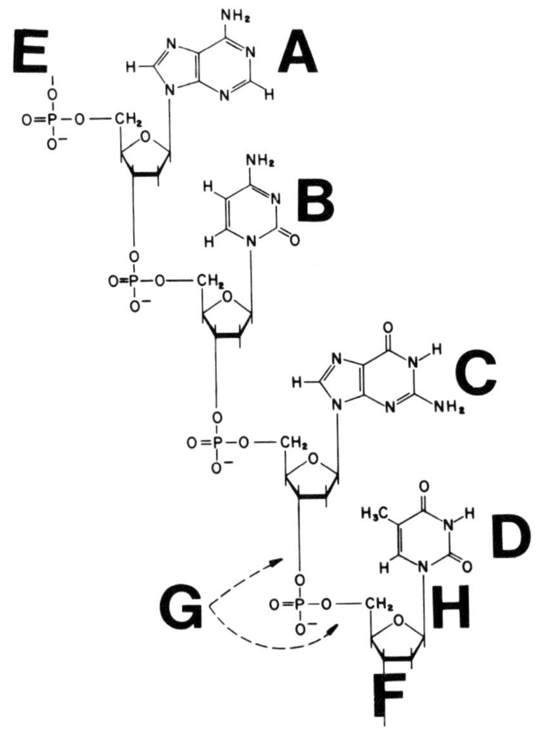

Figure 5.4

98. This structure would pair with cytosine on the opposite strand.

99. This structure would pair with guanine on the opposite strand.

100. This structure would pair with adenine on the opposite strand.

101. This structure would pair with thymine on the opposite strand.

102. This is the end of the chain where new nucleotides are added to the nascent chain.

103. This bond is formed during synthesis of polynucleotides.

104. The glycosidic bond between sugar and base.

Items 105-107

A 13-year-old boy has symptoms of frequent urination and thirst associated with fatigue, dizziness, headache and blurred vision. Laboratory tests show that this patient has Type I or juvenile-onset diabetes mellitus.

105. Which is the most common cause of this disease?

(A) dysfunction of pancreatic α cells
(B) dysfunction of pancreatic β cells
(C) dysfunction of adrenal medullary cells
(D) dysfunction of adrenal cortical cells
(E) dysfunction of adenohypophyseal corticotropes

106. The ketoacidosis associated with this disease is a consequence of

(A) hypoglycemia
(B) renal failure
(C) decreased insulin and increased glucagon
(D) hyperglycemia
(E) accelerated fat breakdown

107. The key intermediate in releasing ketone bodies from the liver in diabetic ketoacidosis is

(A) acetyl CoA
(B) fatty acyl CoA
(C) malonyl CoA
(D) citrate
(E) oxaloacetate

STOP.

YOU HAVE COMPLETED THIS SECTION.

Notes

Biochemistry and Molecular Biology

Answers and Tutorials

ANSWERS AND TUTORIAL ON ITEMS 1-5

The answers are: **1-B; 2-E; 3-A; 4-C; 5-B.** There are three ionizable groups on **glutamic acid**. The steps in the ionization of glutamic acid are shown in **Figure 5.5** below.

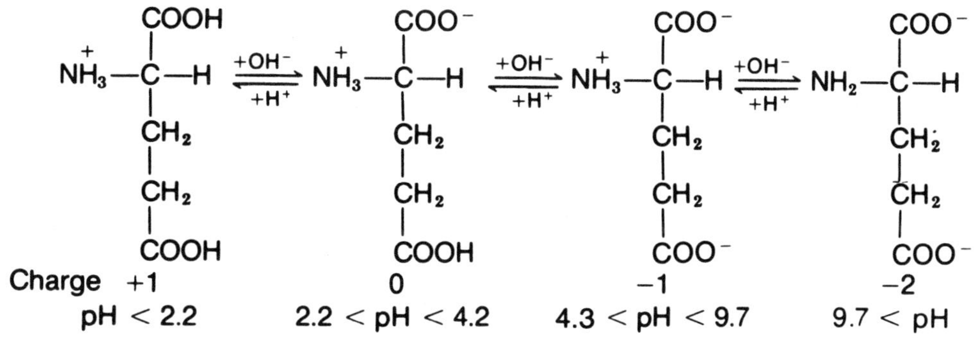

Figure 5.5

The pK of the α-COOH group is 2.2 (A). Below this point, the molecule has a net charge of +1. Addition of further base would cause ionization of the α-COOH producing a zwitterion with a net charge of 0 (B). Electrophoretic mobility depends upon the net charge on a molecule. At the **isoelectric point** of 3.5, polyglutamic acid would have no net charge and would therefore have no electrophoretic mobility. The pK for the γ-COOH is 4.3 (C). At this point, the γ-COOH ionizes, giving a net charge of -1. Addition of further base would finally cause ionization of the NH_3^+ group (D), yielding a net charge of -2. Addition of additional base at E would have no further effects on ionization because the molecule is completely ionized.

ANSWERS AND TUTORIAL ON ITEMS 6-8

The answers are: **6E; 7-B; 8-E**. The classical **Michaelis-Menten curves** are hyperbolic curves where the reaction velocity approaches a theoretical maximal limit with increasing substrate concentration. The K_m is the substrate concentration at which the velocity is half maximal

$$\left(\frac{V_m}{2}\right)$$

The assumptions used to derive the Michaelis-Menten equation are reasonably close to the actual situation which obtains in physiological conditions. For example, the substrate concentration is usually very large when compared to the enzyme concentration because of the extremely low concentration of enzymes. In addition, the product concentration is low enough so that the formation of enzyme-substrate complex from enzyme and product is negligible. As fast as enzyme-substrate complex is formed, it is converted to enzyme and product, so the enzyme-substrate complex concentration is held in a steady state.

The **Lineweaver-Burk equation** was derived because it is difficult to determine accurate values for K_m from a hyperbolic curve. The Lineweaver-Burk plot of the reciprocal of velocity as a function of reciprocal of substrate concentration is a linear curve with a positive slope. The Y-intercept is the reciprocal of V_m and the X-intercept is a negative reciprocal of the K_m. Both competitive and non-competitive inhibitors increase the slope of the Lineweaver-Burk plot with increasing inhibitor concentration. With competitive inhibitors, all curves have the same Y-intercept, ie, the V_m does not vary but the apparent K_m increases. In contrast, with non-competitive inhibitors, the K_m remains unchanged only if $k_I = k_{I-}$, but the apparent V_m decreases.

ANSWERS AND TUTORIAL ON ITEMS 9-14

The answers are: **9-A; 10-H; 11-I; 12-G; 13-J; 14-C. Glycine** is the simplest amino acid. Its -R group = -H and thus it is a neutral amino acid. It is abundant in collagen, making up one third of the total of all amino acids in this ubiquitous fibrous extracellular matrix protein. Alanine is also a simple neutral amino acid with an -R group = $-CH_3$.

Serine and threonine are hydroxy amino acids. Their -R groups respectively = $-CH_2OH$ and = –CH–OH

Arginine and **lysine** are both basic amino acids. They have positively charged (protonated) -R groups at physiological pH (**Figure 5.6**). Lysine residues in adjacent collagen chains can participate in cross-link formation. If lysyl amino oxidase creates an allysyl derivative in only one lysine of closely spaced lysine pairs on adjacent chains, a Schiff base forms, leading eventually to the formation of lysinonorleucine at the interchain cross-link. If lysyl amino oxidase creates two allysyl residues, these will form an aldol cross-link by aldol condensation.

Proline is unusual in that the -R group has the α-imino group in it. Therefore, proline is classified as an α-imino acid rather than an α-amino acid. Collagen contains approximately 10% of its residues as proline and another 10% as hydroxyproline.

Phenylalanine and tyrosine are aromatic amino acids. Their structures are shown in **Figure 5.6**. Phenylalanine is converted to tyrosine by phenylalanine hydroxylase. Tyrosine is then converted to melanin by tyrosinase. Albinos lack tyrosinase and are therefore unable to synthesize melanin.

Glutamic acid is an acidic amino acid with an -R group = $-CH_{2-}CH_{2-}COO-$. This amino acid plays an important role in several aspects of metabolism. For example, glutamate is involved in transamination reactions leading to the formation of α-ketoglutarate, urea cycle intermediates and the synthesis of the nonessential amino acids proline and arginine.

Desmosine is responsible for the elasticity of elastin, an extracellular matrix protein abundant in elastic fibers. In elastin, lysyl residues can be converted to allysyl residues by lysyl amino oxidase. When adjacent elastin chains are close to one another, three allysyl residues and one lysyl residue condense to form an interchain cross-link containing desmosine.

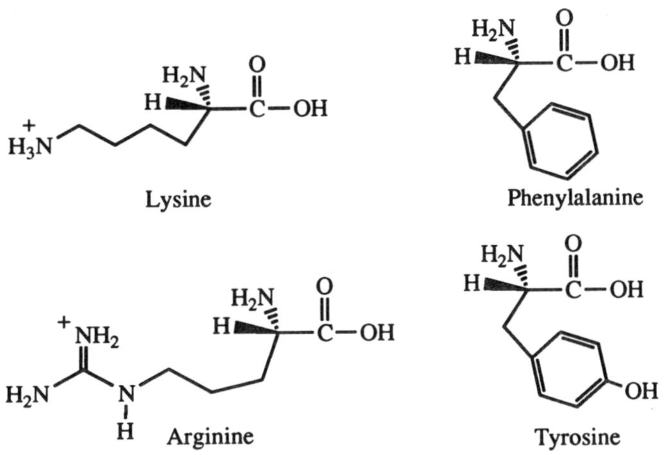

Figure 5.6

Answer and Tutorial on Item 15

The answers is: **15-B**. The **equilibrium constant** for the ionization of a weak acid such as acetic acid is described by the equation

$$K = \frac{[H^+][A^-]}{[HA]}$$

The **Henderson-Hasselbalch equation** is

$$pH = pK + \log_{10}\frac{[A^-]}{[HA]}$$

It describes the relationship between pH and pK. When pH is equal to p*K*, the $\log_{10}\frac{[A^-]}{[HA]}$ is 0, i.e., $\frac{[A^-]}{[HA]} = 1$.

pH is defined as $-\log_{10}[H^+]$. An 0.01 M solution of acetic acid would be essentially completely ionized. Therefore the $[H^+]$ would be 0.01 M = 10^{-2} M. Therefore the pH would equal 2.0.

Answer and Tutorial on Item 16

The answers is: **16-D**. Antibodies are **immunoglobulins** that are synthesized by plasma cells. They are complex macromolecules capable of recognizing foreign antigens and capable of initiating a systemic response that ultimately results in the destruction of foreign antigens. Immunoglobulins are composed of subunits of four polypeptide chains.

In the most abundant immunoglobulin in plasma, **IgG**, there are two heavy (H) chains (MW = 50,000) and two light (L) chains (MW = 25,000), giving a total MW = 150,000. IgG has little covalently coupled carbohydrate. Disulfide bonds are found between H and L chains and also between H chains. The entire molecule is a Y-shaped affair with a hinge region at the neck of the Y. Here, papain splits the molecule into an Fc fragment and two Fab fragments. The Fab fragments have the variable region, where variation in amino acid sequence leads to structural variation at the antigen binding site. The carboxyl terminal of the H chains is in the Fc fragment while the amino terminals of both the H and L chains are in the FAb fragments near the variable region (antigen binding site).

The structures of **IgA** (MW = 170,000-720,000), **IgD** (MW = 160,000), and **IgE** (MW = 190,000) are similar to IgG although the H chains are slightly larger and these immunoglobulins are more glycosylated, yielding correspondingly higher molecular weights. IgA can be polymerized to variable degrees as secretory IgA, an immunoglobulin abundant in exocrine secretions such as mucus and milk. Secretory IgAs are abundant in breast milk and are particularly important for preventing adhesion of bacteria to epithelial cells and thus help control enteric infections and respiratory infections in breast-fed infants. **IgM** is present in plasma as a pentamer with MW = 950,000. IgMs promote phagocytosis of microorganisms by macrophages and are strong activators of the complement system. Little is known about the functions of IgD and IgE although IgE is clearly involved in various allergic reactions.

Answer and Tutorial on Item 17

The answers is: **17-B**. **Lactate dehydrogenase** exists in five electrophoretically distinct isozymic forms. These five variants, LDH_1 to LDH_5, are formed by the five distinct ways of combining two distinct polypeptide chains (H for heart and M for muscle) into tetrameric enzyme molecules. The H and M polypeptides are derived from distinct genes. LDH_1 remains nearest the anode upon electrophoresis. It is abundant in heart muscle and erythrocytes. It consists of four identical H polypeptides. LDH_5 migrates closest to the cathode upon electrophoresis. It is abundant in liver and skeletal muscle. It consists of four identical M polypeptides. **Myocardial infarction** results in damage to heart muscle and release of LDH_1 so that LDH_1 levels become greater than LDH_2 levels, reversing their normal relationship. Often, there is congestive liver involvement secondary to myocardial infarction that leads to an elevation of LDH_5.

Answers and Tutorial on Items 18-21

The answers are: **18-B; 19-A; 20-C; 21-E**. This child suffers from **von Gierke's disease** (Glycogenosis, Type I). This disease can be caused either by a deficiency in **glucose-6-phosphatase** (Type Ia) or in the glucose-6-phosphatase translocase (Type Ib). This is the most common of the glycogen storage diseases (incidence is 1/200,000 live births) and it is caused by an autosomal recessive mutation. Glycogen storage diseases also include **Pompe's disease** (Glycogenosis, Type II) (α-1,4-glucosidase deficiency) and **Cori's disease** (Glycogenosis, Type III (branching enzyme deficiency). The enzyme deficiency of von Gierke's is manifest especially in the liver, kidneys and small intestines and can be diagnosed by enzymatic assays of biopsies of the small intestine.

The fasting hypoglycemia is caused by the lack of production of glucose from glycogen or gluconeogenesis, processes that normally occur in the liver. Similarly, lactic acid accumulates because of inefficient hepatic utilization of lactate for glucose synthesis. The hyperuricemia is caused by stimulation of hepatic degradation of purines.

Answers and Tutorial on Items 22-31

The answers are: **22-B; 23-D; 24-A; 25-G; 26-E; 27-F; 28-I; 29-H; 30-C; 31-D**. **Figure 5.2** illustrates the salient features of the **tricarboxylic acid** (TCA) **cycle**. The basic role of the TCA cycle is to combine pyruvate- or fatty acid -oxidation-derived acetyl CoA with oxaloacetate to form citric acid and then to convert citric acid back into oxaloacetate, releasing CO_2 and producing reduced nucleotides which are subsequently converted to the energy rich compound ATP by the subsequent electron transport-oxidative phosphorylation reactions in the mitochondria.

The **pyruvate dehydrogenase complex** converts pyruvate to acetyl CoA (A). In mammals, this multienzyme complex contains, in addition to 20-30 subunits of pyruvate dehydrogenase, 60 subunits of dihydrolipoyl transacetylase and 5-6 subunits of dihydrolipoyl dehydrogenase, all bound together in a large multi-subunit aggregate with a total MW = 7-8.5 X 10^6. This reaction produces $FADH_2$ and NADH, requires TPP as a cofactor and consumes CoASH. The acetyl CoA produced by this reaction is fed into the TCA cycle.

The first step in the tricarboxylic acid cycle is catalyzed by **citrate synthetase** (B). This enzyme has a MW = 100,000 and is found in the matrix of mitochondria. Acetyl CoA and oxaloacetate condense to form citrate. The equilibrium of this reaction is shifted strongly in favor of citrate.

Aconitase (C) then converts citrate into isocitrate through an unstable intermediate *cis*-aconitate. *Cis*-aconitate is bound to aconitase and is readily converted into isocitrate. This reaction requires ferrous (Fe^{2+}) ions.

Isocitrate dehydrogenase (D) has a MW = 380,000 and consists of eight identical subunits. It catalyses the step that produces the initial NADH of the TCA cycle. It requires NAD^+

as an oxidized acceptor of hydrogen. This enzyme converts isocitrate into an unstable intermediate, oxalosuccinate, which then rapidly releases CO_2 and is converted to α-ketoglutarate. Isocitrate dehydrogenase is inhibited when either ATP or NADH are abundant and is activated when either ADP + P_i or NAD^+ are abundant.

The next enzyme in the TCA, **α-ketoglutarate dehydrogenase** (E), exists as a multienzyme complex structurally similar to pyruvate dehydrogenase. It requires TPP, lipoic acid, CoASH, FAD and NAD^+ as cofactors. The action of this complex results in the production of succinyl CoA, the release of the second CO_2 molecule of the TCA cycle and the formation of the second NADH molecule. The equilibrium of the α-ketoglutarate dehydrogenase complex lies strongly in favor of formation of succinyl CoA.

Succinyl CoA synthetase (F) converts succinyl CoA to succinate by releasing CoASH. Succinyl CoA has an energy-rich thiolester linkage which is preserved during the phosphorylation of GDP to GTP which can subsequently be converted to ATP. Succinate is converted into fumarate by succinate dehydrogenase (G), an enzyme with two subunits MW = 70,000 and 30,000, and it is bound to the inner mitochondrial membrane. The cofactors for this reaction, Fe^{2+} and FAD, are bound to the enzyme. The reducing equivalents released by oxidation of succinate are transferred to FAD and lead to the production of $FADH_2$. Subsequently, these reducing equivalents are passed on the to the coenzyme Q-cytochrome b components of the mitochondrial electron transfer chain.

Fumarase (H) converts fumarate to malate in the next step of the TCA cycle. Fumarate is hydrated to form malate. Then malate dehydrogenase (I) converts malate into oxaloacetate to complete the TCA cycle. Malate dehydrogenase utilizes NAD^+ and removes reducing equivalents from malate to form oxaloacetate and NADH + H^+.

Answer and Tutorial on Item 32

The answers is: **32-D**. **Glycogen synthesis** (glycogenesis) occurs at the nonreducing terminal ends of glucose polymers. The enzyme **glycogen synthase** uses UDP-glucose as a glucosyl donor and glycogen as an acceptor molecule, transferring glucosyl residues one at a time to a growing glycogen molecule. This enzyme results in the formation of $(1 \rightarrow 4)$-α-D-glucosidic linkages. This reaction is useful only for elongation of existing glycogen chains. A second enzyme, called **branching enzyme** (α-D-glucosyl 4:6 transferase), transfers short oligosaccharides from the outer limits of 14 polymers onto position 6 of an α-D-glucosyl residue in a different chain, thus forming an $(1 \rightarrow 6)$-α-D-linkage and forming a branch point. The oligosaccharide is transferred as a group of glucose molecules rather than one glucose molecule at a time. The nonreducing ends form new acceptor for glycogen synthase which then causes further growth of glycogen.

Glycogen degradation (glycogenolysis) is accomplished by the enzyme **phosphorylase a** in the presence of pyridoxal phosphate, an essential cofactor. Phosphorylase a works on the nonreducing terminal of glycogen, removing glucosyl residues one at a time and releasing D-glucose-1-phosphate. Phosphorylase a degrades glycogen to within a few residues of branch points, leaving a limit dextrin. A second enzyme, **$(1 \rightarrow 4)$glycosyltransferase**, then transfers all but one of the glucose residues from chain fragments linked to a glucosyl residue at position 6 to the nonreducing terminal of other fragments, producing additional substrate for phosphorylase a. A third enzyme, α-D-1,6-glucosidase, now releases D-glucose from the former branch point and releases blockage for further degradation by phosphorylase a. Essential glycogen stores remain even in fasted or starved animals. This reserve glycogen probably is required as an acceptor for glycogen synthase.

The regulation of glycogen synthesis and degradation is a complex process which is essentially dependent on the phosphorylation and dephosphorylation of regulatory proteins. For example, phosphorylase in the phosphorylated form (a) is active in glycogen degradation but its dephosphorylated form (b) is inactive. Conversely, the phosphorylated form of glycogen synthase is inactive while the dephosphorylated form adds glycosyl residues to glycogen.

Phosphorylase kinase has four different subunits α, β, γ and δ. cAMP-dependent protein kinase phosphorylates the α and β subunits and activates the enzyme. The γ subunit has catalytic activity and the δ subunit is calmodulin. Activated phosphorylase kinase phosphorylates phosphorylase b and activates it to phosphorylase a, leading to glycogen breakdown.

Glycogen synthase occurs in two different forms, D and I. Glycogen synthase D is formed from glycogen synthase I by a phosphorylation step that is controlled by three different kinases: 1) cAMP-dependent protein kinase; 2) phosphorylase kinase; and 3) glycogen synthase kinase. These three enzymes accomplish the phosphorylation of six different serine residues, all of which must be phosphorylated for the complete inactivation of glycogen synthase I to glycogen synthase D.

Protein phosphatase-1 is a single enzyme capable of dephosphorylating phosphorylase a, glycogen synthase D and phosphorylase kinase. Protein phosphatase-1 in inhibited by protein inhibitor-1 when protein inhibitor-1 is phosphorylated by a cAMP-dependent protein kinase.

Answer and Tutorial on Item 33

The answers is: **33-E. Galactosemia** is caused by a defect in the enzyme **galactose-1-phosphate uridyl transferase**, leading to an accumulation of galactose-1-phosphate in tissues. Galactose and galactose-1-phosphate accumulate in tissues and can cause damage. Often, galactose accumulation in the liver leads to jaundice and neurological symptoms. Placing the patient on a galactose-free diet will lead to rapid amelioration of symptoms if liver damage is not too far advanced.

Galactose is an important monosaccharide in many glycoproteins. It can be derived from glucose in patients on a galactose-free diet. Glucose is converted to glucose 1-phosphate and then to UDP-glucose. An epimerase then converts UDP-glucose to UDP-galactose. Galactosyltransferases then convey the galactosyl moiety of UDP-galactose to the carbohydrate side-chains of glycoproteins.

Answers and Tutorial on Items 34-37

The answers are: **34-D; 35-D; 36-E; 37-D**. This child suffers from **Pompe's disease** (Glycogenosis, Type II A). This is a rare (1/400,000 live births) fatal disease with no known cure. Most children show onset of symptoms in the first 2 months of life and rarely live beyond 2 years. Pompe's disease is caused by an autosomal recessive mutation causing absence or severe reduction in the amount of the lysosomal enzyme **α-1,4-glucosidase**. Under normal conditions, this enzyme is responsible for degradation of glycogen which is destined to be used for energy production. When glycogen can not be degraded, it accumulates inside membrane bound vesicles that are derived from lysosomes. Massive deposits of glycogen eventually compromise muscular function, leading to weakness, cardiac myopathy and death, usually from heart failure.

Answers and Tutorial on Items 38-42

The answers are: **38-B; 39-D; 40-K; 41-C; 42-I**. The **glycolytic (Embden-Meyerhof) pathway** is one of the key pathways of carbohydrate metabolism. This pathway results in the anaerobic degradation of glucose to lactate. It occurs without oxygen and can result in the net production of 2 moles of ATP for each mole of glucose. Glycolysis is also important in the presence of oxygen but the pyruvate produced by glycolysis is then completely oxidized to CO_2 and H_2O in mitochondria by oxidative phosphorylation, resulting in the production of large amounts of ATP. If glycolytic production of pyruvate from glucose and mitochondrial production of CO_2 and H_2O from pyruvate is considered as a whole, 1 mole of glucose results in the formation 6 moles of CO_2, 6 moles of H_2O and 38 moles of ATP.

The first stage of the glycolytic pathway is the **priming stage**. Initially, glucose is phosphorylated to glucose 6-phosphate by **hexokinase** (A). At this step, the first ATP is used to phosphorylate. Next, **glucose phosphate isomerase** (B) converts glucose 6-phosphate to fructose 6-phosphate and then a second ATP is hydrolysed in the phosphorylation of fructose 6-phosphate to fructose 1,6-biphosphate by **6-phosphofructo-1-kinase** (C).

The second stage of the glycolytic pathway is the **splitting stage**. Here, fructose 1,6-biphosphate is cleaved into dihydroxyacetone phosphate and glyceraldehyde 3-phosphate by **fructose-biphosphate aldolase** (D). The splitting stage is completed as **triose phosphate isomerase** (E) catalyses the interconversion of dihydroxyacetone phosphate and glyceraldehyde 3-phosphate.

The third stage of the glycolytic pathway is the **oxidoreduction-phosphorylation stage**. **Glyceraldehyde 3-phosphate dehydrogenase** (F) is a complex enzyme that both reduces NAD^+ to NADH and also produces the high energy phosphate compound 1,3-biphosphoglycerate. Next, the high energy phosphate bond of 1,3-biphosphoglycerate is transferred to ADP to produce ATP and 3-phosphoglycerate. This step is catalyzed by **phosphoglycerate kinase** (G).

Next, **phosphoglycerate mutase** (H) converts 3-phosphoglycerate to 2-phosphoglycerate and then enolase (I) causes a dehydration and formation of a high energy phosphate bond in phosphoenolpyruvate. **Pyruvate kinase** (J) then cleaves the high energy phosphate bond of phosphoenolpyruvate, resulting in the production of ATP and pyruvate. Finally, under anaerobic conditions, **lactate dehydrogenase** (K) converts pyruvate to lactate.

Answers and Tutorial on Items 43-47

The answers are: **43-I; 44-A; 45-D; 46-G; 47-H**. **Mitochondria** are complex intracellular organelles consisting of an outer membrane, an intermembrane space, an inner membrane with numerous folds called cristae and an internal amorphous matrix. There is some evidence that mitochondria have evolved from endosymbiotic organisms. Mitochondria are the powerhouses of the cell. They have the enzyme systems for the oxidation of pyruvate and fatty acids, TCA cycle enzymes, and systems for oxidative phosphorylation and electron transport. The most important metabolic product of mitochondria is the energy rich compound ATP. There is a tremendous variation in the number and structure of mitochondria in different cell types. For example, erythrocytes have no mitochondria at all. Liver parenchymal cells have 1,000 or more mitochondria per cell, reflecting their complex catabolic functions. Cardiac muscle cells have many mitochondria producing ATP required for continuous cardiac muscle contraction.

The **outer mitochondrial membrane** is relatively simple on a structural and functional level. It consists of approximately 50% lipid and 50% protein and has relatively few transport or enzymatic functions. The enzymes monoamine oxidase (A), phospholipase A (B) and kynurenine hydroxylase (C) are all found in the outer mitochondrial membrane. The intermembrane space lies between the outer and inner mitochondrial membranes. Adenyl kinase (D) and nucleoside diphosphate kinase have been found here.

The **inner mitochondrial membrane** is much more complex than the outer mitochondrial membrane and contains approximately 75% protein. Here, one finds succinate dehydrogenase (E); all three components of the electron transport chain: NADH dehydrogenase (F), and cytochrome c oxidase (G); and enzymes for ATP synthesis (ATP synthase) and ADP-ATP transport (ADP-ATP translocase). In addition, the inner mitochondrial membranes have enzymes for transport of carboxylates, glutamate-aspartate and Ca^{2+}.

The **mitochondrial matrix** contains pyruvate dehydrogenase (H), citrate synthase, isocitrate dehydrogenase (I), all of the other enzymes of the TCA cycle except for succinate dehydrogenase (E), succinyl CoA synthetase, fatty acid β-oxidation enzymes, glutamate dehydrogenase, glutamate-oxaloacetate transaminase and ornithine transcarbamoylase (J).

Answers and Tutorial on Items 48-49

The answers are: **48-A; 49-D**. **Orotic acidemia** is a rare disorder presumably occurring with equal frequency is both males and females due to the fact that it is caused by an autosomal recessive mutation altering the activity of **orotodylic pyrophosphorylase-orotodylic decarboxylase**, a key enzyme in the pyrimidine synthesis pathway. These two distinct enzymatic activities are found in a single gene product with a MW = 51,000. Administration of uridine or cytidine bypasses the blockage and supplies nucleotides for RNA and DNA synthesis in rapidly growing hematopoietic tissues. In addition, these nucleosides lead to increased production of UTP, a feedback inhibitor of carbamoyl phosphate synthetase II, which in turn leads to decreased orotic acid production.

De novo synthesis of pyrimidines occurs via a six-step set of reactions. The C2 and N3 of the pyrimidine ring are formed when glutamine and CO_2 form carbamoyl phosphate. ATP is consumed in this reaction which is catalyzed by carbamoyl phosphate synthetase (CPS) II, an enzyme of the cytosol, distinct from the mitochondrial CPS I. The N1 and C4-6 of the pyrimidine ring are added when carbamoyl phosphate combines with aspartate to form N-carbamoylaspartate, due to the action of aspartate carbamoyltransferase. The pyrimidine ring is then closed by dihydroorotase to form dihydroorotate which is then oxidized by dihydroorotate dehydrogenase, an NAD^+ requiring flavoprotein. The N-riboside bond is formed next when orotate phosphoribosyltransferase catalyzes the combination of orotate with PRPP to form orotidine 5-monophosphate (OMP). OMP-decarboxylase completes the formation of UMP. The synthesis of cytidine nucleotides occurs at the triphosphate level. The enzyme CTP synthetase converts UTP to CTP and requires glutamine and ATP. The steps in pyrimidine synthesis are shown in **Figure 5.7**

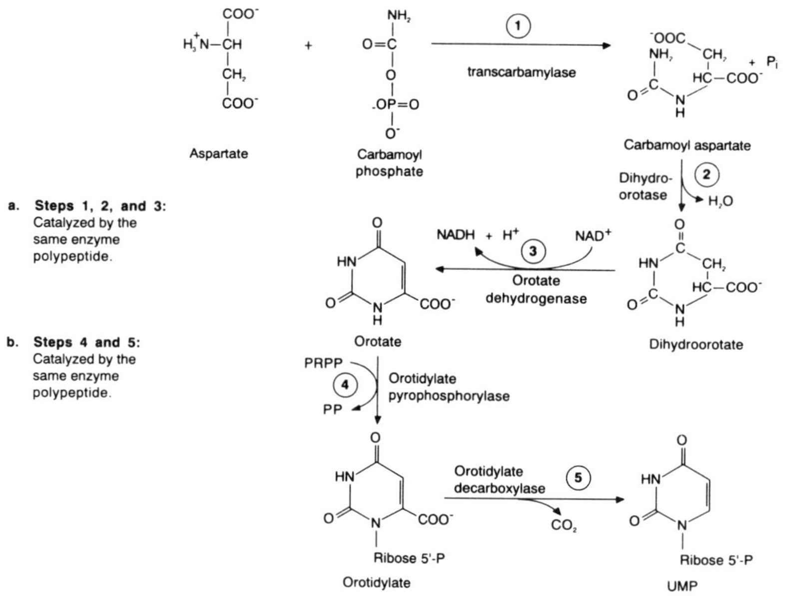

Figure 5.7

ANSWERS AND TUTORIAL ON ITEMS 50-52

The answers are: **50-D; 51-B; 52-D**. **5-Fluorouracil** (5-FU) is a pyrimidine analog. After activation to the nucleotide level by the salvage pathways, 5-FU is converted into FdUMP which is a potent inhibitor of thymidylate synthetase. When thymidylate synthetase is inhibited, DNA synthesis is blocked and cell division is not possible. 5-FU can also be converted to FUTP which will subsequently be incorporated into RNA, perhaps explaining some of the nonspecific cytotoxicity of 5-FU. Thymidine and uridine are both required to rescue 5-FU treated cells.

ANSWERS AND TUTORIAL ON ITEMS 53-54

The answers are: **53-A; 54-B**. The **essential amino acids** are those that can not be synthesized from other compounds and are thus required in the diet. These include methionine, phenylalanine, histidine, isoleucine, leucine, lysine, threonine, tryptophan, and valine. Arginine can be synthesized from ornithine in the urea cycle but not in large quantities. Therefore, arginine is usually included in the list of essential amino acids.

Alpha-ketoglutarate can be derived from glutamate. Proline and arginine can be converted to glutamate and therefore to α-ketoglutarate. When histidine is degraded, it forms glutamate and can therefore be converted into α-ketoglutarate. Phenylalanine is converted to tyrosine by phenylalanine hydroxylase. Tyrosine is then converted to homogentisate which is subsequently degraded to fumarate and acetoacetate.

Succinyl CoA can be produced from methionine, threonine, isoleucine and valine. Each of these amino acids can be converted to propionyl CoA which becomes methylmalonyl CoA in a biotin-dependent carboxylation step. Finally, methylmalonyl CoA is converted to succinyl CoA by a vitamin B_{12}-dependent step. Tryptophan is degraded in a unique pathway, most active in the liver, leading to the formation of nicotinic acid and a host of other byproducts including kynurenate, anthranilate and xanthurenate. Tryptophan can also be converted into serotonin. Oxaloacetate can be produced from aspartate by the glutamate-oxaloacetate transaminase reaction. The oxaloacetate is then used in the TCA cycle for energy production.

ANSWERS AND TUTORIAL ON ITEMS 55-58

The answers are: **55-D; 56-C; 57-A; 58-B**. **Primary gout** is caused by accumulation of abnormally high levels of **uric acid** due to a family of metabolic disorders leading to excessive *de novo* synthesis of purine nucleotides. The elevated synthesis and degradation of purine nucleotides leads to an increase in excretion of uric acid, an end product of purine nucleotide degradation. The painful swelling in the joints of the extremities are one of the hallmarks of primary gout. The essential clinical features of this disease are directly related to the relatively low solubility of uric acid. Formation of sodium urate crystals in the joints leads to painful arthritic swelling and various renal symptoms as well. Chronic gouty arthritis can lead to destruction of the bone at affected articular surfaces. Excessive excretion of uric acid can also commonly lead to urolithiasis (formation of stones in the renal system).

In primary gout, several distinct biochemical lesions can cause elevation of uric acid. For example, mutations have been detected that result in the synthesis of aberrant forms of **PRPP-synthetase**. These aberrant forms are not sensitive to feedback inhibition by GDP and ADP and thus intracellular pools of PRPP rise, leading to excessive production of purine nucleotides.

Several years ago, colchicine or anti-inflammatory drugs were widely used in the treatment of gout. Colchicine was presumed to ameliorate migration of leucocytes into inflamed joints but because it also inhibits cell division due to its effects on microtubules, its use has been discontinued. At the present time, **allopurinol** is widely used in the treatment of primary gout. **Xanthine oxidase** converts allopurinol to alloxanthine which binds tightly to xanthine oxidase, inhibiting conversion of xanthine and hypoxanthine to uric acid. This drug lowers uric acid production by inhibiting xanthine oxidase, simultaneously decreasing uric acid production and increasing hypoxanthine and xanthine excretion. Since uric acid production is reduced, symptomatic relief is often observed after administration of allopurinol.

ANSWER AND TUTORIAL ON ITEM 59

The answer is: **59-C**. The enzyme **aspartate transaminase**, also known as glutamate:oxaloacetate transaminase, requires **pyridoxal phosphate** as a cofactor. Pyridoxal phosphate is formed from vitamin B_6. This enzyme catalyses the transamination reaction in which oxaloacetate and glutamate are converted to aspartate and α-ketoglutarate. Transamination reactions are fully reversible. Thus, they can be used for either synthesis or degradation of amino acids.

Alanine transaminase, also known as glutamate:pyruvate transaminase is another reversible transamination reaction. It converts pyruvate and glutamate to alanine and α-ketoglutarate. This reaction also requires pyridoxal phosphate as a cofactor.

Glutamate dehydrogenase is an enzyme that catalyses the oxidative deamination of glutamate, converting it into α-ketoglutarate and releasing NH^4+. This readily reversible reaction requires either NAD^+ or $NADP^+$, cofactors that are reduced to NADH or NADPH, respectively.

ANSWER AND TUTORIAL ON ITEM 60

The answer is: **60-A**. **Urea** has two N atoms. Urea is formed in the liver by the urea cycle from NH_4^+ (source of first N atom), CO_2 and aspartate (source of second N atom). In the first step of the urea cycle, a reaction catalyzed by the mitochondrial enzyme **carbamoylphosphate synthetase I**, NH_4^+, CO_2 and two ATPs combine to form carbamoyl phosphate, 2 ADP and P_i. Carbamoylphosphate synthetase I activity is stimulated by N-acetyl-glutamate. Carbamoyl phosphate and ornithine are then joined to form citrulline. This reaction is catalyzed by the mitochondrial enzyme **ornithine transcarbamoylase**. Citrulline is then transferred to the cytoplasm of liver parenchymal cells and combined with aspartate, the source of the second N atom in urea. This reaction is catalyzed by **argininosuccinate synthetase**. One mole of ATP is also converted to AMP and PP_i at this step. The product of this reaction is argininosuccinate. Next, fumarate is cleaved from argininosuccinate by the cytosolic enzyme **argininosuccinase**. The product of this reaction is arginine. Finally, **cytosolic arginase** cleaves urea by hydrolysis from arginine, yielding ornithine. The urea is eliminated from the blood via the kidneys. The ornithine produced by arginase is transported back into the mitochondria of liver parenchymal cells where it participates in another round of **citrulline** synthesis.

ANSWER AND TUTORIAL ON ITEM 61

The answer is: **61-A**. **Acetylcholine** binds to the cholinergic receptors in the motor end plates of skeletal muscles and causes contraction. **Acetylcholinesterase** then destroys acetylcholine, stopping contraction. Acetylcholine is synthesized from serine which is first decarboxylated to ethanolamine and then methylated by S-adenosyl methionine to choline. Choline is then converted to acetylcholine by the enzyme cholineacetylase by consumption of acetyl CoA.

Dopamine, **norepinephrine** and **epinephrine** are all derived from **tyrosine**. L-tyrosine is converted to L-dopa by tyrosine hydroxylase using H_4-biopterin as a cofactor. Dopa decarboxylase converts L-dopa into dopamine. Dopamine hydroxylase then converts dopamine to norepinephrine. A **transmethylase**, using S-adenosyl methionine as a methyl donor, then converts norepinephrine to epinephrine.

Serotonin is derived from tryptophan. L-tryptophan is converted to 5-hydroxy-L-tryptophan (5-HT) by tryptophan hydroxylase using H_4-biopterin as a cofactor. 5-HT decarboxylase then converts 5-HT into serotonin.

Parkinson's disease is commonly found in elderly patients. The substantia nigra and locus coeruleus contain neurons that synthesize and secrete dopamine under normal circumstances. For unknown reasons, in Parkinson's disease, these neurons loose their functional capacity. Dopamine deficiencies lead to tremulousness. **L-dopa**, a precursor of dopamine, can ameliorate some of the symptoms of this disease but can cause unpleasant side effects such as nausea, cardiac arrhythmias, hypotension and variable CNS symptoms.

ANSWER AND TUTORIAL ON ITEM 62

The answer is: **62-D**. **Prostaglandins** are a complex family of unsaturated cyclic fatty acids. There are three major groups of primary prostaglandins based on differences in the structure of functional groups in the cyclopentane ring: (1) A series are α,β-unsaturated ketones; (2) E series are β-hydroxy ketones; (3) F series are 1,3-diols. Cyclooxygenase causes the formation of the cyclopentane ring and is a critical enzyme in the synthesis of prostaglandins. PGE_1 and PGF_1a are derived from dihomo-linoleic acid (C_{20}-Δ8,11,14). PGE_2 and PGF_{2a} are derived from arachidonic acid (C_{20}-Δ5,8,11,14). PGE_3 and PGF_{3a} are derived from eicosapentaenoic acid C_{20}-Δ5,8,11,14,17 (**Figure 5.8**).

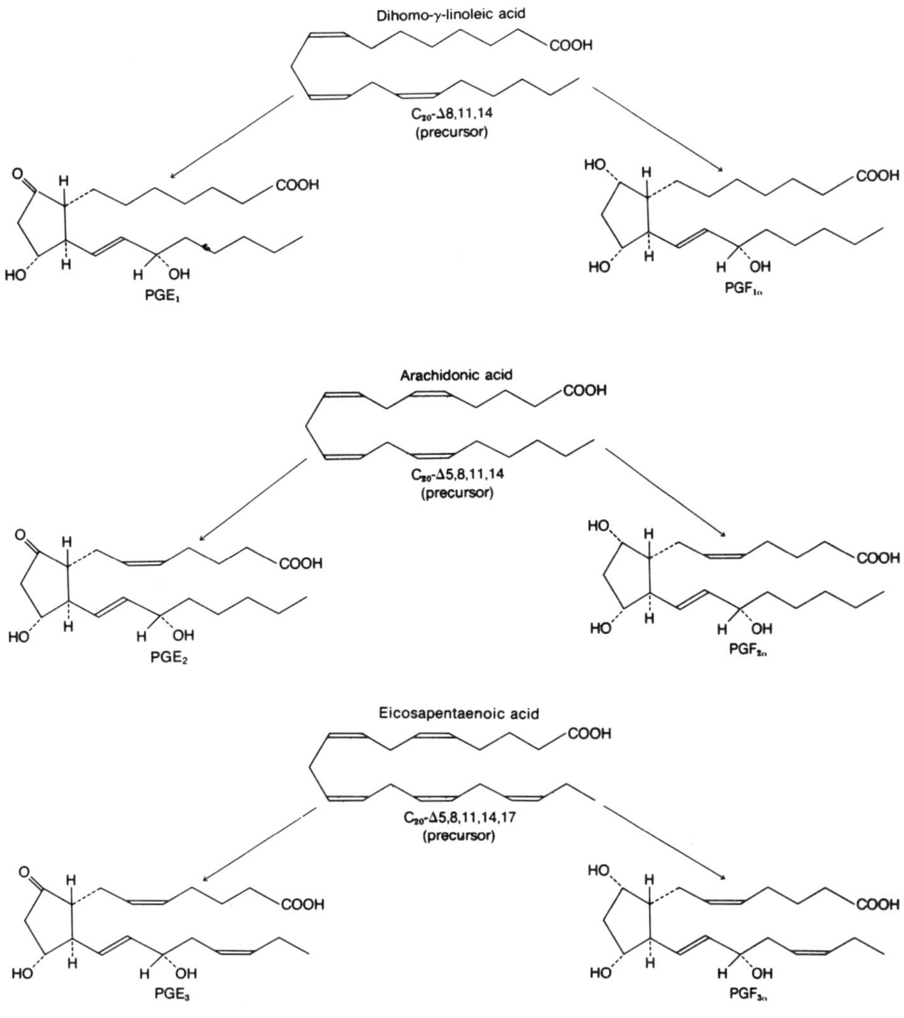

Dihomo-γ-linoleic acid
COOH
C20-Δ8,11,14
(precursor)
O
H
COOH
HO
H
H
OH
PGE1
HO
H
COOH
HO
H
H
OH
PGF1α
Arachidonic acid
COOH
C20-Δ5,8,11,14
(precursor)
PGE2
PGF2α
Eicosapentaenoic acid
C20-Δ5,8,11,14,17
(precursor)
PGE3
PGF3α

Figure 5.8

Prostaglandins are involved in the mediation of inflammation, pain, fever, uterine contractility, healing of gastric ulcers, regulation of blood pressure and platelet aggregation. The wide utility of **aspirin** is due to the fact that it is a **cyclooxygenase inhibitor**. It inhibits prostaglandin synthesis. Thus, it is effective as a mild analgesic, antipyretic and even appears to reduce the risk of heart attack and stroke due to its mild inhibitory effects on thrombus formation.

Indomethacin is a potent cyclooxygenase inhibitor along with other non-steroidal anti-inflammatory drugs such as aspirin, phenylbutazone and **ibuprofen**. Anti-inflammatory steroids such as **hydrocortisone** and betamethasone inhibit phospholipase A_2 which supplies arachidonic acid from phospholipids in cellular organelles. Prostaglandins are involved in maintaining the patency of the ductus arteriosus prior to birth. In cases of postnatal patent ductus arteriosus, indomethacin will inhibit prostaglandin synthesis via cyclooxygenase and thus promote closure of the ductus arteriosus.

Answer and Tutorial on Item 63

The answers is: **63-B**. In **β-oxidation of fatty acids**, energy is released by the sequential removal of two carbon units from the carboxyl end of long-chain fatty acids by dehydrogenation, hydration and finally oxidation to form -keto acids which are subsequently split by thiolysis. The first reaction in this process is the activation of the fatty acid to an acyl CoA derivative, a reaction occurring in the endoplasmic reticulum or on the outer mitochondrial membrane. Further processing of acyl CoA derivatives occurs on the inner mitochondrial membrane. There is an enzyme system in the mitochondrial membranes which transfers fatty acyl CoAs across the mitochondrial membrane (carnitine palmitoyl transferase I and II and carnitine carrier protein). Once inside mitochondria, the fatty acyl CoAs can undergo β-oxidation.

The first step in β-oxidation involves a group of flavoproteins called acyl CoA dehydrogenase which result in the production of reduced flavoproteins and enoyl CoA with a double bond between carbons 2 and 3. The reducing equivalents in the reduced flavoproteins are passed through ubiquinone and eventually result in the production of 2 ATPs for each double bond formed. Enoyl CoA hydratase hydrates the double bond to form an L-3-hydroxyacyl CoA. Next, L--hydroxyacyl CoA dehydrogenase (requiring NAD+) oxidizes the CHOH to a C = 0 at the 3 position, producing NADH reducing equivalents. Finally, a β-ketothiolase cleaves a two-carbon fragment and, utilizing CoASH, produces acetyl CoA and an acyl CoA that is now two carbons shorter.

The oxidation of lipids produces more ATP per gram than carbohydrates or proteins. For each two carbon fragment produced, one acetyl CoA (12 ATP) is produced. Thus, the acetyl CoA from palmitic acid yields 96 ATP. In addition, 7 equivalents of reduced flavoprotein (2 ATP/ equivalent) and 7 NADH (3 ATP/equivalent) are produced by palmitic acid, yielding 96 + 35 = 131. Two ATP equivalents are consumed in the production of palmitoyl CoA from palmitic acid, yielding **129** net ATP.

Answer and Tutorial on Item 64

The answers is: **64-C**. Dietary triacylglycerol is emulsified by **bile acids** secreted from the liver into the duodenum. Here, **pancreatic lipase** converts triacylglerol into 2-monoacylglycerol and two free fatty acids (FA). The monoacylglycerol and free fatty acids diffuse across the membranes of intestinal epithelial cells where they are resynthesized into triacylglycerol (with the consumption of 2 mol of ATP/mol of triacylglycerol). Monoacylglycerols are combined with FA-SCoA on the intracellular membranes on intestinal epithelial cells and accumulate as triacylglycerols in lipid droplets. Next, these droplets are released through the lateral boundaries of epithelial cells as chylomicrons which enter the lymphatic drainage of lacteals and finally make there way into the systemic circulation. **Lipoprotein lipase**, an enzyme on the surface of capillary endothelial cells, then hydrolyses free fatty acids from lipoproteins. The free fatty acids then enter tissues where they are utilized for energy production, eg, by β-oxidation. Free fatty acids in white adipose tissue are then resynthesized into triacylglycerols and stored.

Lipid-derived energy-rich compounds are transported in the blood in several different forms. **Chylomicrons** are micelles of triacylglycerol, cholesterol, phospholipids and lipoprotein. They are transported from the lymph to the blood and then distributed to various organs for further processing. Plasma lipoproteins and fatty acids bound to serum albumin are other prominent features of the vascular transport of lipids. Acetoacetone, α-hydroxybutyrate and acetone (ketone bodies) are products released from the liver when fatty acid is the main metabolic substrate, e.g., during starvation. Free fatty acids are not found in substantial quantities in the blood.

Answers and Tutorial on Items 65-66

The answers are: **65-B; 66-E**. **Cellular membranes** are lipid-protein bilayers. The plasma membrane surrounds each cell. It serves as the boundary between the external and the internal environments of the cell. Deep within cells, there are other membranous systems including the rough and smooth endoplasmic reticulum, the Golgi apparatus and the nuclear envelope. Individual intracellular organelles such as lysosomes are also surrounded by membranes. Mitochondria have an outer membrane which compartmentalizes the organelle from the cytoplasmic domain. The outer mitochondrial membrane surrounds an inner mitochondrial membrane.

The **red cell membrane** is one of the most well characterized plasma membranes. In general, integral membrane proteins span the entire thickness of the plasma membrane and can not be released from their associated lipids without strong detergent treatment or solvent extraction of membranes. They often have a carbohydrate-rich portion on the external surface, a middle region rich in hydrophobic amino acids which interact strongly with the hydrophobic domain of membrane lipids and a second hydrophilic domain on the internal (cytoplasmic) surface. The inner hydrophilic domain often interacts with cytoskeletal proteins in the cytoplasmic domain. In the red blood cell, glycophorin is an integral membrane glycoprotein of unknown function. Band 3 is a second integral membrane protein. It interacts strongly with the cytoskeletal protein ankyrin and may be involved in facilitating diffusion of anions. Glucose translocase is a third integral membrane protein which actively transports glucose into red blood cells. Spectrin is a cytoplasmic protein that interacts with both glycophorin and band 3 protein. It is thought to have a cytoskeletal function, strengthening the cortex of erythrocytes. Ankyrin stabilizes the interaction between spectrin and band 3 protein.

Membrane lipids consist largely of phosphoglycerides, sphingomyelin, cholesterol and "other" lipids, e.g., carbohydrate-containing glycolipids such as cerebrosides and gangliosides. The phosphoglycerides, sphingomyelin and glycolipids are extended amphipathic molecules with hydrophilic charged portions containing phosphate and other water soluble moieties such as choline, ethanolamine, serine and inositol esterified to long, hydrophobic, aliphatic hydrocarbon chains. The amphipathic membrane lipids form a bilayer where the polar heads of one layer interact with the aqueous external milieu and the polar heads of the other half of the bilayer interact with the aqueous cytoplasmic environment. The hydrophobic portions of each half of the bilayer face one another and interact strongly with one another, with cholesterol and with the hydrophobic portion of integral membrane proteins.

Cholesterol is a compact, hydrophobic, planar compound. It is an important constituent of many membranes even though it is less abundant that phosphoglycerides in the plasma membrane. Cholesterol plays a significant role in maintaining membrane fluidity. At physiological concentrations, cholesterol limits membrane fluidity. Abnormally high plasma membrane cholesterol levels significantly decrease membrane fluidity. In red blood cells, when the membrane fluidity decreases, these cells become more susceptible to splenic destruction, leading the anemia.

Different cellular membranes have striking differences in their chemical composition. For example, the **myelin sheath** of nerve fibers (a highly modified plasma membrane) is about 80% lipid and 20% protein. The high lipid content of myelin relates to its insulation function in nerve conduction. In contrast, the inner mitochondrial membrane is about 80% protein and 20% lipid. Here, there are large numbers of enzymes dedicated to electron transport. Most other plasma membranes are just under 50% lipid and just over 50% protein. Similarly, the lipid composition of different membranes varies considerably.

Answer and Tutorial on Item 67

The answers is: **67-A**. The **plasma membrane** is a **selective barrier** between the inside and the outside of individual cells. Solutes can cross the membrane by diffusion or by mediated transport. Diffusion is relatively slow for molecules such as glucose because of their low lipid solubility. Steroids and fatty acids, in contrast, have a relatively high lipid solubility and are able to cross the plasma membrane by diffusion. For **simple diffusion**, there is a linear relationship between rate of transport and external concentration of solute, ie, the higher the external concentration the greater the rate of transport. **Mediated transport** shows saturation kinetics, with high rates of movement at low solute concentrations. As solute concentration increases, the rate will reach a maximal velocity when the carrier for mediated transport becomes saturated with solute. Ions such as Na^+, K^+, Ca^{2+} (cations), HPO_4^{2-}, Cl^- and HCO_3^-(anions) as well as amino acids and sugars are transported by mediated transport.

Mediated transport is facilitated by transporter membrane proteins (translocases) and can be either passive or active. Both **passive-mediated transport** and **active-mediated transport** show saturation kinetics, show specificity for solute transport and can be inhibited. In passive mediated transport, solute moves from a high external concentration to a low internal concentration without the expenditure of energy. In active mediated transport, solute can move against a concentration gradient by coupled energy input.

ANSWERS AND TUTORIAL ON ITEMS 68-74

The answers are: **68-I; 69-F; 70-E; 71-E; 72-D; 73-A; 74-K.** **Phosphatidylcholine** (A), **phosphatidylethanolamine** (B), **phosphatidylserine** (C) and **phosphatidylinositol** (D) are all phospholipids. They consist of a glycerol backbone with two fatty acid chains esterified to two of the alcohol groups of glycerol and the third alcohol group forming an ester linkage to phosphate and choline, ethanolamine, serine or inositol respectively. Phosphatidyl choline is the predominant phospholipid of pulmonary surfactant.

Phosphatidylinositol (D) can be converted to phosphatidylinositol-4,5-biphosphate, the hydrolysis of which leads to the formation of 1,2-diacylglycerol and inositol 1,4,5-triphosphate. The 1,2-diacylglycerol stimulates protein kinase C and the inositol 1,4,5-triphosphate causes release of Ca^{2+} from intracellular membranes. Increased intracellular Ca^{2+} also leads to an increase in protein kinase C activity.

Sphingomyelin (E) is a sphingolipid containing ceramide and choline. It is one of the most important membrane lipids in the nervous system. Sphingomyelin is an important component of myelin and is therefore most abundant in the white matter of the CNS and in the myelin sheaths formed by Schwann cells of the peripheral nervous system. It accumulates in Niemann-Pick disease due to a deficiency in the lysosomal enzyme sphingomyelinase.

Glucocerebroside (F) and **sulfatide** (G) are monohexosyl ceramides. In this regard, they are sphingolipids. Glucocerebroside is a neutral sphingolipid, glucosylceramide. It accumulates in Gaucher's disease due to a deficiency in the lysosomal enzyme glucocerebrosidase. Sulfatide is an acidic sphingolipid, sulfated galactosylceramide. It accumulates in metachromatic leukodystrophy due to a deficiency in the lysosomal enzyme arylsulfatase A.

Gangliosides are acidic glycosphingolipids which contain N-acetyl neuraminic acid (sialic acid) (NANA). Ganglioside G_{M1} (H) accumulates in generalized gangliosidosis. Ganglioside G_{M2} (I) accumulates in **Tay-Sachs disease** due to a deficiency in the lysosomal enzyme hexosaminidase A.

Cholesterol (K) is a hydrophobic planar lipid. It is an important membrane constituent involved in regulation of membrane fluidity.

ANSWERS AND TUTORIAL ON ITEMS 75-82

The answers are: **75-C; 76-H; 77-G; 78-A; 79-B; 80-D; 81-F; 82-E.** **Thiamine** (Vitamin B_1)(A) is converted into the coenzyme thiamine pyrophosphate (TPP) which is essential for the important reactions catalyzed by pyruvate and α-ketoglutarate dehydrogenase. Thus, in thiamine deficiency, energy generation is severely compromised. TPP is also required for the enzyme transketolase of the pentose shunt pathway, an important source of ribose used in the synthesis of nucleic acid precursors. Finally, thiamine plays an important role in acetylcholine synthesis.

Riboflavin (B) is metabolized rapidly into two important coenzymes, FAD or flavin adenine dinucleotide and FMN or flavin mononucleotide. These two coenzymes are widely used in redox reactions, eg, the hydrogen acceptor for succinate dehydrogenase of the TCA cycle is FAD.

Niacin (C) is usually classified as a vitamin even though humans are capable of synthesizing small amounts from tryptophan. Niacin is converted to NAD^+ and $NADP^+$, important hydrogen acceptors in many cellular redox reactions, eg, isocitrate, α-ketoglutarate and malate dehydrogenase of the TCA cycle.

Pyridoxine (Vitamin B_6) (D) is readily converted into pyridoxal phosphate, an essential cofactor for the synthesis, breakdown and interconversion of amino acids. For example, pyridoxal phosphate is a cofactor for transamination reactions such as glutamate-oxaloacetate transaminase, whereby glutamate and oxaloacetate are converted to aspartate and α-ketoglutaric acid.

Pantothenic acid (E) is required for the synthesis of CoA and thus plays a central role in the regulation of fat, protein and carbohydrate metabolism. Acetyl CoA is produced by the β-oxidation of fatty acids and is utilized in the TCA cycle, eg, citrate synthase combines Acetyl CoA and oxaloacetate to produce citrate.

Folic acid (folacin) (F) is converted to tetrahydrofolate (THF) acid by dihydrofolate reductase and then methylated to form, eg, N5-methyltetrahydrofolate and other methylated varieties of THF which then serve as methyl donors in the synthesis of a wide variety of compounds including purines, serine, glycine, methionine, choline and deoxythymidylate.

Vitamin B_{12} (cobalamine) (G) is required in several reactions related to THF turnover. For example, methyl B_{12} is required for conversion of homocysteine to methionine, a reaction which is coupled to the N_5-methyl THF to THF conversion. In B_{12} deficient states, there is an accumulation of N_5-methyl THF and a concomitant reduction in THF derivatives required for purine and deoxythymidylate synthesis, leading eventually to megaloblastic anemia.

Ascorbic acid (Vitamin C) (H) serves as a reducing compound in hydroxylation reactions, eg, lysine and proline in collagen are hydroxylated as a prerequisite for cross-linking. Collagen cross-linking is important for increasing the tensile strength of this fibrous protein of the extracellular matrix. In ascorbic acid deficiency (scurvy), wound healing is retarded, bones are fragile and repair poorly and capillaries are easily damaged.

Answers and Tutorial on Items 83-84

The answers are: **83-D; 84-D**. **Adipose tissue** is the most significant source of stored energy in the human body. The average person has about 85% of their stored fuel as fat. Protein represents less than 15% of this total, while glycogen in the muscle (0.4%) and liver (0.2%) make up the rest.

The **basal metabolic rate** (BMR) is the energy utilization in the fasted state. BMR is measured when the person is awake and resting. It varies with body weight and is approximately 20-25 kcal/kg/day.

Glucose utilization varies from tissue to tissue. In red blood cells, where there are no mitochondria, glucose is oxidized to pyruvate and lactate. Brain and liver cells are rich in mitochondria and therefore oxidize glucose completely to CO_2 and H_2O. Under anaerobic conditions, muscle oxidizes glucose to pyruvate and lactate. When stimulated by insulin, adipocytes take up glucose and utilize it for energy production and for glycerol synthesis for triglyceride storage.

During **fasting**, blood glucose levels will fall. In an attempt to increase blood glucose values, insulin levels fall and glucagon levels rise. Blood glucose levels are maintained initially by hepatic glycogenolysis followed by gluconeogenesis.

Answers and Tutorial on Items 85-87

The answers are: **85-C; 86-E; 87-C**. All steroids, including the androgens and estrogens are derived from **cholesterol** by a complex series of biochemical reactions. Most cholesterol is synthesized in the liver from acetyl CoA (2 C) through HMGCoA (6 C), Δ^3-isopentenyl pyrophosphate (5 C), geranyl pyrophosphate (10 C), farnesyl pyrophosphate (15 C) and squalene (30 C).

There is good evidence that **sex steroids** play an important role in the embryonic development of the internal genitalia, external genitalia and some elements of secondary sexual characteristics and behavior. For example, the development and functional maturation of the mesonephric duct derivatives in the male (ductus epididymidis, ductus deferens and seminal vesicles) are all testosterone-dependent. Sex steroids are produced predominantly in the testes or ovaries, adrenal cortex and placenta during pregnancy.

Cleavage of the cholesterol side chain and subsequent hydroxylation reactions, collectively known as the **desmolase reaction** (A), result in the conversion of cholesterol to pregnenolone. Pregnenolone is then converted to progesterone by **3β-ol-dehydrogenase** (B) or 17α-hydroxypregnenolone by **17α-hydroxylase** (C). Patients with 17α-hydroxylase deficiency are unable to synthesize cortisol, androstenedione, testosterone and estrogens and thus have hypertension and primary amenorrhea in females. Corticosterone can be synthesized from progesterone via 11-deoxy-corticosterone in these patients. 17α-hydroxypregnenolone can then be converted to dehydroepiandrosterone by **17-20-desmolase** (D).

Dehydroepiandrosterone is then converted to androstenedione by 3β-ol-dehydrogenase (B). Androstenedione is then converted to testosterone, the chief male sex steroid, by **17 β-hydroxysteroid dehydrogenase** (E). Deficiencies in this enzyme result in accumulation of androstenedione but failure of formation of testosterone and dihydrotestosterone, both required for the development of normal male secondary sexual characteristics. Testosterone is converted to dihydrotestosterone (DHT) by the enzyme 5α-reductase. Deficiencies in this enzyme result in male pseudohermaphrodites where the external genitalia are feminized due to the fact that the normal development of male external genitalia is DHT dependent. Development of many male secondary sexual characteristics (a testosterone-dependent process) are frequently seen in such patients, however. Testosterone can be converted to estradiol, a potent estrogenic steroid hormone, by the **aromatase** reaction (F).

Answers and Tutorial on Items 88-93

The answers are: **88-D; 89-B; 90-E; 91-F; 92-C; 93-J**. **Calcium** (A) is required in large quantities in the diet. It is an essential component of the mineralized amorphous ground substance of bone and teeth. Serum calcium levels are regulated by parathormone and calcitonin. Calcium is required for muscle contraction and nerve conduction.

Iron (B) is a micronutrient that serves the essential function of binding oxygen and CO_2 in hemoglobin and myoglobin. It is also an important component of several cytochromes. Transferrin binds iron in the blood. Dietary deficiencies in iron lead to iron deficiency anemia which in the severe state, leads to decreases in hematocrit and decrease in cell-mediated immunity and phagocytosis.

Iodine (C) is concentrated in the thyroid gland. It is required for the synthesis of the glycoprotein thyroglobulin. This colloid is stored in the thyroid follicles. When stimulated by TSH, thyroglobulin is phagocytosed and degraded, releasing the iodinated amino acids T3 and T4. Dietary deficiency of iodine leads to goitrous hypertrophy of the thyroid gland.

Fluorine (D) is incorporated into the extracellular matrix of bone and teeth. It increases the hardness of enamel, decreasing dental caries.

Zinc (E) is a constituent of many metalloenzymes including RNA and DNA polymerase. It is also found in a polypeptide of saliva called gustin which is thought to stimulate development of taste buds in children.

Copper (F) is contained in several important metalloenzymes including cytochrome c oxidase, lysyl oxidase and superoxide dismutase. **Chromium** (G) is a component of glucose tolerance factor (GTF), a complex between chromium, nicotinic acid and several amino acids. GTF enhances the binding of insulin to its receptor in the cell membrane. Chromium deficiency results in increased glucose tolerance due to decreased binding of insulin to its cell membrane receptor.

Other trace elements have also been shown to play a role in nutrition. **Selenium** (H) is active in the metalloenzyme glutathione peroxidase, an enzyme which, along with vitamin E, scavenges peroxides to prevent peroxidation of polyunsaturated fats. **Manganese** (I) is a component of several metalloenzymes including pyruvate carboxylase, the ligase enzyme that converts pyruvate to oxaloacetate. **Molybdenum** (J) is found in xanthine oxidase, the enzyme that converts xanthine to uric acid.

Answers and Tutorial on Items 94-97

The answers are: **94-E; 95-D; 96-A; 97-C**. This child suffers from **sickle cell anemia**, the most common of all hemoglobinopathies. The failure to thrive and ulceration on the distal extremities are suggestive of sickle cell anemia in an African-American child. The low hematocrit (anemia), elevated serum hemoglobin values (due to hemolysis) and presence of sickle cells among normal erythrocytes in the peripheral blood smear confirm the initial clinical impression of sickle cell anemia. This disease is most prevalent in African-Americans. In the United States, about 10% of African-Americans are heterozygous carriers of the gene. It is thought that heterozygotes are partially protected from malaria and thus have a selective advantage over wild-type individuals. In Nigeria, up to 30% of the adult population are heterozygous carriers for the sickle trait. Less than 0.5 % of African-American children in the United States are homozygous recessive for the sickle trait. The incidence among adults is lower due to a severe decrease in the life-expectancy of children with sickle cell anemia. The onset of symptoms is not observed until approximately the sixth month after birth. At birth, fetal hemoglobin (Hb F) is present but is gradually replaced by Hb S. As more and more Hb S containing erythrocytes accumulate in the peripheral blood, symptoms begin to appear and increase in severity.

Sickle cell anemia was one of the first congenital human diseases to become understood on the molecular level. It is caused by a missense mutation which changes the glutamate codon to the valine codon in the sixth residue of the chain of hemoglobin to form **hemoglobin S** (Hb S). This substitution of a hydrophobic for a hydrophilic amino acid renders hemoglobin less soluble, especially at low oxygen tension. Precipitated hemoglobin forms large crystalline deposits of hemoglobin and secondarily generates the crescent-shaped erythrocytes found in the blood smear. These abnormal erythrocytes are destroyed more readily in the spleen, leading to hemolytic anemia. The formation of small and large clots leads to infarcts and these cause damage to many organs such as the spleen. Compromise of splenic function leads to recurrent infections. Vascular damage is also commonly observed in the joints, retina, skin and liver.

Prenatal diagnosis of sickle cell anemia can be accomplished by digesting DNA from the suspected carrier with a restriction endonuclease (MstII) and separating fragments electrophoretically. Next, fragments are transferred to nitrocellulose paper and the resolved fragments are hybridized with radioactive human DNA. Autoradiographic analysis of the sheets of nitrocellulose subsequently reveals a specific DNA fragment found only in association with sickle cell anemia.

Answers and Tutorial on Items 98-104

The answers are: **98-C; 99-B; 100-D; 101-A; 102-F; 103-G; 104-H. Deoxyribonucleic acid** (DNA) and ribonucleic acid (RNA) are polynucleotide chains. Nucleotides consist of a base, a sugar and 1, 2 or 3 phosphate groups. The bases are either purines [adenine (A) and guanine (G)] or pyrimidines [cytosine (C), thymine (T) and uracil (U)]. The purines adenine and guanine and the pyrimidine cytosine are found both in DNA and RNA. the pyrimidine, thymine is found only in DNA while the closely related uracil is found only in RNA. DNA contains deoxyribose while RNA contains ribose.

Polynucleotide chains are linked together by phosphodiester prime bonds between the 5´ carbon of one nucleotide and the 3´ carbon of the next nucleotide. In DNA, the amount of the purine adenine is equal to the amount of the pyrimidine thymine (A = T). Similarly, the amount of the purine guanine is equal to the amount of the pyrimidine cytosine (G = C) (**Chargaff's rules**). In fact, these complementary bases pair with one another by hydrogen bonds across adjacent strands of the double helix, maintaining a constant DNA fiber thickness of 20 Å while base pairs are stacked 3.4 Å apart. The sugar-phosphate backbone of each DNA strand is on the outside of the double helix while the purine and pyrimidine base pairs are on the inside. The complementary strands of the double helix are anti-parallel, ie, one strand is 5´→3´ and its other half is 3´→5´. High temperatures can cause dissociation of DNA strands (melting). G-C base pairs share three hydrogen bonds while A-T base pairs share two hydrogen bonds. Because of the three hydrogen bonds in the G-C pairs, a higher melting temperature is required for G-C rich DNA. Upon slow cooling, the single strands of melted DNA will reanneal guided principally by the complementary purine-pyrimidine base-pairing.

The crucial feature of DNA structure is that it most often consists of two complementary polynucleotide chains twisted together in a right-handed double helix. Each chain contains a polynucleotide polymer comprised of individual nucleotides. Each nucleotide contains a purine or pyrimidine base, a deoxyribose and a phosphate group. The **5´ phosphate** (E) of the deoxyribose of one nucleotide is linked via a **phosphodiester linkage** (G) to the 3´-OH of the next sugar, forming a regular sugar phosphate backbone for DNA. There are four different bases in the nucleotides of DNA. These four bases are comprised of two single ringed pyrimidines, **thymine** (D) and **cytosine** (B); and two double ringer purines, **adenine** (A) and **guanine** (C). The order of these four bases (the DNA sequence) constitutes the unique information content (amino acid coding capacity) of each gene.

The two strands of the double helix are complementary and arranged in an anti-parallel fashion. Adenine and thymine invariably pair with one another, forming two hydrogen bonds. Guanine and cytosine invariably pair with one another, forming three hydrogen bonds. If a nucleotide sequence was ATGCGCTA in one strand, the complementary strand would have the sequence TACGCGAT. In the diagram above, one strand is shown with the sequence ACGT. This sequence would dictate the sequence TGCA in the complementary strand. DNA synthesis proceeds in the 5´→3´ direction with new nucleotides being added onto the **3´-OH end** (F).

Answers and Tutorial on Items 105-107

The answers are: **105-B; 106-D; 107-C**. **Diabetes mellitus** is a complex disorder of carbohydrate metabolism which can be separated into two major classes, **insulin-dependent diabetes mellitus** (IDMM) (Type I, juvenile onset) and **noninsulin-dependent diabetes mellitus** (NIDDM) (Type II, adult-onset). In IDDM, onset is usually seen before age 30 and most commonly in the 11-13 age group, is usually associated with ketoacidosis but not obesity and involves severe deficiency of insulin secretion. In NIDDM, onset is usually seen after age 40, is usually associated with obesity but not ketoacidosis and involves variable insulin secretion from higher than normal to moderate deficiency.

Insulin is secreted by the β **cells** of the pancreatic islets of Langerhans. There is evidence that IDDM is an autoimmune disease. Genetic susceptibility and perhaps viral etiology play a role in IDDM pathogenesis, leading to destruction of cells and release of cell antigens. An immune response leads to further destruction of cells and further exacerbation of the disease. In IDMM we find decreased levels of insulin secretion and increased levels of glucagon secretion, leading to increased production of glucose in the liver and decreased peripheral glucose uptake and hyperglycemia. In addition, decreased insulin and increased glucagon levels lead to an increase in the production of **ketone bodies**. In the fasting state, ketone bodies are produced from oxidation of fatty acids in the liver. These ketone bodies can serve as an energy source for the central nervous system, sparing critical proteins. When this homeostatic mechanism is out of control because of decreased insulin production, diabetic ketoacidosis, a life-threatening situation, often results. The key regulatory intermediate in this pathway is **malonyl CoA**. Malonyl CoA is a competitive inhibitor of acylcarnitine transferase, an enzyme involved in the transport of fatty acyl CoA into mitochondria. Fatty acyl CoA is converted to acetyl CoA and ketone bodies in mitochondria.

Notes

CHAPTER 6

Microbiology and Immunology

DIRECTIONS (Items 1-157): For each of the numbered items that proceed, you must select the single best answer from among the lettered options listed.

Some of the numbered items will pose a question or incomplete sentence that is followed by a list of 4-5 lettered options. In all cases, select the ONE lettered option that best answers the question or completes the sentence given.

Some of the numbered items are preceded by 5-24 lettered options. In these sets, the lettered options will be preceded by a single instruction asking you to match one of the lettered options to each numbered item most closely associated with it. In all matching sets, you may use any of the lettered options once, more than once or not at all, but you should still only select ONE lettered option per numbered item.

If you wish to simulate actual USMLE testing conditions, you should aim to complete all the items in this chapter in 2 hours and 40 minutes.

Do NOT look at the answers and tutorials until you have completed all of the items in this chapter.

Good luck!

Items 1-4

A healthy young woman eagerly expected the birth of her first child. She followed prenatal care instructions and all indications appeared normal. Unfortunately, a still-born fetus with neonatal meningitis was the outcome. The mother was an asymptomatic carrier of the pathogen.

1. Such an occurrence could result from the intrauterine or vaginal colonization by

    (A) *Listeria monocytogenes*
    (B) *Bacteroides fragilis*
    (C) *Clostridium difficile*
    (D) *Clostridium perfringens*
    (E) *Gardnerella vaginalis*

2. If a sample of the CSF from the infant were Gram-stained, observed bacteria would be

    (A) Gram-negative cocci
    (B) Gram-negative rods
    (C) Gram-variable rods
    (D) Gram-positive cocci
    (E) Gram-positive rods

3. The drug of choice in the treatment of this pathogen is

    (A) doxycycline
    (B) penicillin
    (C) cephalosporin C
    (D) streptomycin
    (E) amphotericin B

4. The pregnant woman most likely was exposed to the pathogen through

    (A) the bite of an arthropod vector
    (B) contaminated blood products
    (C) inhalation of aerosol droplets
    (D) ingestion of contaminated foods
    (E) an infected pet

Items 5-6

A migrant farm worker disregarded a tender area in his mouth. It eventually developed into a enlarged abscess requiring medical treatment. Fluid obtained from the abscess revealed numerous Gram-negative rods. Nothing grew on a streaked blood agar plate incubated at 37°C.

5. Which of the following is most likely responsible for the abscess?

    (A) *Bacteroides fragilis*
    (B) *Bacteroides corrodens*
    (C) *Bacteroides melaninogenicus*
    (D) *Escherichia coli*
    (E) *Pseudomonas aeruginosa*

6. Which of the following is the most effective drug of choice used in the treatment of the causative agent?

    (A) kanamycin
    (B) vancomycin
    (C) penicillin
    (D) cephalosporins
    (E) clindamycin

Items 7-11

A 75-year-old man lived in a retirement village. He received periodic medical check-ups and was in relatively good health. During the winter an outbreak of influenza affected many residents of the complex even though all had received vaccinations. The man developed a progressive lower respiratory tract illness with symptoms including abrupt chills, high fever, productive coughs and chest pains. Sputum cultures revealed a large number of Gram-positive diplococci which were also found in blood samples. Chest x-rays showed lobar consolidation. The man's conditioned deteriorated ending with his death.

7. The organism observed in the patient's sputum and blood probably belongs to which of the following genera?

(A) *Staphylococcus*
(B) *Streptococcus*
(C) *Micrococcus*
(D) *Neisseria*
(E) *Candida*

8. The organism streaked on a blood agar plate would produce

(A) β-hemolytic, bacitracin-sensitive colonies
(B) γ-hemolytic, optochin-resistant colonies
(C) α-hemolytic, optochin-sensitive colonies
(D) β-hemolytic, bacitracin-resistant colonies
(E) α-hemolytic, optochin-resistant colonies

9. Serotyping of the bacteria is based on

(A) phage typing
(B) precipitation by antisera
(C) flagella labeling by antisera
(D) antisera swelling of the capsule
(E) DNA fingerprint analysis

10. Vaccines against the organism are prepared against the

(A) cell wall
(B) flagella
(C) capsule
(D) ribosomes
(E) nucleic acid proteins

11. A drug of choice often prescribed in treating infections caused by this organism is

(A) streptomycin
(B) sulfonamide
(C) penicillin
(D) tetracycline
(E) cephalosporin

Items 12-15

A small clinic located in a Texas boarder town receives a high volume of patients suffering from a variety of sexually transmitted diseases. Many of the patients are foreign workers lacking residency documentation and therefore follow up treatment is difficult. Local prostitutes serve both the foreign workers and the local residents, thus providing a critical link for the introduction of a variety of diseases previously not encountered. One male patient complained of a venereal infection which was a 1-cm, irritated, soft chancre-like, penile lesion. He also had regional lymphadenitis.

12. A Gram-negative rod isolated from both the lesion and pus taken from the lymph node could represent an infection caused by

    (A) *Haemophilus ducreyi*
    (B) *Neisseria gonorrhoeae*
    (C) *Treponema pallidum*
    (D) *Chlamydia trachomatis*
    (E) *Treponema carateum*

13. The disease is

    (A) yaws
    (B) chancroid
    (C) pinta
    (D) lymphogranuloma venereum
    (E) gonorrhea

14. Diagnosis is based primarily on

    (A) Giemsa stain
    (B) Tzanck smear
    (C) darkfield microscopy
    (D) culture isolation on chocolate agar supplemented with growth factors
    (E) serum antibody titer

15. Which of the following is the most effective drug of choice used in the treatment of the causative agent?

    (A) kanamycin
    (B) vancomycin
    (C) penicillin
    (D) cephalosporins
    (E) clindamycin

Items 16-18

A female taxidermist for the Smithsonian Institution was on an assignment in Brazil. Her work involved the processing of small mammal skins for transport to her home laboratory in Washington, DC. During the second month of her work in the jungles, she experienced an acute illness consisting of severe headache, chills, fever, sweating, loss of appetite and muscle spasm in the lower back and hip. Ampicillin administered by a local physician did not relieve the symptoms. A week later her condition worsened and she returned to Washington and was examined at The George Washington University Medical Center. Her condition had progressed to include a pain in her right axilla, surrounding edema and a dry cough. A presumptive diagnosis of bubonic plague was made.

16. Aspiration of an affected lymph node would show the presence of

    (A) Gram-positive rods
    (B) Gram-negative bipolar rods
    (C) Gram-positive cocci in pairs
    (D) Gram-negative diplococci
    (E) Gram-variable spirochetes

17. Bacteriological cultivation of the lymph node aspirate would most likely yield colonies of

    (A) *Yersinia enterocolitica*
    (B) *Yersinia pseudotuberculosis*
    (C) *Salmonella typhi*
    (D) *Yersinia pestis*
    (E) *Shigella dysenteriae*

18. The researcher probably encountered the bacterium through the bite of an infected

    (A) tick
    (B) flea
    (C) mosquito
    (D) louse
    (E) fly

Items 19-21

A young college student spent his summer working for a forest service agency in Oregon. One month after returning home to Virginia, he experienced a sudden onset of fever, nausea, muscle aches and headaches. Blood and stool cultures were negative. His symptoms subsided and he assumed he had recovered. Two weeks later the symptoms reappeared, but this time accompanied with a marked splenomegaly. He also noticed a single tennis ball-sized bright red rash on his lower left leg which increased in size and sensitivity. This time a blood smear showed the presence of spirochetes.

19. The symptoms described in this case history are consistent with a preliminary diagnosis of

    (A) Rocky Mountain spotted fever
    (B) Lyme disease
    (C) syphilis
    (D) plague
    (E) leptospirosis

20. The most probable etiologic agent for the above illness would be due to organisms of the genus

    (A) *Spirocheta*
    (B) *Rickettsia*
    (C) *Treponema*
    (D) *Borrelia*
    (E) *Leptospira*

21. The etiologic agent responsible for the infection was most likely acquired by

    (A) a tick bite
    (B) drinking contaminated water
    (C) sexual contact
    (D) consumption of contaminated foods
    (E) inhalation

Items 22-26

A young undergraduate college student, majoring in botany, went on a field trip with her classmates to search the Delaware shoreline for representative plants. The area included both shoreline and a deciduous forest inhabited by small rodents. The students entered both areas. A week following the trip she experienced flu-like symptoms which included high fever, headaches, muscle aches, general malaise and a stiff neck. A large 3-4–cm circular red blotch developed on her lower leg and became sensitive to the touch and gradually increased in size.

22. On the basis of the history, the symptoms closely fit a preliminary diagnosis of

    (A) Weil's disease
    (B) leptospirosis
    (C) Lyme disease
    (D) epidemic relapsing fever
    (E) plague

23. The disease is transmitted by the bite of the

    (A) louse
    (B) gnat
    (C) deer tick
    (D) mosquito
    (E) wood tick

24. The causative agent of the disease is

    (A) *Borrelia burgdorferi*
    (B) *Leptospira interrogans*
    (C) *Leptospira icterohemarrhagiae*
    (D) *Borrelia recurrentis*
    (E) *Rickettsia rickettsii*

25. The untreated disease will usually resolve itself, however several months following the initial infection, a small percentage of infected individuals will experience a "second stage" of infection involving

    (A) visual damage
    (B) renal failure
    (C) neurological abnormalities
    (D) disseminated skin lesions
    (E) synovial infection and arthritis

26. A third stage of the disease, occurring months to years after the initial infection, may occur involving

    (A) visual damage
    (B) renal failure
    (C) neurological abnormalities
    (D) disseminated skin lesions
    (E) autoimmune complexes and arthritis

Items 27-30

A male patient with culture-positive gonococcal urethritis was treated with 5 million units of aqueous procaine penicillin G intramuscularly plus probenecid (1.0 g) orally. Eight days later, he returned complaining of similar symptoms consisting of painful urination, but less urethral discharge. A second pathogen was suspected.

27. The symptoms expressed in the patient indicate that

    (A) reinfection should be suspected
    (B) he may have nongonococcal urethritis
    (C) the bacterial strain has acquired a drug resistance plasmid
    (D) he has a viral infection
    (E) he has a fungal infection

28. If the causative agent responsible for the above infection were a Gram-negative diplococcus, and it had developed antibiotic resistance this could be confirmed by which of the following tests?

    (A) coagulase
    (B) catalase
    (C) Kirby Bauer
    (D) methyl red
    (E) methylene blue

29. The second organism most likely responsible for the above infection is

    (A) *Mycoplasma pneumoniae*
    (B) *Chlamydia trachomatis*
    (C) *Candida albicans*
    (D) human papilloma virus
    (E) *Escherichia coli*

30. An antibiotic which has been shown effective in the treatment of bacterial infections of this type is

    (A) doxycycline
    (B) ampicillin
    (C) cephalosporin C
    (D) streptomycin
    (E) amphotericin B

Items 31-36

A retired auto worker was diagnosed with tuberculosis. He had been ill for about nine months with symptoms which included intermittent fever, night sweats and a productive cough. He noted a marked weight loss of 50 lb. A sputum smear showed the presence of numerous Gram-positive acid-fast bacilli. Several of his co-workers were shown to be skin test positive with the tuberculin (PPD) test.

31. Transmission of the causative agent *Mycobacterium tuberculosis* between humans is primarily through

    (A) sexual contact
    (B) respiratory droplets
    (C) contaminated foods
    (D) soil (environment)
    (E) contaminated blood products

32. It would be advisable for the above patients to undergo further testing with

    (A) another skin test
    (B) a CT scan
    (C) a chest x-ray
    (D) a NMR scan
    (E) a bacterial culture isolation

33. Many virulent strains of the bacterium have been shown to contain

    (A) purified protein derivative (PPD)
    (B) small RNA plasmids
    (C) flagella and pili
    (D) cord factor
    (E) potent exotoxins

34. An example of atypical mycobacteria found frequently in conjunction with immunosuppressed patients such as AIDS patients would be

    (A) *M. kansasii*
    (B) *M. marinum*
    (C) *M. smegmatis*
    (D) *M. scrofulaceum*
    (E) *M. avium-intracellulare*

35. The early stage of *M. tuberculosis* infection is characterized by the formation of which of the following lesions in the lungs?

    (A) granulomatous
    (B) exudative
    (C) tubercle
    (D) eschar
    (E) induration

36. Which of the following drugs is LEAST LIKELY to be effective in the treatment of tuberculosis?

    (A) chloramphenicol
    (B) isoniazid
    (C) rifampicin
    (D) ethambutol
    (E) pyrazinamide

Items 37-38

A 60-year-old patient in the burn ward of a hospital develops an infection in the burned tissue. Initial treatment with chloramphenicol and tetracycline was unsuccessful. Cultures of the infected site revealed Gram-negative rods that grew on blood agar, EMB, and trypticase soy agar. On the latter medium they produced a bluish-green pigmentation and aromatic odor. The organism was susceptible to carbenicillin, gentamicin, amikacin and polymyxin B.

37. This organism is most likely

    (A) *Acinetobacter calcoaceticus*
    (B) *Alcaligenes faecalis*
    (C) *Flavobacterium* sp
    (D) *Pseudomonas aeruginosa*
    (E) *Citrobacter* sp

38. A major organism associated with nosocomial infections of surgical wounds is

    (A) *Staphylococcus aureus*
    (B) *Alcaligenes faecalis*
    (C) *Streptococcus pyogenes*
    (D) *Streptococcus pneumoniae*
    (E) *Bacillus cereus*

Items 39-41

A group of 25 businessmen celebrated at a New Year's Day party. In addition to alcoholic refreshments and a wide assortment of cooked foods, the feast included fresh oysters and clams. On January 2, 23 of them began to experience gastrointestinal illnesses which included diarrhea (86%), nausea (82%), abdominal cramps (65%), fever (56%) and vomiting (35%). In most cases the illnesses lasted 15-17 hours. The affected men ate only the mollusks. Bacteriological cultures taken from the mollusks produced significant colony numbers of Gram-negative rods including *Escherichia coli*, *Vibrio parahaemolyticus*, and *Clostridium perfringens*.

39. A low molecular weight protein enterotoxin, comprising part of a bacterial spore is produced by

    (A) *Clostridium perfringens*
    (B) *Escherichia coli*
    (C) *Campylobacter jejuni*
    (D) *Shigella dysenteriae*
    (E) *Salmonella typhi*

40. The halophilic nature and tendency to induce diarrhea, following colonization of the intestinal tract, makes which of the following organisms a primary candidate for causing the illness described in the mev?

    (A) *Clostridium perfringens*
    (B) *Vibrio parahaemolyticus*
    (C) *Campylobacter jejuni*
    (D) *Bacillus cereus*
    (E) *Salmonella typhi*

41. High levels of *Escherichia coli* recovered from shellfish samples is indicative of

    (A) normal environmental conditions
    (B) improper storage of the shellfish
    (C) sewerage pollution of shellfish beds
    (D) shellfish eating patterns
    (E) poor sample collecting procedures

Items 42-44

A 65-year old woman, previously in excellent health, experienced a moderate intestinal tract infection. She had attended a neighborhood oriental restaurant at lunchtime. Within 5 hours she developed nausea and vomiting. Food poisoning was an obvious possibility. Samples of the different dishes consumed by the woman all contained low levels of different bacteria. A rice dish showed a high concentration of aerobic Gram-positive rods.

42. The appropriate treatment for the woman should consist of

    (A) only symptomatic aid
    (B) antibiotics effective against Gram-positive bacteria
    (C) antibiotics effective against Gram-negative bacteria
    (D) intravenous drug therapy
    (E) administration of an antitoxin

43. A possible causative organism would be

    (A) *Staphylococcus aureus*
    (B) *Bacillus anthracis*
    (C) *Clostridium botulinum*
    (D) *Bacillus cereus*
    (E) *Clostridium difficile*

44. The symptoms experienced by the patient are most probably due to

    (A) toxin production
    (B) bacteremia
    (C) sporulation
    (D) massive intestinal bacterial growth
    (E) an inflammatory response

Items 45-48

A 1-week-old newborn was admitted to the intensive care unit after an apparently normal delivery from a healthy mother. The infant had displayed abnormal eating patterns and reduced levels of behavioral alertness indicative of neurological involvement. The routine bacteriological cultures of both blood and CSF were negative. CSF plated on Eaton's agar yielded minute slow-growing colonies.

45. The observed bacteremia is most likely due to an infection caused by bacteria consisting of

    (A) Gram-positive organisms
    (B) Gram-negative organisms
    (C) Gram-variable organisms
    (D) non-Gram-stainable organisms
    (E) a mixed infection

46. Speciation of the causative agent(s) could be most accurately determined by

    (A) microscopic examination
    (B) carbohydrate fermentations
    (C) immunofluorescence using monoclonal antibody to surface antigens
    (D) growth on differential media
    (E) colony characteristics

47. An antibiotic generally prescribed in the treatment of this type of neonatal infection is

    (A) penicillin
    (B) tetracycline
    (C) chloramphenicol
    (D) erythromycin
    (E) gentamicin

48. Which of the following organisms best fits the isolate recovered from either the blood or CSF specimen?

    (A) *Listeria monocytogenes*
    (B) *Chlamydia trachomatis*
    (C) *Neisseria meningitidis*
    (D) *Haemophilus influenzae*
    (E) *Ureaplasma urealyticum*

Items 49-52

A second-year medical student chose to spend the summer working with a private relief organization. She was sent to a very rural Indian reservation in the western Badlands. Most of the visitors to the small clinic had not received periodic medical examinations. One child entered with symptoms of a tonsillitis; malaise, sore throat and fever. The tonsils and soft palate were covered by a gray-white membrane.

49. A Gram's stain of throat smears would show

(A) large Gram-negative rods
(B) small Gram-positive rods
(C) large Gram-positive cocci
(D) small Gram-negative cocci
(E) small club-shaped, Gram-negative rods

50. The student noted the unusual feature of the bacteria and tonsils and sent throat swabs away for microbial analysis which isolated

(A) β-hemolytic streptococci on blood agar
(B) complete hemolytic golden cocci on blood agar
(C) black colonies on Tinsdale agar
(D) blue-green colonies on blood agar
(E) minute clear colonies on Eaton's agar

51. The child has

(A) a simple strep throat
(B) a staph infection
(C) diphtheria
(D) a *Pseudomonas* infection
(E) mycoplasma pneumonia

52. The causative agent is

(A) *Streptococcus pyogenes*
(B) *Staphylococcus aureus*
(C) *Corynebacterium diphtheriae*
(D) *Pseudomonas aeruginosa*
(E) *Mycoplasma pneumoniae*

Items 53-56

A young woman gave birth to a healthy girl. The mother came from a rural area, was in good health and had received prenatal care. At home the energetic infant scratched herself along the left thigh resulting in a slight reddening which the mother noted and treated with an antibacterial ointment. A week later the skin on the infant's leg and hands started to peel. The infant was taken to a clinic where her infection was examined, cultures were taken and treatment was initiated.

53. The exfoliation of large areas of skin from different areas of the body suggests

(A) a systemic viral infection
(B) scalded skin syndrome (Ritter's disease)
(C) toxic shock syndrome
(D) a fungal infection
(E) parasitic infection

54. Bacterial cultures taken from wounds or abscesses on the infant will most likely show the presence of

(A) *Streptococcus pyogenes*
(B) *Pseudomonas aeruginosa*
(C) *Proteus vulgaris*
(D) *Staphylococcus aureus*
(E) *Staphylococcus epidermidis*

55. The exfoliation associated with the infection is caused by

(A) α-toxin
(B) leukocidin
(C) toxic shock syndrome toxin-1
(D) coagulase
(E) exfoliative toxin

56. Treatment of the infection usually requires

(A) drainage of any abscess and treatment with penicillin
(B) treatment with penicillin
(C) treatment with nafcillin or cloxacillin
(D) drainage of any abscess and treatment with nafcillin or cloxacillin
(E) drainage of the abscess

Items 57-60

Two weeks prior to the Christmas vacation holiday, a sixth-grade student developed a severe pharyngitis. He also complained of fever and tenderness in his joints. A thorough examination of the child revealed that an infection had existed even earlier but was not reported by the child. Pain was experienced in multiple joints. His throat was grossly inflamed and throat swab culture produced small, clear, β-hemolytic colonies on blood agar.

57. The symptoms are consistent with early stages of

    (A) croup
    (B) scarlet fever
    (C) rheumatic fever
    (D) typhoid fever
    (E) Q fever

58. The causative organism is

    (A) parainfluenza viruses
    (B) *Salmonella typhi*
    (C) *Streptococcus pyogenes*
    (D) *Coxiella burnetii*
    (E) *Staphylococcus aureus*

59. Which of the following antigens produced by the organism is an antiphagocytic virulence factor?

    (A) α-hemolysin
    (B) β-hemolysin
    (C) C carbohydrates
    (D) M protein
    (E) Coagulase

60. An antibiotic effective in the treatment of the infection is

    (A) penicillin
    (B) tetracycline
    (C) chloramphenicol
    (D) sulfadiazine
    (E) neomycin

Items 61-65

A group of 25 fifth-grade students had lunch at a fast food restaurant. Most ate hamburgers and french fries prepared quickly for the noontime rush. The next day most of the children experienced severe bloody diarrhea and nausea with several requiring hospitalization. Stool and blood cultures recovered small, Gram-negative, nonmucoid bacilli which fermented lactose, were indole-positive, produced acid and carbon dioxide but produced neither hydrogen sulfide nor urease.

61. The organism most likely responsible for the intestinal infection is

    (A) *Pseudomonas aeruginosa*
    (B) *Proteus vulgaris*
    (C) *Klebsiella pneumoniae*
    (D) *Vibrio cholerae*
    (E) *Escherichia coli*

62. Serotyping of these organisms is based primarily on the

    (A) capsule antigens
    (B) flagella (H) antigens
    (C) somatic (O) and (H) antigens
    (D) cell membrane antigens
    (E) cytoplasmic antigens

63. The K (pili) antigens may bind to a host cell ligand ending in

    (A) glucose
    (B) fructose
    (C) maltose
    (D) mannose
    (E) galactosamine

64. The organism isolated from the children might be best categorized as

    (A) enterotoxigenic
    (B) enteroinvasive
    (C) enterohemorrhagic
    (D) enteropathogenic
    (E) enterogenic

65. The potent toxin expressed by this diarrhea-producing isolate is due to the expression of

    (A) LT (heat labile toxin)
    (B) ST (heat stabile toxin)
    (C) *Shigella dysenteriae*-like toxin type 1
    (D) *Salmonella*-like enterotoxin
    (E) *Vibrio*-like toxin

Items 66-67

A young mother became concerned when her 24-month-old infant daughter developed a mild fever and cried continuously. The infant drooled excessively with difficulty sleeping and eating. The pediatrician, bowing to the mothers's requests, performed bacterial cultures of the infant's blood, saliva, urine and stool specimen. The symptoms continued for several days before slowly subsiding.

Here are the results from the lab tests on the infant's specimens.

Blood: negative

Saliva: viridans streptococci, *Lactobacillus* sp

Urine: negative

Stool: *Escherichia coli*, *Lactobacillus* sp, *Bacteroides* sp, *Clostridium* sp

66. The bacteriological findings are consistent with

    (A) possible enteric infection
    (B) hemolytic streptococcal infection
    (C) bacteremia
    (D) respiratory tract infection
    (E) normal flora

67. All of the following are considered normal microbial flora of the colon EXCEPT

    (A) *Bacteroides* sp
    (B) *Fusobacterium* sp
    (C) *Clostridium* sp
    (D) *Escherichia* sp
    (E) *Vibrio* sp

Items 68-78

Many bacteria are associated with commonly occurring illnesses. Routine microscopic analysis of cultures, in many cases, forms the basis for highly reliable preliminary diagnosis of infections. Match the following brief descriptions of bacteria structure and illnesses with the most commonly associated Gram-negative and Gram-variable bacteria.

(A) *Pasteurella multocida*
(B) *Proteus mirabilis*
(C) *Proteus vulgaris*
(D) *Pseudomonas aeruginosa*
(E) *Pseudomonas pseudomallei*
(F) *Rickettsia prowazekii*
(G) *Rickettsia rickettsii*
(H) *Rickettsia tsutsugamushi*
(I) *Salmonella enteritidis*
(J) *Salmonella typhi*
(K) *Shigella dysenteriae*
(L) *Shigella sonnei*
(M) *Treponema pallidum*
(N) *Treponema pertenue*
(O) *Ureaplasma urealyticum*
(P) *Vibrio cholerae*
(Q) *Vibrio parahemolyticus*
(R) *Yersinia enterocolitica*
(S) *Yersinia pestis*

68. A 32-year-old man experienced diarrhea, cramps and bloody, squirty stools following a business encounter group session in a campsite area. Stool specimen plated on MacConkey agar produced white colonies which Gram-stained as negative rods.

69. A teenage boy developed a urethritis and went to the clinic. The Gram stain, chocolate agar and blood agar were all negative. Specimen plated on Eaton's agar (supplemented with urea) produced minute colonies after 2 weeks incubation.

70. A male hunter noticed a rash on his legs that spread to his hands. The first rash appeared where he had removed ticks after an outing in the woods. A serum sample was positive for all antigens in the Weil-Felix test.

71. A 12-year-old boy stepped on broken glass and received medical attention. However he did not complete the follow-up directions and the wound became infected. A lactose non-fermenting rod was isolated. It was resistant to many antibiotics.

72. A woman received a deep claw gash from her pet cat. The wound became infected within 24 hours. A fast-growing, oxidase-positive rod was isolated.

73. A young boy near Denver, Colorado, was playing with a dead prairie dog. Several days later he became sick and his condition was diagnosed as bubonic plague.

74. The serum of a traveling salesman was positive in the VDRL test and the FTA-ABS test.

75. Construction workers became sick with diarrhea, stomach cramps and vomiting. The isolate was lactose nonfermenting, motile and produced hydrogen sulfide.

76. Bacteria from a urinary tract infection produced swarming colonies on blood agar but not MacConkey agar. The isolate produced hydrogen sulfide, was urease-positive but was indole-negative.

77. A refugee from India developed severe diarrhea which produced rice water stools with no accompanying blood. A comma-shaped bacteria was isolated which grew faster under alkaline conditions.

78. The retired army soldier had fever and headaches, symptoms which were similar to the epidemic typhus he experienced years earlier. He had been confined to a hospital nursing home for the previous 4 years.

Items 79-90

Many bacteria are associated with commonly occurring illnesses. Routine microscopic analysis of cultures, in many cases, forms the basis for highly reliable preliminary diagnosis of infections. Match the following brief descriptions of bacteria structure and illnesses with the most commonly associated Gram-positive bacteria.

(A) *Actinomyces israelii*
(B) *Bacillus anthracis*
(C) *Bacillus cereus*
(D) *Bacillus subtilis*
(E) *Bacillus thuringiensis*
(F) *Clostridium botulinum*
(G) *Clostridium difficile*
(H) *Clostridium perfringens*
(I) *Clostridium tetani*
(J) *Corynebacterium diphtheriae*
(K) *Lactobacillus acidophilus*
(L) *Listeria monocytogenes*
(M) *Staphylococcus aureus*
(N) *Staphylococcus epidermidis*
(O) *Staphylococcus enterocolitis*
(P) *Streptococcus pyogenes* Group A
(Q) *Streptococcus pneumoniae*
(R) *Streptococcus mutans*
(S) *Mycobacterium avium-intracellulare*
(T) *Mycobacterium leprae*
(U) *Mycobacterium tuberculosis*
(V) *Nocardia asteroides*

79. Four members of the same family consumed home-made canned beans and became extremely sick and experienced a slight paralysis. The toxin is produced under anaerobic conditions by these club-shaped organisms.

80. A 10-year-old boy had his semiannual dental cleaning. The dentist found some tooth decay. Which bacteria are frequently associated with dental caries?

81. An 82-year-old man was admitted to a US hospital in the Philippines. He showed numerous cuts, burns and bruises on his hands and face. He appeared insensitive to pain in these areas. Tissue biopsy showed acid-fact bacteria.

82. A group of pre-schoolers attending a day care facility all developed fevers and severe sour throats. Cultures of throat swabs grew up β-hemolytic cocci which were bacitracin-sensitive.

83. A middle-aged woman cut her scalp while working in her attic. The cut was improperly treated and became purulent. White colonies, of clumped cocci, causing no hemolysis, were recovered on blood agar. The organisms failed to clot plasma.

84. Two workers on a small ranch discovered sick and dying cattle in the field. One developed vesicular lesions on his hands which formed into black eschars. A stained specimen showed large rods in chains with some bearing spores.

85. A camper in a remote region was involved in a shooting accident. He dressed his leg wound and attempted a 5-day hike for assistance. The wound became inflamed, developed a foul odor and discoloration. Later, physicians detected club-shaped bacteria.

86. Bacterial spores were isolated from an over-the-counter organic pesticide used to control Japanese beetles. It was shown not harmful to pets, adults or children.

87. An 8-year-old girl was diagnosed with meningitis. A Sample of her CSF was cultured on blood agar and produced minute, catalase-positive, clear colonies with β-hemolysis. Further tests showed motile rod-shaped organisms.

88. Researchers attempted to reestablish the proper pH and normal vaginal flora by introducing this organism. The rod-shaped bacteria produce lactic acid and are found in healthy women.

89. A scalp wound on a 45-year-old indigent woman became infected. A culture of the pus revealed clustered cocci which produced complete hemolysis on blood agar plates. A coagulase test was positive.

90. The x-ray film of a 54-year-old indigent man showed the classic Ghon complex of fibrous lesions. Sputum cultures produced yellowish colonies by the Ziehl-Neelsen procedure.

Items 91-101

Many bacteria are associated with commonly occurring illnesses. Routine microscopic analysis of cultures, in many cases, forms the basis for highly reliable preliminary diagnosis of infections. Match the following brief descriptions of bacterial structure and illnesses with the most commonly associated Gram-negative and Gram-variable bacteria.

(A) *Bacteroides fragilis*
(B) *Bordetella pertussis*
(C) *Borrelia burgdorferi*
(D) *Borrelia recurrentis*
(E) *Brucella abortus*
(F) *Campylobacter fetus*
(G) *Campylobacter jejuni*
(H) *Chlamydia psittaci*
(I) *Chlamydia trachomatis*
(J) *Coxiella burnetii*
(K) *Escherichia coli*
(L) *Klebsiella pneumoniae*
(M) *Gardnerella vaginalis*
(N) *Haemophilus ducreyi*
(O) *Haemophilus influenzae*
(P) *Legionella pneumophila*
(Q) *Leptospira interrogans*
(R) *Mycoplasma hominis*
(S) *Mycoplasma pneumoniae*
(T) *Neisseria gonorrhoeae*
(U) *Neisseria meningitidis*

91. A cervical smear from a 42-year-old-woman with cervicitis was cultured and Gram-stained for *Neisseria*. The culture was Gram-negative. A similar sample plated on mouse fibroblast cells and Giemsa stained, showed cytoplasmic inclusions containing minute cocci.

92. A Chinese-American undergraduate student noticed a large, red blotch on her leg. Two weeks earlier she removed tiny deer ticks from her body following a camping trip. Tissue biopsy showed spirochetes.

93. The raw wool processor developed high fever and loss of concentration. Weil-Felix reaction on serum was negative. Serological tests for the agent of Q fever was positive.

94. A new mother developed a high fever following the birth of her first child. Cord blood cultures where negative on blood agar but positive on Eaton's agar.

95. The Gram's stain of urethral discharge smear showed the presence of pink diplococci inside and surrounding polymorphonuclear leukocytes. Oxidase-positive white colonies grew on Thayer-Martin agar.

96. A 10-year-old boy was diagnosed with meningitis. His CSF showed no growth on blood agar. White colonies grew on chocolate agar. Both X- and V-factors were required for colony growth. The Gram's stain showed rods.

97. A 19-year-old female college student described a vaginal infection to her doctor. White colonies were recovered on blood and chocolate agar. A Gram's stain showed variable coccobacilli.

98. Several children in a first grade class developed diarrhea that lasted 2-5 days. One type of organism grew best under microaerophilic conditions. It was oxidase-positive and showed curved rods in the Gram's stain.

99. A bronchial lavage specimen from a 56-year-old man with pneumonia produced creamy white colonies on blood agar. On Endo agar, mucoid, stringy colonies were found. Gram's stain showed rods with halos surrounding them.

100. An abscess developed following abdominal surgery on an elderly woman. Nothing grew on blood, nutrient or EMB agar. Abscess fluid plated on blood, nutrient and EMB agar grew no colonies. The specimen showed the presence of coccobacilli. Identical media did produce colonies when incubated in a candle jar.

101. A retired army sergeant contracted pneumonia a week after a visit to Pennsylvania. Microabscesses and inflammatory exudates developed as the disease progressed. Bronchial lavages showed a few pleomorphic thin rods, but cultivation on most media failed to produce any colonies.

Item 102-104

A diagnosis of malaria was made in the case of a 23-year old female who recently immigrated to the United States from Vietnam. During treatment of the parasitic infection she developed shaking chills and spiking fever. Several days later, small clusters of vesicles appeared around her mouth and nostrils.

102. The most likely cause of the facial lesions is

(A) Coxsackie B virus
(B) herpes simplex virus
(C) varicella-zoster virus
(D) variola virus
(E) vaccinia virus

103. The most likely site of latency for this virus is the

(A) dorsal root ganglion
(B) sacral ganglion
(C) trigeminal ganglion
(D) adenoid tissue
(E) cornea

104. One method for distinguishing different viruses of the same group could include studying

(A) inclusion formation within infected tissues
(B) neutralizing antibodies
(C) size of the vesicles
(D) location of the vesicles
(E) age of the patient

Items 105-107

A 22-year-old homosexual male had severe colds accompanied by copious bloody sputum with greenish flecks, fever, overall loss of energy and skin rashes. He underwent a physical examination which included a full blood workup. His overall cell count was within the normal range with the exception of his $CD4^+$ cells which was $150/mm^3$ (normal range 300-1200).

105. The heavy sputum may have been due to an opportunist infection caused by

    (A) *Chlamydia pneumoniae*
    (B) *Streptococcus pneumoniae*
    (C) *Mycoplasma pneumoniae*
    (D) *Mycobacterium tuberculosis*
    (E) influenza A virus

106. The patient's profile best fits that of an individual infected with

    (A) HIV
    (B) Epstein-Barr virus
    (C) influenza A virus
    (D) coronavirus
    (E) adenovirus

107. Drugs used in the treatment of the pathogen include all of the following EXCEPT

    (A) AZT
    (B) ddI
    (C) ddC
    (D) interferon
    (E) acyclovir

Item 108-112

A 4-year-old African-American male developed a fever, sore throat and unusual irritability. A physical examination revealed 15-25 small, gray-white, shallow, ulcerative lesions along the posterior margin of his soft palate. The pharyngeal walls were extremely red. There were no lesions on the gum but a few on the anterior part of the oral cavity. The child was dark-complexioned and had no obvious rash.

108. The most likely diagnosis is

    (A) herpetic gingivostomatitis
    (B) measles
    (C) chickenpox
    (D) herpangina
    (E) hand, foot and mouth disease

109. The causative viral agent is most likely a

    (A) herpes simplex virus
    (B) enterovirus
    (C) paramyxovirus
    (D) varicella-zoster virus
    (E) rhabdovirus

110. The lesions found in the child's mouth are called

    (A) pustules
    (B) Koplik's spots
    (C) Negri bodies
    (D) Byran's spots
    (D) pocks

111. Another name for the disease is

    (A) rubella
    (B) roseola infantum
    (C) rubeola
    (D) relapsing fever
    (E) rheumatic fever

112. Transmission of the disease occurs primarily through

(A) intimate contact
(B) inhalation of aerosol droplets
(C) ingestion of contaminated foods
(D) the bite of an arthropod vector
(E) blood transfusions or other blood products

Items 113-117

For each of the numbered human tumors, choose the lettered virus thought to cause the malignant disease.

(A) Human papilloma virus
(B) Hepatitis B virus
(C) Hepatitis C virus
(D) Herpes simplex virus type 2
(E) Epstein-Barr virus
(F) Human T cell leukemia virus
(G) Human immunodeficiency virus
(H) Rous sarcoma virus

113. Cervical carcinoma

114. Hepatocellular carcinoma

115. Burkitt's lymphoma

116. Nasopharyngeal carcinoma

117. Hairy-cell leukemia

Items 118-121

A young child was immunized with the Salk polio vaccine. A month later, he was given a booster shot of the same vaccine. Studies designed to monitor the child's seroconversion, by measuring both IgM and IgG titers against the vaccine antigen, revealed the serum titer profile shown in **Figure 6.1** below

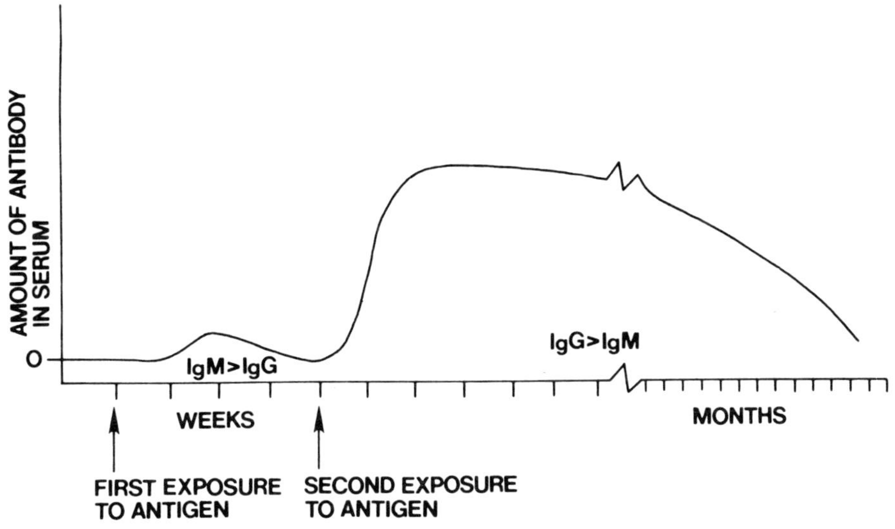

Figure 6.1

118. The heightened level of antibody production following the booster vaccination is commonly referred to as

   (A) differentiation
   (B) stimulation
   (C) memory
   (D) recognition
   (E) activation

119. The immunoglobulin first produced after first exposure to a new antigen is

   (A) IgA
   (B) IgM
   (C) IgE
   (D) IgG
   (E) IgD

120. The longest lived immunoglobulin normally found after the booster vaccination is

   (A) IgA
   (B) IgM
   (C) IgE
   (D) IgG
   (E) IgD

121. Immunoglobulin class switching involves plasma cell clones making

   (A) IgG and IgM of different specificities
   (B) IgM and IgG of the same specificity
   (C) IgM rather than IgG of the same specificity
   (D) IgG, IgA or IgE rather that IgM of the same specificity
   (E) IgM rather than IgG, IgA or IgE of the same specificity

Items 122-125

The mother of an 8-month-old boy noted an unusual recurring illnesses consisting of upper respiratory tract infections, most likely of viral origin. No members of the household had similar infections, however some visiting relatives showed signs of infections. The infant had consistently congested nasal passages and wheezed with each breath. A physical examination detected mild facial hypoplasia. Microbiological studies did not indicate any bacterial infections. Serum immunoglobulin levels were within the average range. Blood chemistry indicated hypocalcemia.

122. A disease which follows this particular pattern of immunodeficiency in infants is

(A) Bruton's agammaglobulinemia
(B) DiGeorge syndrome
(C) Wiskott-Aldrich syndrome
(D) ataxia-telangiectasia
(E) Chédiak-Higashi syndrome

123. The immune dysfunction is due to

(A) congenital viral infection
(B) toxin effect during pregnancy
(C) bone marrow malformation
(D) thymus and parathyroids malformed
(E) defect in stem cell differentiation

124. An examination of the infant's immune functions would most likely indicate a deficiency of

(A) B cell number and function
(B) T cell number and function
(C) macrophage number and function
(D) plasma cell number and function
(E) complement titer and function

125. Which of the following would be most effective in overcoming the deficiency?

(A) blood transfusion
(B) cytokine therapy
(C) thymic transplant
(D) bone marrow transplant
(E) gamma globulin treatment

Items 126-130

The mother of an 8-month-old boy brought him to the pediatrician for the second time in a month. The child appeared to have developed a strep throat infection somewhat similar to one he previously experienced. The child experienced a high fever and extreme irritability due to his condition. Bacterial cultures grew β-hemolytic *Streptococcus pyogenes.* The total level of IgG, IgA and IgM in his serum was only 65 mg/dL. Antibiotics were prescribed to arrest the bacterial infection.

126. The recurrent pyogenic infections experienced by the boy, along with his low overall serum immunoglobulin level suggests

    (A) persistent infections by drug-resistant bacteria
    (B) an immunodeficiency
    (C) the mother is a carrier of the bacteria
    (D) misdiagnosis of earlier infections
    (E) age-related immunodeficiency

127. A disease which results in the markedly reduced levels of all immunoglobulins is

    (A) Bruton's agammaglobulinemia
    (B) DiGeorge syndrome
    (C) Wiskott-Aldrich syndrome
    (D) ataxia-telangiectasia
    (E) Chédiak-Higashi syndrome

128. The defective gene causing this disease is located on which chromosome?

    (A) Chromosome number 13
    (B) Chromosome number 18
    (C) Chromosome number 20
    (D) The X chromosome
    (E) The Y chromosome

129. The basis of the low total immunoglobulin level is a

    (A) T cell deficiency
    (B) B cell deficiency
    (C) complement deficiency
    (D) phagocyte deficiency
    (E) disease acquired deficiency

130. Treatment of the patient, in addition to antibiotics, would include

    (A) passive immunization
    (B) active immunization
    (C) transfusions
    (D) immunosupressive drugs
    (E) cytokine administration

Items 131-134

A 28-year-old Caucasian woman had been diagnosed with tuberculosis based on a positive tuberculin skin test and the presence of acid-fast bacilli in her sputum. Chest x-rays were negative. She was prescribed long-term antibiotic treatment. During her next annual physical examination, the doctor noticed a faint facial rash. Tests of her $CD4^+/CD8^+$ lymphocytes were near normal. Serological test for measles was negative, but positive for certain autoantibodies.

131. The presence of anti-DNA antibody can be used in a preliminary diagnosis of

(A) chronic thyroiditis
(B) allergic encephalitis
(C) rheumatic fever
(D) myasthenia gravis
(E) systemic lupus erythematosus

132. The autoantibodies present in the young woman would most likely react specifically against

(A) thyroid antigens
(B) brain myelin
(C) heart muscle sarcolemma proteins
(D) acetylcholine receptor proteins
(E) H2A-H2B histone proteins

133. Drug-induced autoimmune disease has been observed following long-term treatment with

(A) rifampin
(B) ethambutol
(C) isoniazid
(D) pyrazinamide
(E) streptomycin

134. Management of the disease is done through the use of

(A) gamma interferon (INF-γ)
(B) glucocorticoids
(C) plasmapheresis
(D) irradiation
(E) bone marrow transplants

Items 135-141

A 25-year-old Cambodian refugee in her first trimester of pregnancy developed abnormal symptoms consisting of frequent high fever (104°F) accompanied by malaise, headache, confusion and nausea in three-day cycles. Initially, she attributed the symptoms to her pregnancy but later reported them to her physician. Clinical findings included thrombocytopenia, tachycardia, splenomegaly, hemoglobinuria and anemia. She was admitted to the hospital and shortly went into a coma.

135. The correct presumptive diagnosis would be an infection caused by

(A) *Plasmodium vivax*
(B) *Plasmodium falciparum*
(C) *Toxoplasma gondii*
(D) *Pneumocystis carinii*
(E) *Plasmodium ovale*

136. A confirmation of the diagnosis could be made by

(A) a Giemsa-stained thin blood smear
(B) an indirect fluorescent antibody test (IFA)
(C) culturing a blood sample in an enriched medium
(D) direct microscopic examination of a fresh blood specimen
(E) patient history

137. Administration of the following drug(s) of choice would normally result in a dramatic cure?

(A) quinine sulfate, pyrimethamine and sulfadiazine
(B) chloroquine phosphate
(C) pyrimethamine, sulfadoxine and chloroquine
(D) quinine dihydrochloride, IV
(E) mefloquine

138. Organisms resistant to the first-choice treatment are given

(A) quinine sulfate, pyrimethamine and sulfadiazine
(B) chloroquine phosphate
(C) pyrimethamine, sulfadoxine and chloroquine
(D) quinine dihydrochloride, IV
(E) mefloquine

139. The vector for transmission of this disease is

(A) mosquitos
(B) fleas
(C) gnats
(D) raccoons
(E) parrots

140. The developmental form of the parasite transmitted during the biting process is the

(A) sporozoite
(B) merozoite
(C) hypnozoite
(D) macrogametes
(E) microgametes

141. Microscopic examination of stained, infected red cells would reveal

(A) ring-shaped tropozoites
(B) spherical gametocytes
(C) crescent-shaped gametocytes
(D) rod-shaped gametocytes
(E) beaded gametocytes

Items 142-146

A 28-year-old woman with an extensive prior history of IV heroin abuse, experienced severe headaches, disorientation, high fevers, lethargy and mild seizures lasting two weeks. She did not travel outside her home state of California, lived alone but had three cats and a small dog as house pets. Laboratory studies showed the presence of serum antibody against HIV and a low $CD4^+$ T cell count of 120 cells/mm^3. Chest x-rays appeared normal. Cerebrospinal fluid was negative for bacterial infection, negative for antibody against the picornaviruses and normal for protein. A heterophile test was negative. CT scans showed several small lesions in her frontal lobe.

142. The history and immune state of the individual are consistent to support further serological tests for

(A) malaria
(B) psittacosis
(C) *Pneumocystis carinii* pneumonia
(D) toxoplasmosis
(E) tuberculosis

143. A Giemsa-stained thin blood smear would most likely show

(A) large atypical monocytes
(B) clumped red blood cells
(C) crescent-shaped trophozoites
(D) circular cysts with flattened sides
(E) rod-shaped bacteria

144. Infection was most likely acquired through

(A) sexual contact
(B) IV drug abuse
(C) ingestion of contaminated foods
(D) inhalation of animal feces
(E) an animal bite

145. Drugs of choice used in treating the infection include

(A) trimethoprim-sulfamethoxazole
(B) sulfonamide-pyrimethamine
(C) amphotericin B
(D) sodium stibogluconate
(E) chloroquine

146. Pregnant women should not be exposed to the pathogen because

(A) there is a higher virulence in that population
(B) they are partially immunosuppressed
(C) there is risk of transplacental infection of fetus
(D) there is a greater possibility of CNS involvement
(E) there is a higher frequency of chronic infections

Items 147-150

A 33-year-old woman was diagnosed with an HIV infection two years ago and had undergone aggressive chemotherapy. Her $CD4^+$ T cell count had dropped below 200 cells/mm^3. She developed a pneumonia infection that resulted in the sudden onset of fever, dyspnea, coughs and tachypnea. X-ray images revealed diffuse interstitial pneumonia. Bronchial lavage specimens did not grow bacteria. Other tests ruled out viral pneumonia.

147. The immunocompromised state of the patient makes her a prime candidate for which of the following respiratory pathogens?

(A) *Candida albicans*
(B) *Aspergillus fumigatus*
(C) *Pneumocystis carinii*
(D) *Histoplasma capsulatum*
(E) *Blastomyces dermatitidis*

148. Inhalation of the organism into the lungs initially causes

(A) cell necrosis
(B) massive exfoliation of epithelial cells
(C) inflammation and a frothy exudate that blocks respiration
(D) secondary bacterial infections
(E) granuloma formation

149. Laboratory diagnosis is also based on observation of which of the following in silver-stained bronchial lavage specimens?

(A) mycelia
(B) hyphae
(C) cysts
(D) spores
(E) pigmented microcolonies

150. Drug of choice used in treating the infection include

(A) trimethoprim-sulfamethoxazole
(B) penicillin
(C) amphotericin B
(D) sodium stibogluconate
(E) chloroquine

Items 151-157

Match the parasitic organism in the answers with the most appropriate clinical scenario in the items below.

(A) *Giardia lamblia*
(B) *Taenia saginata*
(C) *Toxoplasma gondii*
(D) *Taenia solium*
(E) *Entamoeba histolytica*
(F) *Trichomonas vaginalis*
(G) *Trypanosoma cruzi*
(H) *Leishmania mexicana*
(I) *Pneumocystis carinii*
(J) *Ascaris lumbricoides*
(K) *Enterobius vermicularis*
(L) *Necator americanus*
(M) *Schistosoma mansoni*

151. A 19-year-old homosexual male developed a progressive pneumonia which did not respond to antibiotics. A silver stain of sputum and bronchial lavage specimens showed small circular cysts containing sporozoites.

152. An underweight 17-year-old girl from Panama was visiting her cousin in Philadelphia. She experienced fever, diarrhea and severe right upper quadrant pain. A fresh stool specimen revealed mobile trophozoites and cysts with four nuclei.

153. A 53-year-old camper developed a case of diarrhea and stomach cramps during the second week of a fishing trip in the Colorado mountains. Trophozoites, with owl-like features, and cysts were observed in his stool specimen. A duodenum string test was also positive for trophozoites.

154. An emaciated 18-year-old female complained of constant headaches and diarrhea. A stool specimen revealed flat proglottids. Microscopic examination showed less than 10 uterine branches per proglottid.

155. A 24-year-old medical student developed an irritating vaginal infection which produced an abundance of watery, whitish discharge. Microscopic examination of a wet mount showed pear-shaped trophozoites.

156. A mother noticed that her 9-year-old son was frequently scratching at his anus. The scratching resulted in a mild bacterial infection. Examination of his perianal region using the transparent tape method revealed tiny worms and small eggs.

157. A 28-year-old female CIA agent gave birth to an infant with splenomegaly and jaundice. Serological tests for the hepatitis viruses were negative. The mother had not traveled during the previous year. She lived with her boyfriend and three cats. Blood smears of the infant showed crescent-shaped trophozoites.

STOP.

YOU HAVE COMPLETED THIS SECTION.

Notes

Microbiology and Immunology

Answers and Tutorials

Answers and Tutorial on Items 1-4

The answers are: **1-A; 2-E; 3-B; 4-D**. ***Listeria monocytogenes*** is a Gram-positive rod and normally only causes asymptomatic transient infections in most adults. Patients infected with *Listeria* may become septic as the bacteria enter the blood. The bacteria may also enter the central nervous system, especially in immunocompromised adults. Pregnant women are most at risk because the organism can either infect the fetus by crossing the placental membrane or infect the neonate during transit through the birth canal. Stillbirths, abortions, premature births and neonates suffering from disseminated abscesses and/or granulomas may result.

A prime source of infection is through contaminated foods. *Listeria* is known to survive both pasteurization processes and refrigeration. Penicillin, ampicillin, erythromycin and chloramphenicol are all effective in treating the disease.

Answers and Tutorial on Items 5-6

The answers are: **5-C; 6-E**. ***Bacteroides*** sp are Gram-negative anaerobic organisms commonly associated with abscesses. They are normally found in the body, but are opportunistic, taking advantage of breaks in the mucosal lining. *Bacteroides melaninogenicus* causes oral, pharyngeal and pulmonary abscesses.

Standard blood agar cultivation will not yield colony growth. Anaerobic conditions are necessary with the inclusion of antibiotics, such as kanamycin and vancomycin present in the culture media, to reduce contamination by other bacteria.

Bacteroides melaninogenicus infections respond favorably to treatment with clindamycin. Penicillin sensitivity varies with different species of *Bacteroides*; *B. fragilis* is resistant, whereas *B. melaninogenicus* is sensitive.

Answers and Tutorial on Items 7-11

The answers are: **7-B; 8-C; 9-D; 10-C; 11-C**. The bacteria isolated from sputum and blood belong to the genus ***Streptococcus***. Some members of the genus such as *Streptococcus pneumoniae*, also called pneumococci, form short chains in which the bacteria appear paired. Each Gram-positive coccus is slightly elliptical. Overgrown cultures will stain variably as the bacteria loose viability. *S. pneumoniae* plated on blood agar forms clear flat colonies surrounded by zones of α-hemolysis. The organism is sensitive to optochin which distinguishes it from the viridans streptococci which also produce α-hemolysis on blood agar.

The quellung (capsule swelling) reaction has been used to serotype the pneumococci. The test uses antisera prepared against known serotypes of *S. pneumoniae*. A positive antibody-antigen reaction results in the swelling of the polysaccharide capsule which surrounds the organisms. There are over 80 capsule types. The antigenic properties of the capsule polysaccharide is the basis of pneumococcal vaccines.

Pneumococcal infections in either elderly or immunosuppressed patients are a major health concern because they are often life-threatening. The traditional drug of choice has been penicillin, however new drug-resistant strains have emerged. Chloramphenicol and erythromycin have been used as secondary drug choices. Virulence factors expressed in the pneumococci include pneumolysin which has enzymatic properties similar to neuraminidase. It cleaves sialic acid residues from glycoproteins and glycolipids, however its role in pathogenesis is still unclear. The ability of the polysaccharide capsule to prevent phagocytosis is an important virulence factor.

Pneumococcal disease in the elderly patient causes respiratory tract failure by rapid growth in the alveoli, causing fluid production and white cell infiltration. Bacteremia may also cause endocarditis, meningitis, arthritis or peritonitis.

Answers and Tutorial on Items 12-15

The answers are: **12-A; 13-B; 14-D; 15-D**. Chancroid is a relatively rare venereal disease limited primarily to North America. It is caused by the bacteria ***Haemophilus ducreyi***. The infection is acquired through direct sexual contact. A non-indurated chancre, also referred to as a soft chancre—which distinguishes it from the indurated hard chancre associated with syphilis—develops on the penis. The bacteria may cause additional genital lesions along with invasion of the lymph nodes. An inflammatory response results in the recruitment of lymphocytes and plasma cells by relatively few bacteria.

Diagnosis in based on clinical symptoms and the isolation of *H. ducreyi* on chocolate agar, supplemented with hematin (X factor). Like some members of the genus *Haemophilus*, it has a natural requirement for hematin for growth. Other species such as *H. influenzae* require both heme and NAD (V factor) for growth. Competing bacteria are reduced during isolation attempts by the inclusion of vancomycin in the growth agar to reduce overgrowth by other organisms.

Antibiotic resistance is a growing concern with *Haemophilus* sp. Many have acquired penicillin resistance through the acquisition of plasmid-derived β-lactamases. Penicillin is therefore prescribed less frequently. The new cephalosporins or sulfonamides are drugs of choice. Combination drug therapy with erythromycin and sulfonamide is also effective.

Answers and Tutorial on Items 16-18

The answers are: **16-B; 17-D; 18-B**. Bubonic plague is caused by the Gram-negative bacteria ***Yersinia pestis***. The bacterial infection is acquired through the bite of an infected flea followed by rapid multiplication in regional lymph nodes and dissemination to other organs. In this case, the right axilla was affected. Localized necrosis results from tissue damage and toxin production. Recovery confers natural immunity against reinfection. The more deadlier pneumonic plague, involving person-to-person transmission, may result from the inhalation of the bacteria.

A primary task of the project was the collection of small mammal pelts. Many such animals harbor parasites including fleas and ticks. The researcher, in an effort to economize on materials required for the study, substituted the usual chloroform used to euthanize animals, for less bulky nembutal. The latter is injected into animals; however, the former kills both the small animals and their harbored fleas. Therefore live fleas could have easily come into contact with the researcher and transmitted the pathogen.

Yersinia pestis has bipolar staining patterns and is easily recovered from bubo aspirate, blood and sputum. Vaccination against plague should be boosted every 1-2 years for those traveling in endemic regions. Treatment with streptomycin for 10 days will usually cure bubonic plague.

Answers and Tutorial on Items 19-21

The answers are: **19-B; 20-D; 21-A**. Lyme disease is a bacterial infection caused by the spirochete ***Borrelia burgdorferi***. It is a zoonotic infection within the deer and rat populations and accidentally transmitted to man through the bite of the deer tick. The extremely small size (<2mm) of the deer tick renders them difficult to detect. A large red petechial rash usually develops at the site of the tick bite. It may grow to over 10 cm in diameter. Different arthropod vectors are instrumental in the transmission of other *Borrelia* sp infections.

Relapsing fever is another disease caused by bacteria of the genus *Borrelia*. Syphilis and leptospirosis are diseases also caused by spirochetes. Leprosy is caused by the Gram-positive, acid-fast bacillus *Mycobacterium leprae*.

Answers and Tutorial on Items 22-26

The answers are: **22-C; 23-C; 24-A; 25-C; 26-E**. **Lyme disease** is caused by the bacteria *Borrelia burgdorferi*. The pathogen is transmitted through the bite of an arthropod vector, namely the deer tick *Ixodes dammini* and *I. pacificus*. The ticks are very small, measuring less than 2 mm, rendering them easily overlooked when they attach and feed. The ticks have been found on other animals including mice, rats, skunks, opossums and dogs.

The primary lesion grows into an enlarged rash as the spirochete proliferates and invades the blood and lymphatics. The lesion usually disappears after several weeks. Some individuals progress into a second stage of infection involving neurologic or cardiac abnormalities. An arthritic response may develop months to years after the initial infection, probably due to an autoimmune response. This is indicative of the third stage of Lyme's disease.

Answers and Tutorial on Items 27-30

The answers are: **27-B; 28-C; 29-B; 30-A**. Most ***Neisseria gonorrhoeae*** isolates respond to penicillin. Multiple drug resistant strains are becoming more frequent. Therapy against such organisms would not necessarily cause a diminution of symptoms. Drug resistance can be determined diagnostically using the classical agar plate antibiotic sensitivity tests (eg,

Kirby Bauer) and minimal inhibitory concentration (MIC) determination.

The overall response is best explained by a dual infection with another organism of different antibiotic sensitivity. Sexually transmitted disease clinics report high (>40%) instances of such dual infections consisting of *N. gonorrhoeae* and *Chlamydia trachomatis*, a major agent of nongonococcal urethritis. Chlamydiae do not respond to penicillin therapy. The tetracyclines, erythromycin and azithromycin are effective in treating chlamydial infections.

Answers and Tutorial on Items 31-36

The answers are: **31-B; 32-C; 33-D; 34-E; 35-B; 36-A**. There has been a reemergence of **tuberculosis** in the United States affecting a broad spectrum of the population. This is in part due to the increase of immune deficiency diseases, multiple drug resistance and noncompliance with prescribed antibiotic therapy regimen. ***Mycobacterium tuberculosis***, the causative agent of the disease, is acquired by the inhalation of respiratory droplets from infected individuals. Initial infection therefore takes place in the lungs with the formation of exudative lesions which progress into granulomatous and finally tubercle lesions consisting of walled-in bacteria, giant and epithelioid cells surrounded by fibrosis and calcification.

The highly immunogenic nature of the mycobacterial cell wall elicits a strong cell-mediated immune response. Purified protein derivative (PPD), administered intradermally, produces induration (thickening) and erythema (reddening) in the area of injection in previously exposed individuals. Induration in excess of 10 mm within 48-72 hours indicates a positive skin test. Virulence in the bacteria is closely correlated with the presence of cord factor (trehalose dimycolate) in the organisms. Most *Mycobacteria* sp display slow growth rates. The cell-mediated immune response attempts to restrict the spread in healthy individuals, therefore immunocompromised individuals are more prone to infections. *M. avium-intracellulare* is an atypical mycobacterium and has been observed with high frequency in such patients.

Antibiotic therapy usually consists of a combination of isoniazid, rifampicin, ethambutol (or streptomycin) or pyrazinamide, sometimes for more than 6 months. The extended period is necessary because of the slow-growing nature of the bacteria and to enable the drugs to permeate granulomatous and tubercle lesions.

Answers and Tutorial on Items 37-38

The answers are: **37-D; 38-A**. Hospital-acquired, or **nosocomial**, infections require continued surveillance and adherence to proper hygiene practices on the part of all health care providers. ***Pseudomonas aeruginosa*** is among the most common nosocomial pathogens and most difficult to treat due to its broad range of antibiotic resistance. Burn patients are among those at high risk from this pathogen due to its ability to survive under conditions of low nutrient requirement on surfaces and stagnant water. Growth properties on EMB, colony pigmentation and the aromatic compounds they produce make them easy to identify. Contamination of hospital solutions (eg, IV fluids or antibiotics) by *Pseudomonas* is less likely than floors, walls, drinking water, dialysis machinery, whirl pools and machinery. Medical personnel may harbor the bacteria and pass it, unknowingly, during routine patient examinations.

Staphylococcus aureus, a Gram-positive coccus, is a major nosocomial agent infecting surgical wounds and injuries. Many individuals carry staphylococcal organisms on their skin and upper respiratory tract. It is the most prevalent of the Gram-positive cocci causing hospital-acquired infections, followed by *Streptococci* sp.

All hygienic measures such as washing, disinfection and sterilization of potential sources of contamination will reduce the probability of pathogen spread. The indiscriminate use of antibiotics, in the long run, will only result in the selection of more fastidious antibiotic-resistant microbes.

Answers and Tutorial on Items 39-41

The answers are: **39-A; 40-B; 41-C**. Public Health Departments in most states closely regulate the sale of shellfish. Some guidelines include the tagging and tracing of such foods especially those crossing interstate lines. Gastroenteritis is not always traced to a specific causative agent, but rather several potential pathogens.

A variety of bacterial, viral and parasitic pathogens are associated with the consumption of raw shellfish. ***Serratia*** sp are not normally associated with the high salt conditions of shellfish-associated diseases, but rather nosocomial infections.

Clostridium perfringens is a spore forming bacterium listed in item 39. The enterotoxin is associated with the spore wall. It is released during germination.

Many ***Vibrio*** organisms are water-borne. They have a high tolerance to sea water, thus they are commonly isolated from shellfish and fish. Disease results from colonization of the bacteria in the intestines and release of exotoxins. Diarrheal infections caused by *Vibrio parahemolyticus* respond to antibiotic therapy which also diminishes the likelihood of secondary infections and shortens the duration of diarrhea. Tetracycline, ampicillin and chloramphenicol are among the drugs used for this purpose.

The abruptness of the symptoms following consumption of the foods imply the presence, in the foods, of significant toxin. However, rapid colonization of the gastrointestinal tract and toxin production are characteristics of certain bacteria such as *V. parahemolyticus.* Improper storage and extended shipping intervals may provide additional favorable conditions for bacterial growth and toxin production. High colony counts of ***Escherichia coli*** are indicative of fecal contamination. The waters of shellfish collection may have been polluted with human sewage.

Answers and Tutorial on Items 42-44

The answers are: **42-A; 43-D; 44-A**. The spores of Gram-positive aerobes such as the ***Bacillus*** sp can cause gastrointestinal illnesses which mimic food poisoning caused by other organisms. Grains may harbor spores not destroyed by routine cooking and reheating. This allows the vegetative bacteria to colonize and release toxins into prepared foods. This is most true of the aerobic bacilli such as *Bacillus cereus.*

The **gastroenteritis** usually lasts briefly without the development of bacteremia. Transient colonization of the gastrointestinal tract occurs without the necessity of any specific antibiotic treatment. Antidiarrhetics are usually sufficient remedy for the infection which will resolve itself.

Answers and Tutorial on Items 45-48

The answers are: **45-D; 46-C; 47-D; 48-E**. An increasing number of women are asymptomatic carriers of *Mycoplasma* sp in the genital tract. ***Ureaplasma urealyticum*** is the slowest-growing of *Mycoplasma* sp. They are isolatable on special nutrient media, such as Eaton's agar, which contains highly purified ingredients and antibiotics which prevent the overgrowth of most conventional bacteria. As with all mycoplasmas, *Ureaplasma* sp do not contain a cell wall, thus do not react with Gram's stain. The absence of a cell wall also precludes the choice of the penicillins. The organisms are surrounded only by a cell membrane, which contains species-specific antigens and others which cross-react with human antigens. Many are pleomorphic. *Ureaplasma* sp differ from *Mycoplasma* sp by their urea requirement. All mycoplasmal organisms require sterols for growth.

There are approximately 14 recognized serovars of *Ureaplasma urealyticum.* Most have invasive abilities and are not normally found in either the blood or cerebrospinal fluid of healthy people; however, there are reported cases involving the latter, as presented in this case history. Generally they are confined to the surface colonization of epithelial cells of the genital tract of infected individuals. *Ureaplasma* sp are easily distinguished by the presence of unique membrane antigens detectable using immunofluorescence and monoclonal antisera.

Erythromycin is an effective antibiotic in the treatment of *Ureaplasma* infections. It is active in the inhibition of bacterial protein synthesis, as is tetracycline, but without the deleterious side effects on developing bones in the newborn.

Answers and Tutorial on Items 49-52

The answers are: **49-E; 50-C; 51-C; 52-C**. Most children are immunized against ***Corynebacterium diphtheriae***, a club-shaped, Gram-negative bacterium that causes **diphtheria**. In isolated populations, where immunization practices are not stringently applied, children are susceptible to rapidly-spreading outbreaks. The tonsils of infected children are usually covered by a gray-white membrane consisting of bacteria, dead epithelial cells, fibrin and white cells resulting from the actions of the potent diphtheria toxin. The bacteria, *Corynebacterium diphtheriae*, display a characteristic appearance of club-shaped, Gram-negative rods.

A major priority in the treatment of diphtheria is the neutralization of the toxin by antitoxin through passive immunization and inactivation of bacteria by antibiotics. The ready-made immune globulin inactivates unbound toxin while antibiotics such as erythromycin, penicillins, cephalosporins or tetracycline kill the bacteria.

The diphtheria toxin, produced by toxigenic strains, consists of plasmid-encoded gene products composed of two subunits. The B-subunit is required for adherence to susceptible host cells. The A-subunit enters the cell and disrupts transcription by inactivating the transcriptional elongation factor 2 (EF2). The inhibition is irreversible, but results in cell death. Immunity is established by administering vaccine consisting of toxoid and booster injections.

Answers and Tutorial on Items 53-56

The answers are: **53-B; 54-D; 55-E; 56-D**. Scalded skin syndrome or **Ritter's disease** is one of many diseases caused by ***Staphylococcus aureus***. The organisms are Gram-positive cocci which appear randomly scattered in stained smear preparations. They colonize different portions of the skin and take opportunistic advantage of access into the body through cuts, wounds or confined locations such as certain vaginal tampons. Staphylococci in abscesses produce a variety of exotoxins which have profound pathological actions in distal parts of the body.

Exfoliative toxin causes the exfoliation of the epidermal skin layer commonly seen in scalded skin syndrome. The bacterial infection is commonly acquired by the infant, from the mother, during birth. The infant experiences a minor cut allowing the bacteria to establish an abscess. The toxin is absorbed into the blood stream and acts on the skin far from the abscess. *Staphylococcus aureus* produce many other toxins such as enterotoxin, which induces diarrhea and vomiting; toxic shock syndrome toxin-1, which can cause muscle cramps, fever and diarrhea; and α-toxin, which may cause skin necrosis and hemolysis.

Antigenic differences in the surface receptors are used to distinguish the different strains of staphylococci. Phage typing is based on the presence of such receptors demonstrated by the ability of different phage to attach, infect and lyse specific *Staphylococcus aureus* isolates.

Treatment of staphylococcal infections usually involves drainage of any prominent abscesses and antibiotic therapy. Many *Staphylococcus aureus* isolates produce penicillinase and are therefore resistant to penicillin. Beta-lactamase-resistant penicillins such as nafcillin, methicillin or cloxacillin have been effective.

Answers and Tutorial on Items 57-60

The answers are: **57-C; 58-C; 59-D; 60-A**. **Rheumatic fever** develops as a result of a prior pharyngitis caused by ***Streptococcus pyogenes***. The organism causes an initial sore throat which progresses into a major pharyngitis with fever, exudate, leukocytosis and tender regional lymph nodes. An autoimmune reaction develops against joint tissue. A scarlet fever rash may develop in susceptible individuals if the bacteria produces an erythrogenic toxin. Penicillin G is the drug of choice in the treatment of *Streptococcus pyogenes* infections.

Other toxins produced by *Streptococcus pyogenes* includes streptokinase, a plasminogen activator; hyaluronidase, which dissolves connective tissue; streptolysin O, which lysis red blood cells and is used as a diagnostic parameter for streptococcal infections; streptodornase, a DNA nuclease; and streptolysin S, another hemolysin.

Streptococci sp are grouped based of the carbohydrate characteristics of the surface antigens called the Lancefield groupings. Group A are β-hemolytic and, by definition, sensitive to bacitracin. Other members of the genus are resistant to bacitracin and vary in bile solubility and ability to grow in high NaCl media. M protein found on the surface of the bacteria has antiphagocytic activity and therefore serves as a virulence factor. The Group A streptococci are positive for the M protein.

Answers and Tutorial on Items 61-65

The answers are: **61-E; 62-E; 63-D; 64-C; 65-C**. Intestinal infections caused by pathogenic strains of ***Escherichia coli*** have remained a major public health concern due to the like-threatening nature of some infections. *E. coli* are easily identified by their ability to grow on a number of synthetic media. Lactose fermentation with the production of acid and gas are characteristic identifiers. These organisms produce neither urease nor hydrogen sulfide which distinguishes them from many *Proteus* species.

Typing of *E. coli* isolates is dependent on the somatic O antigens and flagellar H antigens. The pili (K) antigen may act as an adhesin which enables the organism to adhere and colonize the intestinal tract. A terminal mannose sugar residue on the mucosal surface is an important ligand in the attachment of bacteria to host cells.

The virulence of the many different strains is dependent on the type of plasmid or virus-controlled toxin. The heat-labile (LT) and heat-stabile (ST) toxins are both involved in diarrhea. They are found in the enterotoxigenic *E. coli* (ETEC) strains. The enteroinvasive *E. coli* (EIEC) strains rarely cause diarrhea. The enteropathogenic *E. coli* (EPEC) strains produce diarrhea and both ST and LT.

The most virulent of these organisms belong to the enterohemorrhagic *E. coli* (EHEC) strains. These express LT, ST and a very potent *Shigella dysenteriae*-like type 1 toxin. Bloody diarrhea is a characteristic of this group of bacteria. Advanced infection may prove fatal. The O157:H7 serotype is the most virulent EHEC because it expresses all three toxins. The *Shigella dysenteriae*-like type 1 toxin inhibits host cell protein synthesis resulting in cell death.

Rapid typing of *E. coli* isolates has been advanced through the use of DNA probes which identify those strains expressing the O157:H7 antigens. Aggressive treatment with antibiotics is important with individuals infected with EHEC strains.

Answers and Tutorial on Items 66-67

The answers are: **66-E; 67-E**. Occasionally the disposition or transient irritability of an individual, especially of infants, might be interpreted as symptoms of microbial infection. The bacteriological findings in specimens taken from the infant are consistent with normal flora. Many body sites are colonized by avirulent organisms or opportunistic bacteria. These organisms are blocked from entering the body by epithelial barriers such as the epidermis. ***Staphylococcus aureus*** isolated from the surface of the skin is not an unusual finding; however, its presence in wounds, blood or inner ear infections is cause for alarm and warrants antibiotic treatment.

All of the bacteria isolated from the stool specimen are normal, however organisms such as *Vibrio* sp could represent possible enteric infection. Bacteria account for approximately 25% of the mass of human adult feces. Infants, because they consume human or animal milk, often harbor large numbers of *Lactobacillus* sp in their saliva and stools.

Body specimens such as blood, urine, CSF and tissues are normally free of bacteria. Tears, however contain low numbers of bacteria even in the presence of lysozyme. Constant exposure to the environment accounts for the ever present low number of bacteria in tears.

The infant was free of bacterial infection based on the specimens tested. Factors such as her general disposition, teething or family tensions may have accounted for the observed symptoms. Similarly, a nonbacterial factor could have been responsible. This seems unlikely because the symptoms abated soon after examination and required only supportive treatment from the pediatrician.

Answers and Tutorial on Items 68-78

The answers are: **68-L; 69-O; 70-G; 71-D; 72-A; 73-S; 74-M; 75-I; 76-B; 77-P; 78-F.** ***Pasteurella multocida*** (A) is associated with dog or cat bites or scratches. The fast growing organism produces toxic effects within 24 hours of the encounter. The bacteria ferments many sugars and gives an oxidase-positive reaction.

Proteus mirabilis (B) infects the urinary tract. It has a characteristic swarming growth pattern that is inhibited by the bile in MacConkey agar. It is urease- and hydrogen sulfide-positive, but indole-negative (which distinguished it from *Proteus vulgaris* which is indole-positive).

Pseudomonas aeruginosa (D) is a lactose nonfermenting rod. It is an opportunist which is resistant to many antibiotics and capable of growing in superficial and deep wounds. It is also responsible for major nosocomial infections.

Rickettsia prowazekii (F), the agent of epidemic typhus, also causes Brill's disease which is a re-emergence of a milder form of the disease, years later, in the absence of new vector (louse) contact.

Rickettsia rickettsii (G) is the cause of Rocky Mountain spotted fever. The characteristic rash is more pronounced on the extremities than on the trunk. Antibody reacts to all of the *Proteus* antigens of the Weil-Felix test. Transmission occurs via tick bite.

Salmonella enteritidis (I) causes profound diarrhea and vomiting within hours of consuming contaminated foods. Groupings are based on surface O-antigens and H-antigens located on the flagella. Hydrogen sulfide production distinguishes it from the *Shigella* sp.

Shigella sonnei (L) can cause diarrhea in which the watery stools change from clear to bloody as the disease progresses. *S. sonnei* (Group D) is more frequently encountered than *S. dysenteriae* (Group A).

Treponema pallidum (M) causes syphilis. The VDRL test is a flocculation test which indirectly detects anti-treponemal antibody using nonspecific antigen. The fluorescent treponemal antibody absorption test (FTA-ABS) tests for antibody directed against the bacterial antigen.

Ureaplasma urealyticum (O) is a mycoplasmal organism which causes venereal infections. It is the slowest-growing of the mycoplasmas and requires urea and cholesterol for growth. Eaton's agar is an enriched nutrient system with inhibitors of faster growing bacteria.

Vibrio cholerae (P) causes classical cholera. The comma-shaped rods grow on many nutrients agars but faster under alkaline conditions with citrate, bile and thiosulfate

Yersinia pestis (S) is the agent of bubonic plague. The disease is transmitted in the prairie dog population, carried by fleas. Accidental infection to humans occurs through contact with infected animals. The infected swollen lymph node (bubos) commonly occurs in the groin area.

Answers and Tutorial on Items 79-90

The answers are: **79-F; 80-R; 81-T; 82-P; 83-N; 84-B; 85-H; 86-E; 87-L; 88-K; 89-M; 90-U.** ***Bacillus anthracis*** (B) is often associated with bovine and equine disease. Spores germinate in open wounds or lungs after being inhaled. Vegetative rods produce potent exotoxin that causes tissue necrosis.

Bacillus thuringiensis (E) is commonly used as a biological insecticide. The bacteria produce toxins which prevent the morphogenesis of a variety of insect larvae. The bacteria are harmless to humans.

Clostridium botulinum (F), under alkaline anaerobic conditions, produces a potent toxin in improperly prepared foods. Untreated food poisoning can cause paralysis or death. Heat at 100°C for 10 minutes will inactivate the toxin.

Clostridium perfringens (H) causes gas gangrene. The spores germinate in uncleaned wounds and produce α-toxin which kills tissue cells. The effects are treatable with antitoxin.

Lactobacillus acidophilus (K) is found in the normal vaginal flora in most women. It produces lactic acid from vaginal glycogen. The resultant lowered pH helps to maintain the proper vaginal flora.

Listeria monocytogenes (L) is a motile rod which produces hemolysin detectable on blood agar. It is associated with meningitis and neonatal infections. A positive catalase reaction and morphology distinguishes it from *Streptococci.*

Staphylococcus aureus (M) is often found in uncleaned wound infections. It produces grape-like clusters on Gram's stain and form complete hemolytic, golden-yellow colonies on blood agar. A positive coagulase test distinguishes it from *Staphylococcus epidermidis.*

Staphylococcus epidermidis (N) produces white colonies on blood agar. It is coagulase negative. Found on many body surfaces, it is morphologically identical to *Staphylococcus aureus.*

Streptococcus pyogenes Group A (P) causes strep throat, scarlet fever, rheumatic fever, impetigo and other diseases. Bacitracin sensitivity distinguishes it from other streptococci. The presence of antistreptolysin O in serum is diagnostic.

Streptococcus mutans (R) is a primary cause of dental caries. Colonization is dependent on adherence to enamel by polyglucan synthesis.

Mycobacterium leprae (T) causes leprosy. Advanced stages of leprosy result in the loss of nerve function leading to self-mutilation. The acid-fast bacilli grow slowly on Ziehl-Neelsen medium.

Mycobacterium tuberculosis (U) is the agent of tuberculosis. Primary infection in lungs is confirmed by x-ray. Granulomas occur in both lungs with walled-in bacteria. Reactivation may occur due to malnutrition, alcoholism, diabetes or other life-changing events.

Answers and Tutorial on Items 91-101

The answers are: **91-I; 92-C; 93-J; 94-R; 95-T; 96-O; 97-M; 98-G; 99-L; 100-A; 101-P**. ***Bacteroides fragilis*** (A) is the most commonly encountered anaerobic rod-shaped bacterium. It is frequently recovered from abscesses of the intestinal and genital tracts. Some strains will tolerate low oxygen levels.

Borrelia burgdorferi (C) is the spirochete which causes Lyme disease. It in microaerophilic and visualized with the Giemsa and silver stains. Human infection may involve the joints and heart.

Campylobacter jejuni (G) is a major cause of diarrhea associated with the consumption of poorly processed poultry. It produces an enterotoxin. The bacteria are shaped like curved rods.

Chlamydia trachomatis (I) causes sexually transmitted disease along with pneumonia (spread by inhalation) and conjunctivitis (spread by direct contact). It is an obligate intracellular bacteria which requires a eucaryotic host cell in which to grow.

Coxiella burnetii (J) causes Q fever. This rickettsial organism does not require an arthropod vector for transmission. Transmission is by inhalation of contaminated wool or dried fomites.

Klebsiella pneumoniae (L) produces a large amount of capsule polysaccharide. Many serotypes (>70) exist. The capsular properties distinguish it from other bacteria.

Gardnerella vaginalis (M) often causes secondary vaginitis. It is a slow-growing bacteria with growth properties similar to those of *Haemophilus* sp.

Haemophilus influenzae (O) is a slow-growing bacillus which requires both X (hematin) and V (NAD) factor. *Staphylococcus aureus* excretes V-factor and will therefore support satellite colonies of *H influenzae* on blood agar.

Legionella pneumophila (P) is the cause of Legionnaires' disease. It is a facultative intracellular pathogen of macrophages and monocytes. Colonies grow on charcoal yeast extract agar.

Mycoplasma hominis (R) is the cause of postpartum fever experienced by new mothers. The organism is an opportunist which may infect during child birth. The absence of a cell wall renders the Gram's stain uninformative. Speciation is by serotype differences.

Neisseria gonorrhoeae (T) causes gonorrhea. Kidney bean-shaped Gram-negative cocci within white cells is diagnostic. Sugar fermentation is used to distinguish different *Neisseria* species. Thayer-Martin agar restricts growth of other bacteria by the inclusion of various selective antibiotics.

Answers and Tutorial on Items 102-104

The answers are: **102-B; 103-C; 104-B**. Most individuals have been exposed to a **herpes simplex virus** by their early teen years. The virus, and other members of this group, often enter a latency phase whereby the virus remains dormant within neuronal cells. A variety of circumstances may assist in the activation of the virus and result in the production of lesions, usually within an area of prior lesion expression. Chemotherapy, sunlight, trauma and even menstrual cycle changes have been reported to have affects of the expression of a latent herpes virus infection. Viruses expressed on the face establish latency within the trigeminal ganglion because its nerve branches innervate the face.

The size, location and patterns of herpes virus lesions are indicative of different infections. Broad variations occur among individuals. Likewise, their ultrastructures are similar and not easily distinguished. A simple distinguishing procedure would be the use of a neutralizing antibody. Recently, the use of nucleic acid probes and DNA fingerprinting techniques have been used to identify herpes viruses.

Answers and Tutorial on Items 105-107

The answers are: **105-D; 106-A; 107-E**. Infection by **HIV** and the disease **AIDS** are not easily diagnosed because the incubation period may vary from months to years. Most diagnostic procedures for the virus detect circulating antibodies which emerge slowly in some cases. **Opportunistic infections**, such as *Mycobacterium tuberculosis* occur at a higher rate in immunocompromised individuals. Deep, productive coughing with blood are indications of possible mycobacterial infection and therefore warrants further confirmatory tests.

Surrogate markers for AIDS take into account several factors because the CD4+ (helper) T cell count fluctuates among individuals. A count of less than 300 cells/mm^3 is considered a sign of immunosuppression. 2-microglobulin, a component of the major histocompatibility complex; neopterin, produced by white cells; and interferon are all elevated in HIV-infected people. Delayed-type hypersensitivity (DTH) is suppressed. Fever may be a result of pathology due to opportunistic infections and therefore is not a reliable surrogate marker for HIV infection.

AZT, ddI, ddC and interferon have all been used in different treatment protocols for AIDS. Acyclovir is effective against certain DNA viruses such as herpes simplex, but not effective against HIV.

Answers and Tutorial on Items 108-112

The answers are: **108-B; 109-C; 110-B; 111-C; 112-B**. **Measles virus** is a highly infectious childhood virus usually attacking youngsters 6 months and over. The virus belongs to the paramyxovirus group which consists of enveloped RNA viruses which possess strong hemagglutinin activity on their surfaces. Infection usually occurs through the inhalation of contaminated aerosols; however, youngsters are also likely to place contaminated articles (such as toys or shared foods) into their mouths and assist in the transmission of the virus.

Measles undergoes several viremic stages which disseminate the virus throughout the body. The skin rash may vary in intensity in different individuals and even go unnoticed in dark-complexioned individuals. However, characteristic oral lesions, called Koplik's spots develop in the posterior of the mouth and inner cheeks. These represent focal areas of viral infection, cell necrosis and infiltrating white cells. Another name for the measles is rubeola, which is different from rubella (caused by a togavirus) and roseola (caused by a herpes virus).

Complications associated with measles include neurological damage (encephalitis), inner ear infections (otitis media), sterility (especially in older individuals), and bacterial superinfections. The latter may be due, in part, to a transient immunosuppression associated with measles infections. The virus does not propagate in the gastrointestinal tract and therefore diarrhea is not a common symptom directly associated with the infection.

Answers and Tutorial on Items 113-117

The answers are: **113-A; 114-B; 115-E; 116-E; 117-F**. The relationship between cancer and tumor viruses in lower animals was established long before similar cancer\virus relationships were established in humans. The presence of several human viruses showed high correlations with certain cancers but causal relationships were difficult to prove. This was due, in part, because of the ethical difficulty of testing Koch's postulates using human subjects. Several causal relationships have been established indirectly.

Human papilloma viruses (A), known to cause benign warts, also cause human cancer. One form of cervical carcinoma is caused by the human papilloma virus 16. DNA sequences from the virus have been identified in certain cervical cancers. A similar relationship has been established between DNA sequences of the **hepatitis B virus** (B) and hepatocellular carcinoma. The hepatitis B virus shows a preference for human hepatocytes in culture. Individuals suffering from Burkitt's lymphoma and certain nasopharyngeal carcinomas show the presence of DNA sequence homology with the **Epstein-Barr virus** (E). Certain hairy cell leukemias show the presence of DNA sequences of the **human T cell leukemia virus** (HTLV-1) (F).

A feature common to all cancers is the integration of the viral genomic DNA into the host chromosome. RNA tumor viruses have **reverse transcriptase activity** which converts the single-stranded RNA into a double-stranded DNA circular form enabling it to insert into the host chromosome and affect cell transformation. The mechanism of cell transformation is complex and requires multiple events involving viral products altering cellular regulatory factors, many of which have DNA-binding properties.

Answers and Tutorial on Items 118-121

The answers are: **118-C; 119-B; 120-D; 121-D**. The initial **humoral response** to a specific antigen is usually small because cells of the immune system have no previous exposure to the antigen. IgM is characteristically produced initially followed by an IgG response in the case of serum antibody. A second exposure to the same antigen usually results in a more rapid humoral response with a higher level of IgG versus IgM produced. The IgG level is usually long lived. The difference in humoral responses to the same antigen illustrates immunological memory and the influence of memory cells. **Memory cells**, either B cells or T cells, are clonally selected cells which have been sensitized by a particular antigen. The residual presence of the antigen in the animal, rather than the location of the exposure is important in maintaining a small population of sensitized cells which, when re-exposed to the same antigen, quickly amplify and produce immunoglobulins. Memory cells are essential in providing natural immunity against reinfections by the same pathogen.

Antigenic switching is the consequence of chromosomal rearrangements in B cells yielding clones which convert from producing specific IgM into producing either IgG, IgA or IgE, with the same specificity. DNA rearrangements and RNA splicing results in the positioning of the variable region of the heavy chain of IgM onto the constant region of the IgG heavy chain. IL-2, IL-4 and IL-10 are important signals in determining which immunoglobulin will be expressed by activated B cells.

Answers and Tutorial on Items 122-125

The answers are: **122-B; 123-D; 124-B; 125-C**. This child suffers from **DiGeorge syndrome**. This immunodeficiency disease is caused by congenital hypoplasia of IIIrd and IVth pharyngeal arch derivatives. Hypoplasia of the face, the thymus and the parathyroid glands are all associated with DiGeorge syndrome.

Patients with DiGeorge syndrome often have near normal levels of immunoglobulins for their age but significant decreases in T cell numbers and a concomitant relative increase in the percentage of B cells. The expression of this disease is highly variable ranging from mild to profound. Thymic hypoplasia or complete lack of a thymus results in a decrease in T cell numbers and a reduction in the cell-mediated immune response. In some instances, thymus-dependent areas of the lymph nodes and spleen also show variable T cell depletion. The hypocalcemia is caused by depressed secretion of parathormone by the hypoplastic or absent parathyroid glands

The eradication of protozoal, fungal and viral infections depends on the function of an adequate **cell-mediated immune** (CMI) **response**. The essential T cells of the CMI mature in the **thymus**. Malformation of the thymus and parathyroid results in a major immune dysfunction resulting in negligible T cell populations. Cytotoxic T cells and helper T cells act to kill host cells infected with intracellular pathogens. Both cell populations also produce essential cytokines which stimulate clonal expansion of stimulated (activated) T cells and B Cells.

Transplants of thymic tissue have had some limited success in correcting this deficiency. Claimed benefits from thymic transplants are difficult to evaluate, given the highly variable nature of the initial immunodeficiency state in DiGeorge syndrome.

Answers and Tutorial on Items 126-130

The answers are: **126-B; 127-A; 128-D; 129-B; 130-A**. Recurrent pyogenic bacteria infections in infants from organisms such as *Streptococcus* may indicate an underlying immunodeficiency. **Bruton's agammaglobulinemia**, also called X-linked agammaglobulinemia, results from a B cell deficiency. B cell deficiency results in a reduction in B cell function and concomitant reduction in immunoglobulins, secreted by plasma cells which are derived from B cells. It is X-linked and therefore expressed only in males (XY). The serum of infants show a uniform reduction in all immunoglobulin levels. Infections, starting around 6 months of age, occur with increasing frequency as maternal IgGs, transferred across the placenta during the fetal period, are depleted from the infants circulatory system after birth.

In a related disorder, **X-linked hyperimmunoglobulin M syndrome** (HIM), patients produce normal levels of IgM. B cells fail to "switch" into producing other immunoglobulins. HIM is believed to be due to a defective CD40 ligand on T cells. CD4 ligand is essential for activated helper T cell interaction with B cells.

One treatment used in cases of agammaglobulinemia is pooled **γ-globulin**. This form of passive immunization provides the infant with higher levels of mixed antibody, some of which may cross react with a variety of commonly occurring pathogens, resulting in a reduction of infections. The genetic nature of the disease currently precludes any permanent cure. Future advances in gene therapy may one day provide alternative approaches.

Answers and Tutorial on Items 131-134

The answers are: **131-E; 132-E; 133-C; 134-B**. Patients exposed to certain drugs experience a higher probability of developing an autoimmune disease. Patients undergoing treatment for tuberculosis with the drug **isoniazid** show an increased incidence of **systemic lupus erythematosus** (SLE). Other drugs such as procainamide, acebutolol and penicillamine have also been associated with a higher frequency of SLE. The target of the autoantibodies is similar even though the drugs differ. The underlying reasons for the effect are not known. Not all drug-induced autoimmune responses develop into SLE.

Patients with SLE may experience a transient facial flush or rash prior to the development of autoantibodies. The antibodies react with the H2A/H2B histone proteins which serve to organize eucaryotic chromosomal nucleic acid into nucleosomes, the fundamental structural subunit of the chromosome. Advanced cases of SLE may result in damage to the kidneys or the central nervous system. There is no cure for SLE, but the disease has been successfully managed with glucocorticoids.

There are many different autoimmune diseases which result in autoantibodies of different specificities. Examples of other common autoimmune disease and the targeted antigens are shown below.

Autoimmune Disease	Target Antigens
Chronic thyroiditis	Thyroid antigens
Allergic encephalitis	Brain myelin
Rheumatic fever	Heart muscle sarcolemma
Myasthenia gravis	Acetylcholine receptor

Answers and Tutorial on Items 135-141

The answers are: **135-B; 136-A; 137-B; 138-A; 139-A; 140-A; 141-C**. This woman is suffering from **malaria** caused by an infection by ***Plasmodium falciparum***. Malaria affects over 200 million people worldwide. Endemic regions include tropical and subtropical regions of Asia, Africa, South and Central America. *Plasmodium falciparum* is the most virulent of the four species which cause the disease. *P. vivax*, *P. ovale*, and *P. malariae* are the other members of the group. Fatalities are less frequent in cases involving *P. vivax* and *P. ovale*. Both produce recurrent episodes of latent infections.

Initial transmission of the disease begins with the injection of sporozoites from the mosquito vector. *Anopheles*, *Aedes*, and *Culex* mosquitos may transmit the disease. Individuals infected with *P. falciparum* have pronounced parasitemia in all stages of red cell maturity and a higher level of parasitemia than other malaria organisms. Identification of *P. falciparum* is obtained from the examination of Giemsa-stained blood smears. Crescent-shaped gametocytes are present in many red blood cells.

The drug of choice in treating malaria is chloroquine. Resistant organisms are treated with a combination of drugs consisting of quinine sulfate, pyrimethamine and sulfadiazine. New malaria vaccines which incorporate antigen incorporated into liposomes have been used in limited human trials.

Answers and Tutorial on Items 142-146

The answers are: **142-D; 143-C 144-C; 145-B; 146-C**. The patient suffers from toxoplasmosis caused by ***Toxoplasma gondii***. Cats serve as a primary reservoir for these parasites. Infections in humans are incidental, but more pronounced in immunocompromised individuals. In the latter population, especially in HIV positive patients, infections of the CNS are common.

Human infection occurs by the ingestion of foods contaminated by cat feces. Cysts mature and release sporozoites which may enter the blood stream and infect red blood cells. Eventually, the organisms reach the brain and form cysts which induce inflammatory responses and tissue damage. Infections of the eye, such as chorioretinitis, resulting in severe visual impairment, may also result.

Pregnant women infected with the parasite during the third trimester show a high (>60%) probability of passing the parasite to the fetus. Stillbirth or mental retardation may result. If a pregnant woman washes her hands frequently and avoids cat feces, she can greatly reduce the incidence of infections and disease. Treatment for toxoplasmosis includes the use of sulfonamides and pyrimethamine in adults.

ANSWERS AND TUTORIAL ON ITEMS 147-150

The answers are: **147-C; 148-C; 149-C; 150-A**. Immunocompromised patients are prime candidates for infection by the fungus ***Pneumocysistis carinii***. Cysts are inhaled in to the lungs where they germinate and release 2-8 trophozoites. Each trophozoite eventually develops into a cyst. Antigens produced by the organism initiate an inflammatory response resulting in the production of frothy mucous material which interferes with normal oxygen transport, thus the observed difficulty in breathing.

A bronchial lavage or sputum specimen from a patient usually contains numerous cysts which are easily recognized in silver-stained preparations or Giemsa-stained smears. The cysts are nearly spherical but have flattened sides and usually appear in small clumps.

The fatality rate in untreated *Pneumocystis* pneumonia approaches 100%. Vigorous therapy with trimethoprim-sulfamethoxazole reduces the rate to 50%. The drugs inhibit parasite dihydrofolate reductase and dihydropteroate synthase activities. Most individuals have been exposed to the fungus but experience only asymptomatic infections. This fungus is profoundly opportunistic in immunocompromised patients.

ANSWERS AND TUTORIAL ON ITEMS 151-157

The answers are: **151-I; 152-E; 153-A; 154-B; 155-F; 156-K; 157-C**. ***Giardia lamblia*** (A), giardia. It has both trophozoite and cyst forms. The binucleate trophozoite has two basal bodies, is shaped like a sting ray with prominent "owl-like eyes." The organisms are 5-15 µm in wide and 9-21 µm long. Four pairs of long flagella border the body. Each cyst contains two trophozoites.

Taenia solium (B), pork tapeworm. The head, or scolex, has 4 suckers and a circle of hooks which anchor it. The long series of proglottids have 8-12 lateral branches in the uterus. A mature organism may grow as long as 5 meters with hundreds of aligned proglottids. Infected individuals may appear anorexic.

Toxoplasma gondii (C). The elliptical 10 µm oocyst may have two sporocysts, each with four sporozoites. The crescent-shaped tropozoites, 3×7 µm, have a large nucleus and asymmetric organelle distribution. Cats carry the organism and transmit it to humans. Infected mothers can infect their unborn fetuses, resulting in congenital damage to the brain, liver and/or spleen.

Taenia saginata (D), beef tapeworm. The head has four suckers all on the same plane. There are no circular hooks. The proglottids have 15-25 lateral branches in the uterus. May reach 10 meters in length with several hundred proglottids.

Entamoeba histolytica (E). The circular cyst, 15 µm, have four nuclei and two cigar-shaped chromatoid bodies. The Trophozoite, 12-20 µm, is elliptical with pseudopod-like projections, and vacuolated. The cysts of *Entamoeba coli* have eight nuclei. Transmission occurs through contaminated drinking water.

Trichomonas vaginalis (F). The trophozoite, 7×15 µm, is pear-shaped with a single nucleus, five flagella, with one appearing attached to the body. A long rod, called the axostyle, traverses and extends past the body longitudinally. The organism is transmitted through sexual contact.

Trypanosoma sp (G). These long ,15-30 µm, hemoflagellates differ in shape but most have a single flagellum running longitudinally, a central nucleus and kinetoplast.

Leishmania sp (H). Amastigote forms are small, 1-2 µm, with a single nucleus and kinetoplast. Many found in cytoplasm of infected white cells. The promastigotes are flagellated.

Pneumocystis carinii (I). The cysts, 5-8 µm, are nearly circular but often have flattened sides, contain 2-8 small sporozoites and may appear with a honeycomb-like surface. The mature trophozoites are pleomorphic with a single eccentric nucleus. This is an opportunistic organism commonly found infecting immunocompromised patients.

Ascaris lumbricoides (J). Largest of the intestinal helminths, 150-350 mm, with a creamy cuticle and blunted anterior end.

Enterobius vermicularis (K), pinworm. Females, 1×10

mm, creamy colored with blunt anterior end. The oval egg is flattened on one side. These organisms are difficult to detect in stool specimens. The transparent tape test captures worms and eggs from the skin of the perianal areas for easy microscopic examination.

Necator americanus (L), hookworm. Adults measure 1x10 mm with blunt anterior head and 'hook' shaped body. Eggs measure 20 x 60 μm with 4-8 cells visible.

Schistosoma mansoni (M). Eggs appear reddish-brown, 50 x 90 μm, with a characteristic large lateral spine near the posterior end. A rigid capsule surrounds the egg.

Notes

CHAPTER 7

Pharmacology

DIRECTIONS (Items 1-101): For each of the numbered items that proceed, you must select the single best answer from among the lettered options listed.

Some of the numbered items will pose a question or incomplete sentence that is followed by a list of 4-5 lettered options. In all cases, select the ONE lettered option that best answers the question or completes the sentence given.

Some of the numbered items are preceded by 5-24 lettered options. In these sets, the lettered options will be preceded by a single instruction asking you to match one of the lettered options to each numbered item most closely associated with it. In all matching sets, you may use any of the lettered options once, more than once or not at all, but you should still only select ONE lettered option per numbered item.

If you wish to simulate actual USMLE testing conditions, you should aim to complete all the items in this chapter in 1 hour and 40 minutes.

Do NOT look at the answers and tutorials until you have completed all of the items in this chapter.

Good luck!

Item 1

1. To achieve a loading dose of a drug where the volume of distribution of the drug is 35 L and the clearance rate is 70 ml/min, and the desired dose is 3.5 mg/L, one should administer how many mg of drug initially?

    (A) 70 mg
    (B) 122 mg
    (C) 175 mg
    (D) 200 mg
    (E) 225 mg

Items 2-5

Figure 7.1 below shows the concentration of a drug as a function of time. Match the lettered part of the graph with the most appropriate description of steady-state conditions in the items.

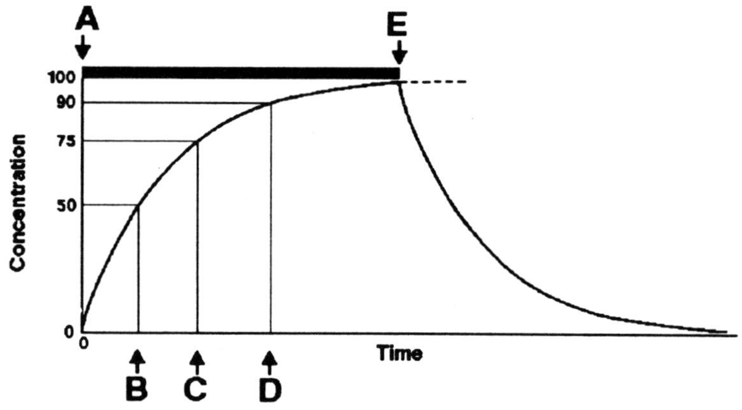

Figure 7.1

2. Drug administration stopped here.

3. Half of the steady-state level is achieved here.

4. Three-quarters of the steady-state level is achieved here.

5. This level is reached at 3.3 times $t_{1/2}$.

Item 6

6. To calculate the loading dose of a drug, when you have a desired steady state concentration intended, one would need to know

    (A) the steady state concentration
    (B) the rate of clearance
    (C) the rate of elimination
    (D) the volume of distribution
    (E) the rate of infusion

Items 7-10

Figure 7.2 below shows the effect of the drug as a function of drug concentration under different circumstances. Match the lettered curve with the most appropriate description of the circumstances in the items below.

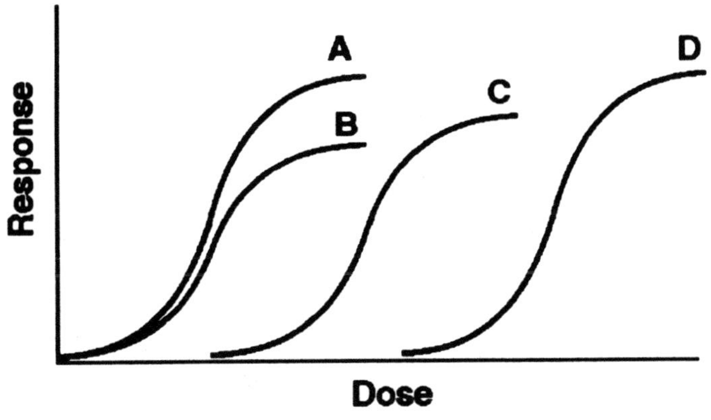

Figure 7.2

7. Drug with competitive antagonist

8. Drug with noncompetitive antagonist

9. Drug alone

10. Drug with partial agonist

Item 11

11. Of the following drugs, which has the largest therapeutic index?

    (A) penicillin
    (B) warfarin
    (C) digoxin
    (D) vincristine
    (E) cisplatin

Item 12

12. In a patient suffering from phenobarbital poisoning, which compound administered intravenously would increase elimination of the drug by decreasing distal tubular resorption?

    (A) HCO_3^-
    (B) epinephrine
    (C) NH_4Cl
    (D) glucose
    (E) inulin

Item 13

13. If a drug has a half-life of 1 day and a volume distribution of 40 L, the total body clearance would be approximately

    (A) 8 ml/min
    (B) 10 ml/min
    (C) 19 ml/min
    (D) 29 ml/min
    (E) 35 ml/min

Items 14-20

Match the lettered expression from the list below with its most appropriate definition in the items below. Answers may be used once, more than once, or not at all.

(A) Apparent volume of distribution
(B) Half-life
(C) Clearance
(D) Bioavailability
(E) Area under the curve
(F) Minimum therapeutic concentration
(G) First-pass effect
(H) Extraction
(I) Effectiveness
(J) Phase I reaction
(K) Phase II reaction

14. This parameter would be most directly and drastically altered in a patient with chronic renal failure.

15. This parameter is an expression of the time required for a drug concentration to be reduced to 50% of an initial value.

16. This parameter will vary depending upon the affinity of peripheral tissues for the drug and lipid solubility.

17. Depends on chemical changes in drug due to cytochrome P-450 modification, especially in the liver.

18. UDP-glucuronate often involved in this process which increases drug solubility.

19. The fraction of a drug removed from the circulation of blood through an organ.

20. This parameter is usually less than 1 for orally administered drugs.

Item 21

21. Which of the following compounds would have the highest selective affinity for β-adrenoreceptors?

    (A) isoproterenol
    (B) epinephrine
    (C) norepinephrine
    (D) dopamine
    (E) ATP

Items 22-24

22. A depressed patient on MAO inhibitors enters your ED complaining of tachycardia, high blood pressure and headaches. These symptoms developed rapidly after eating cheese and drinking red wine. Which agent in these foods caused this crisis?

    (A) quinine
    (B) methamphetamine
    (C) tyramine
    (D) atropine
    (E) dopamine

23. A 45-year-old woman presents with sinus bradycardia (heart rate of 36 beats per minute) and symptoms of fatigue. She is not currently taking any medications. Which drug could reverse the parasympathetic tone in this woman?

    (A) atropine
    (B) carbachol
    (C) succinylcholine
    (D) hexamethonium
    (E) prazosin

24. A 40-year-old patient presents with an acute hypertensive crisis. Which agent will act to block the increased blood pressure by acting at sympathetic ganglia?

    (A) propranolol
    (B) hexamethonium
    (C) nitroglycerin
    (D) digoxin
    (E) nicotine

Items 25-35

Match the receptor type in the list of answers below with the most appropriate corresponding tissue reaction in response to receptor activation. Answers may be used once, more than once, or not at all.

(A) α_1
(B) α_2
(C) β_1
(D) Muscarinic
(E) Nicotinic
(F) Dopamine
(G) β_2

25. Mydriasis

26. Relaxation of ciliary muscle

27. Miosis, constriction of pupillary sphincter muscle

28. Constriction of bronchial smooth muscle

29. Relaxation of bronchial smooth muscle

30. Retention of urine in bladder

31. Expulsion of urine from bladder

32. Constriction of veins

33. Dilation of veins

34. Activation of sympathetic ganglia

35. Relaxation of smooth muscle in media of renal afferent arterioles

Items 36-39

Examine **Figure 7.3** below. It is a diagrammatic representation of the nervous system. Match the lettered structure with the most appropriate descriptive phrase in the items below the diagram. Answers may be used once, more than once, or not at all.

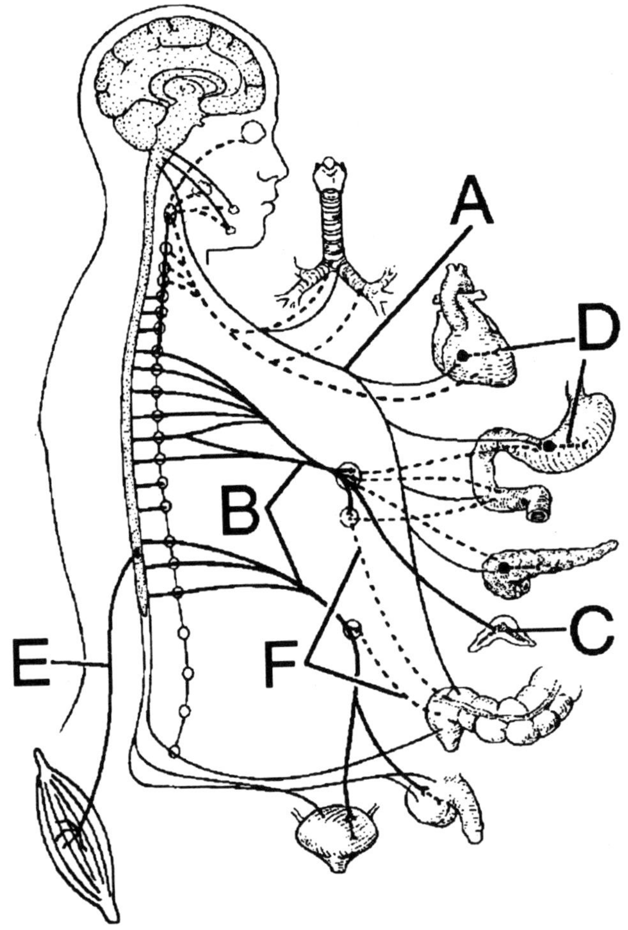

Figure 7.3

36. These parasympathetic postganglionic fibers use acetylcholine as a neurotransmitter.

37. These somatic efferent fibers innervate receptors coupled to ion channels.

38. Preganglionic sympathetic fibers trigger release of catechol amines from chromaffin cells located here.

39. These autonomic preganglionic fibers synapse with ganglionic fibers that release a neurotransmitter that uses inositol triphosphate as a second messenger.

Items 40-44

Match the drug listed in the answers below with the most appropriate description of its therapeutic application or pharmacologic effects in the items below. Answers may be used once, more than once, or not at all.

(A) Isoflurophate
(B) Neostigmine
(C) Physostigmine
(D) Carbachol
(E) Pralidoxime
(F) Atropine
(G) Hexamethonium

40. Reversible inhibitor of acetylcholine, used for myasthenia gravis.

41. A direct cholinergic agonist with muscarinic activity.

42. Counteracts effects of irreversible cholinesterase inhibitors.

43. Irreversible cholinesterase inhibitor.

44. Produces immediate mydriasis but could exacerbate glaucoma.

Item 45

45. Which of the following neuroleptics has the lowest likelihood of producing tardive dyskinesia?

(A) imipramine
(B) chlorpromazine
(C) haloperidol
(D) clozapine
(E) droperidol

Items 46-50

A 72-year-old man exhibits progressive tremors, bradykinesia, and muscular rigidity. He is slow to initiate movements and shows other motor abnormalities.

46. The most likely diagnosis of his disease is

(A) amyotrophic lateral sclerosis
(B) Duchenne's muscular dystrophy
(C) Parkinson's disease
(D) Huntington's chorea
(E) Niemann-Pick disease

47. The most likely cause of this disease is

(A) loss of dopaminergic neurons in substantia nigra
(B) metabolic demyelination
(C) death of motor neurons in ventral motor horns
(D) viral infection
(E) inherited membrane abnormalities

48. Which drug is most useful in the treatment of this disease?

(A) dopamine
(B) carbidopa
(C) haloperidol
(D) L-dopa
(E) apomorphine

49. Which drug mimics the effects of this disease and should be avoided in patients with this disease?

(A) lithium
(B) haloperidol
(C) diazepam
(D) phenobarbital
(E) L-dopa

50. The efficacy of drug therapy for this disease can be increased by co-administration of which of the following drugs?

(A) aspirin
(B) antacids
(C) carbidopa
(D) diazepam
(E) ibuprofen

Items 51-53

51. Benzodiazepines allosterically enhance the actions of

(A) dopamine receptor
(B) acetylcholine receptor
(C) GABA receptor
(D) muscarine receptor
(E) nicotine receptor

52. Their physiological mode of action is based on

(A) increased nerve conduction rate
(B) decreased nerve conduction rate
(C) opening chloride channels
(D) decreasing cAMP levels
(E) increasing cAMP levels

53. Benzodiazepine toxicity can be reversed using

(A) chlorpromazine
(B) morphine
(C) phenobarbital
(D) flumazenil
(E) naloxone

Items 54-55

54. Which of the following opioids has the lowest potential for addiction?

(A) morphine
(B) heroin
(C) meperidine
(D) codeine
(E) fentanyl

55. In an unconscious patient, which characteristic is most useful in differential diagnosing of coma due to heroin overdose?

(A) blood pressure
(B) respiratory rate
(C) pupillary constriction
(D) muscle spasms
(E) nuchal rigidity

Items 56-58

A 25-year-old woman with a history of seizures becomes unconscious, and later exhibits tonic and then clonic seizures. After she regains consciousness, she is confused and extremely tired. Her vital signs were essentially normal before and after the seizures.

56. The most likely diagnosis of her disease is

    (A) generalized epilepsy-grand mal seizure
    (B) febrile seizure
    (C) simple partial epilepsy
    (D) generalized absence seizure
    (E) eclampsia

57. Which drug would be effective in treatment of her disease?

    (A) lithium
    (B) haloperidol
    (C) phenytoin
    (D) clonazepam
    (E) captopril

58. This drug is contraindicated in pregnancy because

    (A) it is a known teratogen
    (B) it produces hypertension
    (C) it is an abortifacient
    (D) it reduces placental perfusion
    (E) it stimulates uterine smooth muscle contraction

Items 59-62

Match the CNS stimulant in the list below with the most appropriate description of it in the items below.

(A) Amphetamine
(B) Caffeine
(C) Cocaine
(D) Tetrahydrocannabinol
(E) Lysergic acid diethylamide
(F) Nicotine
(G) Nikethamide
(H) Theophylline
(I) Theobromine
(J) Doxapram
(K) Phencyclidine
(L) Methylphenidate

59. This drug can be used to counteract the respiratory depressive effects of barbiturates. It acts primarily by stimulating CNS respiratory centers.

60. This drugs leads to rebound depression due to decreases in brain dopamine after chronic abuse. It acts by inhibiting dopamine re-uptake.

61. This drug triggers strong release of dopamine and norepinephrine and thus has effects on both the brain and sympathetic nervous system.

62. This drug has CNS stimulatory effects at low doses and causes sympathetic ganglionic cell depolarization.

Items 63-66

From the list of answers below, select the one best answer to match the descriptions in the items below. Answers may be used once, more than once, or not at all.

(A) Ethanol
(B) Heroin
(C) Nitrous oxide
(D) Secobarbital
(E) Amphetamine
(F) Mescaline
(G) Marijuana
(H) Cocaine
(I) Diazepam
(J) Ether
(K) Ethambutol
(L) Hashish

63. Most fatal overdoses are caused by respiratory depression.

64. Blocks the neuronal re-uptake of norepinephrine, serotonin, and dopamine.

65. Often used to reduce anxiety during detoxification of alcoholics.

66. Shows similar central and peripheral effects as psilocybin and lysergic acid diethylamide.

Items 67-71

Match the anesthetic listed in the answers below with the most appropriate description of its therapeutic application or pharmacologic effects in the items below. Answers may be used once, more than once, or not at all.

(A) Halothane
(B) Isoflurane
(C) Nitrous oxide
(D) Thiopental
(E) Fentanyl
(F) Ketamine
(G) Procaine
(H) Bupivacaine
(I) Tubocurarine

67. A short-acting nonbarbiturate anesthetic which produces dissociative anesthesia.

68. This gaseous general anesthetic is a halogenated ether with little negative effect on cardiovascular function.

69. This gaseous general anesthetic must be used with other agents for complete surgical anesthesia.

70. A synthetic barbiturate used for induction of anesthesia.

71. An opioid analgesic used in balanced anesthesia.

Items 72-74

72. In a 55-year-old male patient with Prinzmetal's variant angina and moderate hypertension (BP = 150/100 mmHg), which one of the following agents would be best suited to treat both conditions?

    (A) nifedipine
    (B) captopril
    (C) atenolol
    (D) nitroglycerin
    (E) hydrochlorthiazide

73. A 50-year-old male patient presents with hypertension (BP = 150/95 mmHg) and atrial flutter. His cardiac output appears sufficient and there is no evidence of coronary artery disease. Which of the following agents might help both his hypertension and his atrial flutter?

    (A) nifedipine
    (B) digoxin
    (C) verapamil
    (D) prazosin
    (E) quinidine

74. A 45-year-old woman presents with moderate hypertension (BP = 165/100 mmHg). Total blood cholesterol (275 mg/dl) and lipid profiles (LDL 220, HDL 35) and past family history indicate risk for coronary artery disease and familial type IIa hypercholesterolemia. Based on this information, which of the following antihypertensives could exacerbate her hyperlipididemia?

    (A) enalapril
    (B) hydrochlorthiazide
    (C) nifedipine
    (D) indapamide
    (E) prazosin

Item 75

75. With respect to side effects of consequence in the elderly, which antihypertensive would be most likely to cause significant orthostatic hypotension?

    (A) propranolol
    (B) chlorthiazide
    (C) atenolol
    (D) clonidine
    (E) captopril

Item 76

76. Which inotrope is best suited for treatment of shock?

    (A) digoxin
    (B) digitoxin
    (C) amrinone
    (D) dopamine
    (E) dobutamine

Item 77

77. A patient presents with acute pulmonary edema secondary to congestive heart failure. She has been treated with digoxin, and is given furosemide to cause acute diuresis. Within several hours post-furosemide, the patient begins to show signs of acute digoxin toxicity. Which serum electrolyte must be monitored under such circumstances?

    (A) Ca^{2+}
    (B) Na^{+}
    (C) Mg^{2+}
    (D) K^{+}
    (E) HCO_3^-

Item 78

78. Which ion efflux is associated with Phase III repolarization seen in cardiac tissue?

(A) Na^+
(B) Mg^{2+}
(C) K^+
(D) Ca^{2+}
(E) Cl^-

Item 79

79. Class IC antiarrhythmics greatly prolong cardiac action potentials and can be proarrhythmogenic in a significant percentage of patients. Which of the following represents such a drug?

(A) lidocaine
(B) quinidine
(C) tocainide
(D) propofenone
(E) sotalol

Items 80-81

80. Which antiarrhythmic drug controls ventricular arrhythmias, increases AV nodal conduction and thus, is useful for digoxin toxicity?

(A) phenytoin
(B) procainamide
(C) tocainide
(D) atropine
(E) verapamil

81. A 35-year-old asthmatic woman is diagnosed with atrial flutter. Which agent should be avoided in treating atrial flutter in this patient?

(A) verapamil
(B) propranolol
(C) quinidine
(D) digoxin
(E) diltiazem

Item 82

82. Which fibrinolytic binds directly to fibrin clots, leading to local activation of plasminogen?

(A) streptokinase
(B) urokinase
(C) tissue plasminogen activator (t-PA)
(D) heparin
(E) warfarin

Item 83

83. Which of the following agents is especially useful in treating hyperlipidemias that are accompanied by high levels of triglycerides?

(A) gemfibrozil
(B) probucol
(C) lovastatin
(D) cholestyramine
(E) colestipol

Items 84-88

Based on the hypertensive patient subtypes in the items below, choose which antihypertensive drug would be best suited for initial monotherapy. Answers may be used once, more than once, or not at all.

(A) Furosemide
(B) Hydrochlorthiazide
(C) Diltiazam
(D) Captopril
(E) Minoxidil
(F) Guanethidine
(G) Diazoxide
(H) Reserpine
(I) Esmolol
(J) Methyldopa

84. Caucasian female, aged 75, with no coronary artery disease

85. African-American male hypertensive, aged 45, with diabetes mellitus

86. Caucasian male, aged 33, with high renin levels

87. Caucasian male, aged 55, with acute hypertensive crisis

88. Acute intraoperative hypertension with tachycardia, requiring short-acting agent

Items 89-93

Side effects occur with many cardiovascular agents. Match the side effect which is best associated with a given drug. Answers may be used once, more than once, or not at all.

(A) Amrinone
(B) Amiodarone
(C) Propranolol
(D) Quinidine
(E) Lidocaine
(F) Procainamide
(G) Dopamine
(H) Epinephrine
(I) Atenolol
(J) Dobutamine
(K) Sotalol
(L) Captopril
(M) Streptokinase

89. High doses can cause CNS effects, including convulsions

90. Can aggravate diabetes, heart failure, asthma

91. Causes cinchonism – tinnitus, headache, deafness, anaphylactoid shock

92. Causes renal artery dilation, increased cardiac output, but increases total peripheral resistance at high doses.

93. Unusual and long-lived pharmacokinetics, drug deposits in eyes.

Items 94-96

A patient visits your office and reports that she is about to leave the US for a bird watching expedition to the Amazon River basin in Brazil. She expresses concern about receiving some prophylaxis for malaria.

94. Which drug would you prescribe for her?

    (A) mefloquine
    (B) quinine
    (C) chloroquine
    (D) primaquine
    (E) chloroguanide

95. All of the following are true for this drug EXCEPT

    (A) used for chloroquine resistant forms
    (B) effective as a tissue schizonticide
    (C) effective as a blood schizonticide
    (D) effective against *Plasmodium falciparum*
    (E) ineffective against gametocytic form

96. Which side effects of this drug are most common?

    (A) gastrointestinal upset
    (B) hallucinations and depression
    (C) tachycardia
    (D) cinchonism
    (E) urticaria

Item 97

97. Which of the following is a reversible inhibitor of cyclooxygenase activity?

    (A) aspirin
    (B) prostacyclin
    (C) leukotriene E_4
    (D) ibuprofen
    (E) prednisone

Item 98

98. Which drug commonly produces cutaneous vasodilation?

    (A) colestipol
    (B) probucol
    (C) niacin
    (D) lovastatin
    (E) gemfibrozil

Item 99

99. Which antacid is contraindicated in a patient being treated with tetracycline?

    (A) aluminum hydroxide
    (B) nizatidine
    (C) sodium bicarbonate
    (D) omeprazol
    (E) pirenzepine

Items 100-101

100. Which of the following drugs would counteract the hypokalemia produced by a loop diuretic?

    (A) indapamide
    (B) furosemide
    (C) bumetanide
    (D) acetazolamide
    (E) spironolactone

101. Antidiuretic hormone has is primary effect on which structure?

    (A) adrenal cortex
    (B) proximal convoluted tubule
    (C) distal convoluted tubule
    (D) loop of Henle
    (E) collecting tubule

STOP.

YOU HAVE COMPLETED THIS SECTION.

Notes

Pharmacology

Answers and Tutorials

Answer and Tutorial on Item 1

The answers is: **1-B**. The **loading dose** of a drug is defined as the [volume of distribution] X the [desired therapeutic plasma concentration]. The loading dose is independent of the clearance rate. Loading doses can be given intravenously and because the plasma concentration is reached almost immediately, the clearance rate can be ignored. If the volume of distribution is large, due for example to peripheral binding of the drug, then the volume of distribution is relatively high and the loading dose may be correspondingly high, requiring that the loading dose be administered more slowly to avoid toxicity. In the example in Item 1, the loading dose would be 35 L (volume of distribution) X 3.5 mg/L (therapeutic concentration) = 122.5 mg.

The maintenance dose of a drug is dependent upon the clearance rate. The dosing rate can be calculated by multiplying the clearance rate by the desired therapeutic plasma concentration. For this calculation, one does not need to know the volume of distribution for the drug.

Answers and Tutorial on Items 2-5

The answers are: **2-E; 3-B; 4-C; 5-D**. **Figure 7.1** shows the concentration of a drug as a function of time. The **steady state** level is approached asymptotically because drug concentration as a function of time shows first-order kinetics. The $t_{1/2}$ value is the time required to reach 50% of maximal steady state concentration. Because of the first-order kinetics, 2 x $t_{1/2}$ is required to reach 75% of steady state and 3.3 x $t_{1/2}$ is required to reach 90% of the steady state concentration. Once the infusion of drug is stopped, the steady state concentration falls with the same kinetics as it rose.

Answer and Tutorial on Items 6

The answer is: **6-D**. The steady state concentration of a drug is best described by the following equation

$$C_{ss} = R_o/k_eV_d$$

Where:
C_{ss} = steady state concentration
R_o = the rate of infusion
k_e = rate constant for drug elimination
V_d = volume of distribution

From this equation, it is apparent that doubling the rate of infusion, R_o, would effectively double the steady state concentration. An alcoholic with a cirrhotic liver would have a significant decline in rate of elimination of a hydrophobic drug. Many of the enzymes for elimination of hydrophobic drugs are found in hepatic parenchymal cells which are destroyed by cirrhosis. Single IV injection of a loading dose of a drug that you wanted to make rapidly available to a patient, you would only need to know the volume of distribution (V_d)

Answers and Tutorial on Items 7-10

The answers are: **7-D; 8-B; 9-A; 10-C**. **Noncovalent drug-receptor** interactions are concentration dependent phenomena. For many drugs, the shape of the dose-response curve, when plotted on a semi-logarithmic scale, is **sigmoidal** (A). The shape of this curve is basically related to the fact that the receptors for many drugs become saturated at high doses. Thus, an increase in dose above saturation has little effect. Drug potency is usually defined as the dose that gives 50% of the maximal response (ED_{50}). **Noncompetitive antagonists** (B) bind to the receptor but at a different site from that occupied by the drug. Noncompetitive antagonists decrease the response by preventing drug binding or by reducing cellular responsiveness. **Competitive antagonists** (D) interact with the receptor at the same site as the drug itself (agonist) and thus shift the response to higher drug concentrations (to the right), ie, they act to lower drug potency. **Partial agonists** (C) decrease the potency of the full agonist and also reduce the response to the drug. Thus, drug efficacy is determined by the ability to achieve a full biologic response, irrespective of concentration. Drug potency compares relative concentrations of two drugs needed to produce an equivalent response.

Answer and Tutorial on Item 11

The answer is: **11-A**. The **therapeutic index** of a drug is the ratio of the dose producing toxicity to the dose producing useful clinical therapy. Some drugs such as penicillin are not often toxic in doses used therapeutically. A very high dose of penicillin is required before toxic side effects are observed (assuming that the patient is not allergic to penicillin). Therefore, penicillin has a high therapeutic index. The other drugs have various undesirable side effects which reduce their therapeutic index. For example, anticoagulants such as warfarin will increase blood clotting time at therapeutic doses but slightly higher doses can lead to serious side effects such as hemorrhage. Thus, the therapeutic index of warfarin is lower then penicillin. Similarly, the other drugs are anti-cancer drugs which can have severe side effects such as depression of bone marrow, gastrointestinal disorders, and hair loss. Digoxin is a cardiac glycoside with a notoriously narrow therapeutic window. An increase in any physiologic response that would lead to toxicity would naturally decrease the therapeutic index of a drug. An increase in clearance would have no effect on the therapeutic index.

Answer and Tutorial on Item 12

The answer is: **12-A**. In many clinical settings, it is important to determine how the health of the patient would alter the half-life of a drug. The **half-life of a drug** is directly proportional to its volume distribution and inversely proportional to its total body clearance. If the volume distribution of a drug is increased, then the half-life would also be increased. Heart failure and loss of blood would decrease the circulation of a drug and therefore increase its half-life. Similarly, renal failure would reduce renal clearance and would thus increase half-life. Hepatitis would decrease hepatic metabolism of the drug and thus would reduce its clearance, resulting in an increase in half-life.

Renal and hepatic elimination of drugs are crucial for determining the **clearance of a drug** and therefore its half-life. Factors increasing glomerular filtration rate, such as vasoconstriction of the efferent arteriole or increase in renal plasma flow, would significantly increase renal elimination and therefore significantly decrease half-life. Vasoconstriction of the afferent arteriole would decrease glomerular filtration rate and therefore increase the half-life of a drug.

In phenobarbital (a weak acid) poisoning, administration of HCO_3^- would increase the pH of the urine which would increase the ionization of phenobarbital. As a result, there would be a decrease in poison reabsorption and increase in its elimination from the body. NH_4Cl would be used to speed elimination of a weak base. Epinephrine would cause constriction of the afferent arteriole of the glomerulus and thus decrease glomerular filtration rate, leading to a decrease in clearance.

Answer and Tutorial on Item 13

The answer is: **13-C**. At a constant infusion rate, a drug with a half-life ($t_{1/2}$) of 10 hrs would reach 50% of its steady-state level in 10 hours. In 2 X $t_{1/2}$ or 20 hours, the drug would reach 75% of its steady-state level. The steady-state level of a drug is directly proportional to the infusion rate. It has nothing to do with the loading dose. Therefore, halving the infusion rate would halve the steady-state level.

The following equation can be used to calculate **total body clearance** (TBC) when you know the half-life and volume distribution of a drug

$$t_{1/2} = 0.693\ V_d / \text{total body clearance}$$

Where: $t_{1/2}$ = half-life of drug

V_d = volume of distribution

Total body clearance is usually expressed in ml/min.

Substituting

$$1440 \text{ min} = 0.693 \text{ X } 40{,}000 \text{ ml/TBC}$$

$$\text{TBC} = 27{,}720 \text{ ml/ } 1440 \text{ min}$$

$$\text{TBC} = 19.25 \text{ ml/min}$$

Answers and Tutorial on Items 14-20

The answers are: **14-C; 15-B; 16-A; 17-J; 18-K; 19-H; 20-D**. The **apparent volume of distribution** (A) of a drug can be estimated by dividing the amount of drug in the body by the plasma concentration of the drug. This value will obviously be altered by the exact mode of distribution of the drug in the body. For example, if a drug binds avidly to some peripheral tissue such as adipose tissue, its volume of distribution will be quite high. In contrast, if it remains largely in the plasma, the volume of distribution will nearly approximate the blood volume.

The **half-life** (B) of a drug is the amount of time required for the amount of drug in the plasma to decrease to 50% of the level determined at an earlier time. This is a reflection of the rate of clearance and rate of metabolism of the drug. It is dependent upon the volume of distribution and the clearance rate.

The **clearance** (C) is the rate of elimination of the drug divided by the blood concentration of the drug. Clearance varies with the drug and also with the state of perfusion and health of the organs of elimination, eg, the kidneys and the liver. Clearance can be altered drastically in patients with diseased organs, in patients with systemic diseases that influence rate of perfusion, and in patients treated with drugs that alter organs of clearance.

Bioavailability (D) is the ratio of the administered drug reaching the systemic circulation to the total dose of drug. For intravenous drugs administered as a bolus, the bioavailability is 1. For other routes of administration, bioavailability is usually less than 1. For example, if a drug is administered orally, its bioavailability will be decreased by partial absorption from the GI tract, binding to GI and hepatic cells, and first-pass effect (G) hepatic metabolism. To calculate the total dose received, it is necessary to plot a plasma concentration as a function of time curve and then integrate the area under the curve (E)(AUC).

The **minimum therapeutic concentration** (F) is the smallest plasma concentration of a drug which has some therapeutic benefit for the patient. In drugs with low toxicity, therapeutic doses are generally higher than the minimum therapeutic concentration. If the effectiveness (I) of a drug is high, they are therapeutically useful at relatively low concentrations and below the toxic dose of the drug.

Extraction (H) is the fraction of the drug that is removed from the plasma as the drug moves through a particular organ. In many instances, the extraction of drugs is relatively high in the liver and the kidneys, assuming that these organs are healthy and well perfused.

Phase I reactions (J) are used to convert hydrophobic (lipophilic) molecules into more hydrophilic molecules by the introduction or uncovering of ionizable or charged groups such as $-NH_2$ and $-OH$. These reactions are present in many cells of the body but are an especially prominent feature of hepatic parenchymal cells. These reactions are catalyzed by the cytochrome P-450 (mixed function oxidase) system of the smooth endoplasmic reticulum.

Phase II reactions (K) are conjugation reactions which speed the elimination of drugs by increasing their aqueous solubility. Glucuronic acid (from UDP-glucuronate), acetate (from acetyl CoA), and amino acids are commonly conjugated to drugs in Phase II reactions to inactivate them and speed their elimination from the body.

Answer and Tutorial on Item 21

The answer is: **21-A**. The receptors for γ-aminobutyric acid (GABA) are intrinsic ion channels and are found on the postsynaptic membranes of many central nervous system neurons. The **$GABA_A$ receptor complex** has α subunits, β subunits (GABA binds here), and δ subunits in unknown stoichiometry forming a Cl^- ion channel. Stimulation of inhibitory pathways releases this neurotransmitter which binds to the GABA receptor in the postsynaptic membrane. This opens ion channels, allowing Cl^- to enter cells and K^+ to leave cells, resulting in inhibitory hyperpolarization of cells. There is no second messenger involved in the function of GABA receptors.

The **β-adrenoreceptors** come in several varieties, called β_1, β_2 and β_3. This classification is based on differences in affinities for adrenergic agonists. For example, β_1-receptors have nearly equivalent affinities for norepinephrine and epinephrine. In contrast, β_2-receptors have a lower affinity for norepinephrine than epinephrine. Thus, when epinephrine is secreted by adrenal medullary cells, it has a strong effect on causing dilation of skeletal muscle blood vessels because the smooth muscle cells of these vessels have a large number of β_2-adrenoreceptors. β_1-adrenoreceptors are abundant in cardiac muscle. β_1-agonists increase contractility of cardiac myocytes and increase the rate of heart beat. When agonists bind to β-adrenoreceptors, the intracellular concentration of the second messenger cAMP increases due to an activation of adenylate cyclase. The affinity of agonists for β-adrenoreceptors is related to the degree of substitution on the amine. Larger groups convey a greater affinity. Consequently, the relative affinities are isoproterenol [$-CH(CH_3)_2$] >

epinephrine (–CH_3) > norepinephrine (–H) > dopamine. ATP has no affinity for β-adrenoreceptors.

The cardiovascular effects of epinephrine and norepinephrine are distinctly different. Epinephrine increases rate and forcefulness of cardiac contraction (β_1 effect). It increases systolic but decreases diastolic blood pressure. It also decreases peripheral resistance by causing β_2-mediated vasodilation. In contrast, norepinephrine increases the heart rate, increases both systolic and diastolic blood pressure, and causes a striking generalized increase in the resistance of peripheral blood vessels. The effects of norepinephrine are countered by a strong baroreceptor reflex, leading to bradycardia.

Answers and Tutorial on Items 22-24

The answers are: **22-C; 23-A; 24-B**. The **sympathetic** and **parasympathetic nervous system** innervate the heart; whereas, the arteries and veins of the body are innervated predominately by the sympathetic nervous system. The postganglionic sympathetic fibers to the heart and blood vessels release norepinephrine, while postganglionic parasympathetic fibers release acetylcholine. Released norepinephrine acts on cardiac β_1 receptors to speed heart rate, while parasympathetically-released acetylcholine slows the heart via muscarinic receptors. Cardiac β_1 receptors are found throughout the heart, while muscarinic receptors are only found in atrial and nodal tissues.

Sinus tachycardia is caused by excessive activation of cardiac β_1 receptors by norepinephrine, while bradycardia is caused by excess acetylcholine at the muscarinic receptors. A β_1 blocker such as metoprolol will slow sinus tachycardia caused by excess norepinephrine. Atropine, a muscarinic antagonist will block the bradycardic effects of acetylcholine on the SA and AV nodes. Excess norepinephrine can be indirectly released by the agent tyramine, which is found in aged cheeses and red wines. This effect is particularly dangerous in patients who are on monoamine oxidase inhibitors for depression. In hypertensive crises, agents which block autonomic ganglia, such as hexamethonium, can be used to blunt the response of the sympathetic nervous system.

Answers and Tutorial on Items 25-35

The answers are: **25-A; 26-C; 27-D; 28-D; 29-G; 30-A; 31-D; 32-A; 33-G; 34-E; 35-F**. The key to understanding this set of items is to recognize which autonomic receptors are present in which end organs. Agonists of each receptor would be expected to activate the listed process. In the eye, **mydriasis** and **miosis** are controlled by α_1 and **muscarinic receptors** respectively. Thus, norepinephrine would lead to mydriasis, which would be blocked by an alpha blocker such as prazosin. Acetylcholine would cause miosis, and this would be blocked by atropine.

A parallel system occurs in other tissues such as the smooth muscle in the urinary bladder. Sympathetic nervous system stimulation leads to urinary retention; whereas, parasympathetic activation leads to urination. Agents which block sympathetic responses can block sympathetic-induced retention, while atropine will cause urinary retention. **Nicotinic receptors** are on sympathetic ganglia, and are activated by drugs such as nicotine; this response is blocked by drugs such as hexamethonium.

Finally, **dopamine receptors** in the periphery are found in the renal and mesenteric veins. Activation of these receptors by dopamine leads to a selective relaxation. This is one reason why dopamine is useful in shock.

Answers and Tutorial on Items 36-39

The answers are: **36-D; 37-E; 38-C; 39-A**. **Acetylcholine** is the neurotransmitter for **cholinergic neurons**. The preganglionic fibers of the **sympathetic** (B) and **parasympathetic** (A) nervous systems, the sympathetic fibers to the **adrenal medulla** (C), and the voluntary motor neurons of the somatic innervation of **skeletal muscles** (E) are all cholinergic. As such they secrete acetylcholine which binds to a nicotinic receptor located in the ganglionic cell bodies of sympathetic and parasympathetic nerves, or in adrenal medullary chromaffin cells, or in skeletal muscle fibers. **Postganglionic parasympathetic neurons** (D) similarly use acetylcholine as their neurotransmitter. In this case, acetylcholine binds to muscarinic receptors in effector organs.

Epinephrine and **norepinephrine** are the neurotransmitters for a**drenergic neurons**. The adrenal medulla chromaffin cells and other **sympathetic postganglionic neurons** (F) release catecholamines into the blood and these bind to adrenergic receptors in effector organs.

The receptors located on effector organs act by several different mechanisms. For example, **cholinergic nicotinic receptors** (and GABA receptors) alter permeability in ion channels, causing changes in membrane potential. **Cholinergic muscarinic receptors** and α_1-adrenoreceptors utilize diacylglycerol and inositol triphosphate as a second messenger to intervene between the neurotransmitter and cellular effect, while **α_2-adrenoreceptors** and β-adrenoreceptors use **cAMP** as a second messenger.

Answers and Tutorial on Items 40-44

The answers are: **40-B; 41-D; 42-E; 43-A; 44-F. Isoflurophate** (A) (isopropylfluorophosphate) is an organic phosphate which is an irreversible inhibitor of acetylcholinesterase. It binds covalently to acetylcholinesterase, irreversibly inactivating the enzyme. This inactivation can be reversed by **pralidoxime** (E) which binds to the isoflurophate and removes it from the acetylcholinesterase. Pralidoxime must be used quickly after administration of isoflurophate due to the fact that the isoflurophate-acetylcholinesterase complex slowly releases an isopropyl group, making it impossible to break the complex.

Neostigmine (B) (a synthetic compound) and **physostigmine** (C) (a plant alkaloid) are reversible acetylcholinesterase inhibitors. Neostigmine has been used in the treatment of myasthenia gravis. In this disease, antibodies are formed against the acetylcholine receptor in skeletal muscles. It is characterized by progressive muscle weakness because the acetylcholine that is released presynaptically at the neuromuscular junction has little effect because of inactivation of the receptor in the postsynaptic membranes. Neostigmine increases the concentration of acetylcholine by reversibly inhibiting cholinesterase.

Carbachol (D) is a cholinergic agonist. It effects primarily muscarinic cholinergic receptors.

Atropine (F) is a plant alkaloid and although it is chemically unrelated to acetylcholine, it nevertheless has a high affinity for cholinergic muscarinic receptors. Atropine produces pupillary dilation (mydriasis) and prevents contraction of the ciliary muscles (leading to inability to focus on near objects) and would counteract the effects of pilocarpine and could exacerbate glaucoma. It also blocks contractions of the smooth muscle in the urinary bladder and gastrointestinal tract. Salivary gland secretion is also blocked by atropine, causing dry mouth. **Hexamethonium** (G) is a potent ganglionic blocking agent.

Answer and Tutorial on Items 45

The answer is: **45-D. Clozapine** is a **neuroleptic** that acts by producing blockage of the D_4-dopamine receptor. It is useful especially in patients not responding to other neuroleptics. It has the advantage of producing fewer extrapyramidal side effects and has a lower risk of producing tardive dyskinesia. Unfortunately, there is a significant risk of alteration in peripheral white blood cell counts because of its effects on myelopoiesis.

Neuroleptics are commonly used to treat **schizophrenia**, **mania**, and **drug induced psychoses**. They also have antiemetic effects but are more potent than necessary for treating nausea. **Epilepsy** may be worsened by neuroleptic treatment. The most common side effects of neuroleptics include impotence, parkinsonian tremors, tardive dyskinesia, postural hypotension, dry mouth (xerostomia), constipation, and anuresis (urinary retention).

Answers and Tutorial on Items 46-50

The answers are: **46-C; 47-A; 48-D; 49-B; 50-C**. This patient suffers from **Parkinson's disease**. In individuals over 65 years old, the incidence is approximately 1:100. Although the root cause of Parkinsonism is unknown, most patients show a reduced function in the dopaminergic neurons in the substantia nigra and corpus striatum, parts of the basal ganglia which are important in the control of motor function.

The **substantia nigra** contains dopaminergic neurons which project to the corpus striatum where they make numerous synaptic contacts with many cells and exert an inhibitory function via release of dopamine. Since these neurons fire tonically, they appear to exert a constant influence on motor functions. The neurons of the corpus striatum project to the substantia nigra. The neurotransmitter for these neurons is

GABA. Furthermore, axons from the cerebral hemispheres and thalamus terminate in the corpus striatum where they secrete the excitatory neurotransmitter glutamate which results in voluntary initiation of contraction of skeletal muscle and intentional movements of the body. Striatal interneurons secrete acetylcholine.

In Parkinson's disease, neurons in the substantia nigra atrophy and consequently, the levels of dopamine decline. **Levodopa** (L-dopa) (but not dopa itself) crosses the blood-brain barrier rapidly and can be converted directly into dopamine. Increases in dopamine levels ameliorate the effects of death of dopaminergic neurons in the substantia nigra. Large doses of L-dopa must be administered because it is rapidly decarboxylated in peripheral tissues, leading to increases in peripheral dopamine with unwanted side effects (arrhythmias, hypotension, nausea and vomiting). Co-administration of a dopamine decarboxylase inhibitor such as carbidopa, a drug which does not cross the blood-brain barrier, decreases peripheral production of dopamine from levodopa, thus decreasing unwanted peripheral side effects, allowing a four-fold reduction in the dose of levodopa required to obtain relief of parkinsonian symptoms.

Haloperidol blocks the dopamine receptors in the brain, releasing inhibitory neurons in the corpus striatum. Thus, one of the major side effects of this and other neuroleptics is secondary parkinsonism. These drugs are contraindicated in parkinsonian patients.

ANSWERS AND TUTORIAL ON ITEMS 51-53

The answers are: **51-C; 52-C; 53-D**. The **benzodiazapines** are a complex group of widely used **anxiolytic drugs**. They all contain a heterocyclic ring with two N atoms attached to two aromatic rings (the parent compound is the 5-aryl-1,4-benzodiazepine nucleus) (**Figure 7.4**). The variety of this class of drugs is based on different substitution patterns. For example, diazepam has R_1 = $-CH_3$, R_2 =O, and R_7 = -Cl.

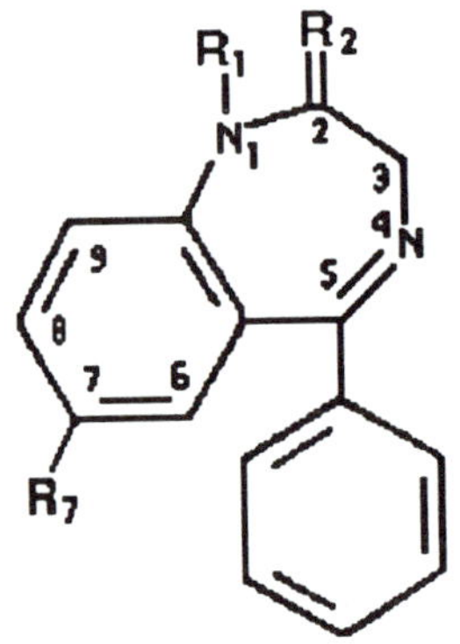

Figure 7.4

The benzodiazepine receptor is part of the $GABA_A$ receptor. When benzodiazepines bind to their receptor, they enhance the **ion channel** opening properties of GABA when it binds to its receptor, leading to a stimulation of entry of Cl^- ions into cells, and inhibitory **hyperpolarization** of neurons. This class of drugs works in the central nervous system (CNS), and can be used not only to alter mood but also in panic attacks, epilepsy, and as muscle relaxants (they have an inhibitory effect on the portions of the CNS which initiate muscle contraction). One of their chief benefits is that they achieve therapeutic results at low doses. The ratio of lethal dose to effective dose is typically about 1000, nearly two orders of magnitude higher than morphine, and also much higher than chlorpromazine and phenobarbital, drugs formerly used as sedatives. Flumazenil is an antagonist, and reverses effects.

Short-acting benzodiazepines (3-8 hours) include oxazepam and triazolam. Onset of withdrawal symptoms can be sudden with these drugs. Intermediate-acting benzodiazepines (0.5-1 day) include alprazolam, lorazepam, quazepam, and temazepam. The long-acting benzodiazepines (1-3 days) clorazepate, chlordiazepoxide, diazepam, and flurazepam are eliminated from the body more slowly. Consequently, withdrawal symptoms usually develop more slowly.

Patients treated with high doses of benzodiazapines over extended periods can develop dependence on these drugs. Withdrawal symptoms include anxiety, tension, insomnia, and restlessness. Other CNS depressants, including especially alcohol, potentiate the effects of benzodiazepines and can lead to fatal overdoses due to respiratory depression.

Answers and Tutorial on Items 54-55

The answers are: **54-D; 55-C. Opioids** are natural or man made compounds that bind to opioid receptors in the brain. The prototype opioid, **morphine**, is a constituent of opium, a dried poppy exudate. **Codeine** is also derived from opium. There are three major opioids receptors, mu (μ), kappa (λ), and delta (δ) each with subtypes. These receptors are most abundant in areas of the CNS involved in pain sensation, eg, the brainstem and spinal cord. A fourth receptor type, sigma (σ), may be related to the euphorigenic and hallucinogenic properties of opioids. The opioids are widely used as analgesics for moderate to severe pain management. Unfortunately, the most effective analgesics are also the most likely to lead to addiction and physical dependence on the drug. Morphine binds predominantly to the μ receptors in the spinal cord and decreases the sensation of pain. The opioids are also useful as cough suppressants (antitussives) but because of their addictive potential, their use has largely been supplanted by over the counter drugs such as dextromethorphan. Opioids are used in the treatment of severe diarrhea. They prevent diarrhea by inhibiting gastrointestinal motility.

Fentanyl acts very rapidly and is nearly 100 times more potent than morphine. It also has a very short duration of effect. It is used in conjunction with droperidol for neuroleptanesthesia. Codeine is a minor constituent of opium. It is less effective as an analgesic than morphine but also has a lower potential for addiction. Heroin is not used medically but is a commonly abused opiate. It is a chemically modified form of morphine that crosses the blood-brain barrier more readily and therefore produces more of a "rush" of euphoria when taken intravenously.

Patients suffering from **opioid overdose** will most often be stuporous or in a coma. These drugs are significant depressants of the respiratory centers. However, opiates have a stimulatory effect on the Edinger-Westphal nucleus, causing extreme pupillary constriction. In most other instances of coma, eg, caused by head injury, the pupils will be dilated. **Naloxone** and **naltrexone** displace opioids from all opioid receptors (they have a higher affinity for μ than receptors) and thus can be used in acute emergency settings to counteract opioid overdose. These antidotes have rapid effects when administered intravenously. Naloxone will also produce withdrawal symptoms when administered to opiate addicts.

Answers and Tutorial on Items 56-58

The answers are: **56-A; 57-C; 58-A**. **Epilepsy** is a common disease of the central nervous system. In the case described, the woman has experienced a **grand mal seizure** due to severe generalized epilepsy. Since her vital signs are normal, she is not experiencing febrile seizures or seizures associated with eclampsia.

Phenytoin is the drug commonly used in the treatment of this severe form of epilepsy. It acts by decreasing neuronal propagation in the CNS, specifically by decreasing Na^+ conductance. It is known to be a teratogenic drug closely associated with craniofacial anomalies such as cleft palate and lip, cardiovascular anomalies, and mental retardation. Therefore, its use is contraindicated in pregnant women.

Answers and Tutorial on Items 59-62

The answers are: **59-G; 60-C; 61-A; 62-F**. **Amphetamine** (A) has a stimulatory effect on the brain because it triggers the release of stored catecholamines, particularly dopamine. It also has a strong effect on the adrenergic system because it causes release of norepinephrine.

Caffeine (B) in coffee, theophylline (H) in tea, and theobromine (I) in cocoa are all methylxanthines. They are mild CNS stimulants that may work by increasing cAMP levels in cells. They all increase heart rate and mental alertness. The methylxanthines also cause relaxation of bronchiolar smooth muscles and thus theophylline is widely used in the treatment of chronic asthma.

Cocaine (C) is a widely abused drug in the US. It is a powerful CNS stimulant that inhibits neuronal re-uptake of dopamine, norepinephrine, and serotonin. Chronic abuse of cocaine leads to depletion of dopamine and can have severe rebound depressive effects.

The main psychoactive alkaloid in marijuana is **Δ^9-tetrahydrocannabinol** (D). Its mechanism of action is poorly understood.

Lysergic acid diethylamide (E) (LSD) is a potent hallucinogen. It has multiple effects on the CNS, due to the fact that it is a serotonin agonist, binding to both the 5-HT1 and 5-HT2 receptors.

Nicotine (F) is the psychoactive ingredient in tobacco. Its high lipid solubility means that it rapidly crosses the blood-brain barrier. In the doses typically delivered by use of tobacco products, nicotine has a stimulatory effect on the CNS and causes depolarization of sympathetic ganglionic neurons.

Nikethamide (G) and doxapram (J) are respiratory stimulants. Nikethamide has its effects primarily by stimulating the CNS respiratory centers. It can be used therapeutically to counteract the respiratory depressive effects of barbiturate overdose and can also be used to counteract the respiratory depressive effects of some anesthetics.

Phencyclidine (K), also know as PCP or "angel dust" on the streets, is an analog of ketamine. Its mechanism of pharmacologic action is mediated in part by inhibition of dopamine, norepinephrine, and serotonin re-uptake. Abusers of PCP often show aggressive and bizarre behavior.

Methylphenidate (L) is an amphetamine derivative. Its mechanism of action is similar to amphetamine. It is used therapeutically in the treatment of attention deficit disorder.

Answers and Tutorial on Items 63-66

The answers are: **63-B; 64-H; 65-I; 66-F**. Drugs of abuse generally fall into six classes:

(1) hallucinogens

(2) inhalants

(3) marijuana

(4) opioids

(5) sedative-hypnotics

(6) stimulants

Hallucinogens include phencyclidine (PCP, "angel dust"), lysergic acid diethylamide (LSD, "acid"), psilocybin, mescaline, and scopolamine. These drugs induce altered perceptual states, often accompanied by bright, colorful, constantly changing visual hallucinations. They also interfere with rational thought processes leading persons under their influence to impaired judgment and sometimes reckless, hostile and/or bizarre behavior that may be dangerous to the abuser or others. These drugs are sometimes classified as "psychotomimetic drugs" because their effects on the CNS mimic some features of psychosis. PCP abuse is widespread and dangerous. It blocks re-uptake of dopamine, norepinephrine, and serotonin, alters glutamate receptor function, causing dissociative anesthesia and analgesia, and also produces staggering gait, numbness in the extremities, muscular rigidity, and slurred speech. Abusers may become extremely violent and aggressive. Overdoses produce marked hypertension, seizures, stupor and potentially fatal coma. LSD binds to serotonin receptors (5-HT_1 and 5-HT_2) and has effects on many different regions of the CNS. It causes vivid hallucinations that may be frightening, hypertension, pupillary dilation, piloerection, and increased body temperature. Adverse effects include nausea, muscular weakness, paresthesia, and panic reactions. Neuroleptics such as haloperidol can reverse the hallucinatory effects of LSD.

Inhalants include gases and volatile liquids that produce euphoria and disinhibition. Organic nitrites ("poppers") such as amyl nitrite and isobutyl nitrite are used to enhance sexual experiences. These inhalants produce flushing, hypotension, dizziness, and tachycardia. Adverse effects to the nitrites have not been widely reported; however, methemoglobinemia is one possible side effect. Chloroform, nitrous oxide, and diethyl ether are anesthetics that are widely abused. In low doses they impair judgment and in higher doses produce unconsciousness. Nitrous oxide used without oxygen produces hypoxia and death. Diethyl ether is extremely volatile and explosive when mixed with air or oxygen. Diethyl ether and chloroform irritate the respiratory tract, causing increased mucus secretion and salivation. Gasoline and other solvents in commercial products such as paint thinner, nail polish, adhesives, and hair spray are easily obtained and therefore widely abused by adolescents. Many of these solvents have severe adverse effects on the kidneys, liver, lungs, bone marrow, and nervous system.

The most commonly abused **opioids** are heroin, morphine, meperidine, fentanyl, oxycodone, propoxyphene, and codeine. These substances are either natural or structurally related synthetic compounds that bind to specific opioid receptors in the CNS, producing effects that mimic the action of endogenous neurotransmitters such as the endorphins. Intravenously administered heroin produces a "rush" or orgasmic sensation followed by euphoria and sedation. Abusers may also consume these drugs orally or by smoking them. Tolerance as well as psychological and physical dependence do develop, with their onset being more rapid with intravenous administration. Respiratory depression is the chief cause of most fatalities due to opioid analgesic overdosing. Physically dependent individuals suffer withdrawal syndrome when they are deprived of opioids. Withdrawal symptoms include sweating, cramps, weakness, lacrimation, rhinorrhea, vomiting, tremors, and hyperpnea. Replacement of the drug with a pharmacologically equivalent substance such as methadone followed by gradual dose reduction is the current form of treatment for opioid addiction.

The most commonly abused **sedative-hypnotics** include ethanol, pentobarbital, diazepam, and methaqualone. These drugs are widely abused in industrialized societies. Overdoses of all of these drugs are usually caused by profound depressive effects on the medullary respiratory centers and cardiovascular centers.

The most commonly abused **stimulants** include caffeine, nicotine, cocaine, and amphetamines. Nicotine abuse in the form of cigarette smoking is widespread and is a leading preventable cause of disease in the US, leading to the premature deaths of hundreds of thousands of people each year from heart attack, stroke, emphysema, and lung cancer. Amphetamines and cocaine produce striking CNS effects leading to a false sense of mental power, euphoria, power, and well-being.

Answers and Tutorial on Items 67-71

The answers are: **67-F; 68-B; 69-C; 70-D; 71-E**. **Halothane** (A) is a halogenated ethane that is an effective general anesthetic when administered as mixtures with air or oxygen. Its effective minimal alveolar concentration is low (0.75%). In a few individuals, halothane is metabolized into hepatotoxic intermediates. Halothane can cause marked cardiovascular effects such as sensitization of the heart to catecholamines.

Isoflurane (B) is a halogenated ethyl methyl ether. Its effective minimal alveolar concentration is higher than halothane (1.15% vs 0.75%). Its use has largely supplanted halothane because it allows rapid adjustments of depth of anesthesia, potentiates the effects of muscle relaxants, does not lead to the formation of hepatotoxic intermediates, and does not sensitize the heart to catecholamines.

Nitrous oxide (C) is a gaseous anesthetic with extremely low solubility in blood and consequently, it results in rapid induction of and recovery from anesthesia. It is commonly used as a 30% mixture with oxygen. By itself, it cannot produce surgical anesthesia but it can be used as a component of balanced anesthesia in combination with a short-acting barbiturate such as the commonly used thiopental (D), the muscle relaxant tubocurarine (I), and the opioid analgesic fentanyl (E). It is also used in minor dental procedures because of its safety.

In **neuroleptanesthesia**, the patient remains conscious. It is the technique of choice when the voluntary cooperation of the patient is required. It involves co-administration of a neuroleptic such as droperidol, an opioid analgesic such as fentanyl, and nitrous oxide/oxygen mixtures.

Ketamine (F) is a short-acting anesthetic which produces dissociative anesthesia. Chemically, ketamine hydrochloride is (2-[o-chlorophenyl]-2-[methylamino] cyclohexanone (non-barbiturate). In dissociative anesthesia, the patient is sedated and immobilized while experiencing analgesia, amnesia, and a peculiar sensation of dissociation from their surroundings.

Procaine (G) and bupivacaine (H) are local anesthetics. They block nerve transmission by interfering with voltage-gated Na^+ channels.

verapamil yes → AV Node
Nifedipine No → Conduction

Answers and Tutorial on Items 72-74

The answers are: **72-A; 73-C; 74-B**. In Item 72, **Prinzmetal's variant angina** is treated by calcium channel blockers; thus **nifedipine** is the correct choice, because it is a calcium channel blocker and will lower blood pressure effectively. In Item 73, atrial flutter is a supraventricular arrhythmia treated by drugs which slow AV nodal conduction. Digoxin, quinidine and verapamil all slow nodal conduction; however, only verapamil will also effectively lower blood pressure. Nifidepine will lower blood pressure, but does not slow AV nodal conduction. In Item 74, all of the agents listed will lower blood pressure; however, thiazide diuretics such as hydrochlorthiazide also raise cholesterol and LDL levels, and would not be a first choice in a hyperlipidemic patient. PAT is a supraventricular arrhythmia and could be treated by agents which slow AV nodal conduction. However, only propranolol will effectively lower blood pressure and slow AV nodal conduction. The key feature of these items is the use of a given drug for hypertension concomitant with other conditions, resulting in alleviation of both diseases.

ANSWERS AND TUTORIAL ON ITEM 75

The answer is: **75-D**. **Orthostatic hypotension** in the elderly is most often associated with the use of centrally-acting sympatholytic drugs, making **clonidine** the best choice. Balanced vasodilators act to simultaneously dilate arterial and venous systems; nitroprusside is an intravenously administered balanced vasodilator, while **captopril** and other **angiotensin converting enzyme** (ACE) **inhibitors** are good examples of balanced vasodilators used in outpatient treatment of **congestive heart failure** (CHF). Balanced vasodilators lower preload (venodilation) and afterload (arteriolar dilation). In CHF, this lessens edema by causing venous pooling while simultaneously reducing the amount of force needed to maintain adequate perfusion (afterload).

ANSWER AND TUTORIAL ON ITEMS 76

The answer is: **76-D**. The two different drugs highlighted in these two items are **dopamine**, a naturally occurring catecholamine, and the synthetic drug **dobutamine**. Dopamine is well-suited for shock because it dilates renal and mesenteric arteries, allowing maintenance of urine output. Dobutamine increases cardiac output via direct actions on cardiac tissues. Unlike dopamine, it's β_2-agonist properties offset α_1 effects. This causes a high cardiac output without direct effects on systemic vascular resistance.

The other choices force discrimination based on increased cardiac output in shock vs. CHF. Thus, digoxin can be used in CHF, but acts too slowly and too variably to have any utility in shock. The other discriminator is increased peripheral resistance. In shock, increased resistance is good, shunting blood to key organs like brain and kidney. In CHF, peripheral resistance is undesirable.

ANSWERS AND TUTORIAL ON ITEM 77

The answer is: **77-D**. **Digoxin** is cleared by the kidney and thus renal failure will increase serum levels, as will quinidine. Maintenance of serum K^+ levels are critical in preventing digoxin toxicity; **furosemide** can cause a rapid hypokalemia, leading to digoxin toxicity. In cases of excess drug administration, specific administration of Digibind FAb fragments will help to effectively lower free drug by binding to excess digoxin.

The toxicity of digoxin is a leading cause of problems in patients needing this drug. Any disease state which decreases clearance will increase the risk of toxicity. The lethal events in digoxin toxicity are generally caused by fatal ventricular arrhythmias in the face of severe A-V block.

ANSWER AND TUTORIAL ON ITEMS 78

The answer is: **78-C**. The predominant ionic fluxes associated with each **phase** of the **cardiac action potential** are Phase I = Na^+, Phase II = Ca^{2+}, Phase III = K^+, and Phase IV diastolic depolarization = Ca^{2+} and Na^+. Diastolic depolarization in pacemaker cells is responsible for generation of normal cardiac rhythms. This item requires a direct knowledge of the ionic movements during the cardiac action potential.

ANSWER AND TUTORIAL ON ITEM 79

The answer is: **79-D**. These items deal with recognition of **antiarrhythmic drug classes**. **Class IC drugs** are unusual in that they cause prominent slowing of Phase O of the cardiac action potential; flecanide, encainide, and propofenone are representative examples. **Class III drugs** block K^+ channels involved in cardiac repolarization; amiodarone, sotalol, and bretylium are examples of this class. Amiodarone is unusual in that it has a very long half life and deposits in ocular tissues. Sotalol is unique in that it also blocks - receptors.

The overall goal of antiarrhythmic therapy is to normalize cardiac impulses. However, some arrhythmias are highly resistant to therapy, and require potent medications, thus, the risks associated with flecanide and amiodarone must be balanced against the benefits.

ANSWERS AND TUTORIAL ON ITEMS 80-81

The answers are: **80-A; 81-B**. These items address issues reflecting appropriate drug choices for treatments of specific **arrhythmias**. **Tocainide** is an orally active congener of lidocaine and is not effective at treating atrial arrhythmias. AV nodal conduction velocity is key for a number of agents; atropine, via blockade of cardiac muscarinic receptors, can block the effects of acetylcholine on the AV node, which leads to increased conduction velocity. One drug which stands out as a theoretical best choice for treatment of **digoxin toxicity** is **phenytoin**. It blocks ventricular arrhythmias and will speed AV conduction directly. In the final case, asthmatic diseases, β-blockers are contraindicated, thus, propranolol would be a poor choice.

The normal control of AV conduction velocity is achieved by sympathetic and parasympathetic neurons. Norepinephrine accelerates AV conduction via β_1-receptors; this is blocked by β_1-blockers like **metoprolol**. Acetylcholine slows AV conduction via muscarinic receptors. **Atropine** will block this effect and thus speed AV nodal conduction.

Answer and Tutorial on Items 82

The answer is: **82-C**. These items address mechanisms and side effects of the **fibrinolytics**. Human-derived **tissue plasminogen activator** (t-PA) binds directly to fibrin in the clot, and activates plasminogen on site; this does not cause a generalized activation of plasmin.

Due to a short half-life, t-PA must be given intravenously, and increases somewhat the possibility of a serious hemorrhagic stroke. Patients who are recovering from major surgery may also bleed profusely following t-PA. This drug does not discriminate against any fibrin-based clot in the body. Thus, bleeding and stroke are potential complications.

Streptokinase is derived from bacteria, and can cause allergic reactions. **Urokinase** is derived from human sources, and is not an allergen; however, it causes a generalized increase in plasmin. Streptokinase and urokinase can also cause excess bleeding in post-surgical patients.

Answer and Tutorial on Items 83

The answer is: **83-A**. **Niacin** is useful at high doses for treatment of a wide range of hyperlipidemias; unfortunately, flushing and pruritus are common, and are often blocked by pre-administration of aspirin. The next two items address specific mechanisms of lipid-lowering agents. Bile acid sequestrants like **colestipol** and **cholestyramine** interrupt enterohepatic reabsorption of bile salts, leading to an acceleration in LDL uptake. More recent agents like **lovastatin**, pravastatin and mevastatin directly inhibit HMG-CoA reductase, leading to increased LDL receptor synthesis. Of particular note are agents which have unique uses for hypertriglyceridemias-**clofibrate** and **gemfibrozil** are well-suited for reductions of triglycerides.

The lipid-lowering drugs reduce cardiac mortality and morbidity resulting from atherogenic plaques. Lipid-lowering protocols are common in patients suffering from angina, in patients with disorders of cholesterol uptake, and **familial hyperlipidemias**.

Answers and Tutorial on Items 84-88

The answers are: **84-B; 85-C; 86-D; 87-G; 88-I**. Elderly hypertensives respond well to **thiazide diuretics**, thus a 75-year-old woman would respond well to hydrochlorthiazide. African-American males respond best to **calcium channel blockers**; diabetes mellitus renders several of the other possible choices unlikely. High renin-based hypertension responds best to and **angiotensin converting enzyme** (ACE) **inhibition**; **captopril** is the only drug of this class listed. Acute hypertensive crisis is best treated with either **diazoxide**, which is listed, or with nitroprusside, which is not. Acute intraoperative hypertension is best treated by the short-acting β-blocker, **esmolol**. **Furosemide** is a potent **loop diuretic**, and not used in initial monotherapy. **Guanethidine** and **reserpine** act centrally, and are reserved for severe, **resistant hypertension**.

Answers and Tutorial on Items 89-93

The answers are: **89-E; 90-C; 91-D; 92-G; 93-B**. This item requires knowledge of specific and mechanism-related toxicity. **Amiodarone** has unusual pharmacokinetics, and deposits in skin and eyes. **Lidocaine** has local anesthetic properties, and can cause CNS toxicity. It is otherwise relatively safe. Cinchonism is a specific toxicity of **quinidine**; whereas, systemic lupus-like effects are seen with **procainamide**. Noncardioselective β_1, β_2-blockers like propranolol aggravate asthma and diabetes mellitus via β_2-blockade. **Dopamine** can greatly increase systemic vascular resistance at high doses. The ACE inhibitors are generally without serious side effects.

Answers and Tutorial on Items 94-96

The answers are: **94-A; 95-B; 96-A**. **Mefloquine** is widely used in prophylaxis of **falciparum malaria**. Its exact mode of pharmacologic action is not well understood but it is only effective as a blood schizonticide. It is effective against strains of *Plasmodium falciparum* that have become resistant to chloroquine. In therapeutic doses, it is well tolerated with few side effects, the most common of which are gastrointestinal distress.

Answer and Tutorial on Item 97

The answer is: **97-D**. **Prostaglandins** (PG) belong to an important group of compounds called eicosanoids. Other members of this family include prostacyclin (PC), thromboxanes (TX), leukotrienes (LT), and hydroperoxyeicosatetraenoic acid (HETE). These compounds are produced in minute quantities by most tissues where they have effects as local hormones. They have a wide range of functions, including inhibition of gastric secretion and uterine contraction, stimulation of steroidogenesis in the adrenal cortex and gonads, lowering of blood pressure, and generation of the inflammatory response. They are rapidly metabolized to inactive products at their site of action and therefore do not circulate in the blood at significant concentrations.

All prostaglandins and related compounds are derived primarily from the 20-carbon polyunsaturated fatty acid **arachidonic acid** (AA). Intracellular free AA concentration is extremely low; however, it is present in membrane phospholipids. AA is released from membrane phospholipids by phospholipase A_2 (PLA_2) and other hydrolases via a closely regulated process involving hormones (eg, bradykinin, angiotensin, and corticosteroids) and other stimuli (see **Figure 7.5**).

In **Figure 7.5**, the letters after the acronyms refer to different substituents while the subscripts indicate the number of double bonds in the side chains. There are two major pathways in the synthesis of eicosanoids from arachidonic acid: 1) ring structures such as PG, TX, and prostacyclins are derived from the cyclooxygenase pathway and 2) the straight chain derivatives such as 5-HPETE and LT are products of the lipoxygenase pathway.

PG and other eicosanoids act primarily by binding to cell surface receptors where they stimulate or inactivate adenylate cyclase, thereby modifying the cAMP cascade. In some tissues they may increase intracellular Ca^{2+} or act via the second messengers IP3 and diacylglycerol (DAG).

Endogenously synthesized eicosanoids act as local chemical signals to fine tune the responses of cells where they are produced. Examples of specific effects are as follows

1) Thromboxane release in platelets signals platelet aggregation, the first step in clot formation.
2) The slow-reacting substance of anaphylaxis (SRS-A) consists of leukotrienes LTC_4, LTD_4 and LTE_4.
3) PGE_2 and prostacyclin may play roles as vasodilators.
4) LTB_4 is a chemotactic factor in the inflammatory process.
5) PGE derivatives show protective effects in the gastric mucosa, probably by increasing mucus and bicarbonate secretion, decreasing acid secretion, or both.
6) PGF_2 may play a role in dysmenorrhea and associated uterine contractions.
7) PGE_2 and PGF_2 may have a physiological role in labor.
8) Leukotrienes may play a role in aspirin hypersensitivity because their synthesis may be increased when aspirin irreversibly inhibits cyclooxygenase thereby shunting arachidonic acid to the lipoxygenase pathway.

The therapeutic uses of eicosanoids are summarized as follows

1) In obstetrics, PGE_2 and $PGF_{2\alpha}$ are used as abortifacients in the second trimester of pregnancy because they stimulate powerful uterine contractions. Misoprostol (a PGE_1 analog) in combination with mifepristone (RU486) has been used in Europe as an abortifacient.
2) Prostacyclin (PGI_2) is occasionally used in dialysis machines to prevent platelet aggregation.
3) Misoprostol and other synthetic PGE derivatives are used or are under investigation as potential treatments for peptic ulcers.
4) In infants with transposition of the great vessels, PGE is infused to maintain patency of the ductus arteriosus until surgical intervention.

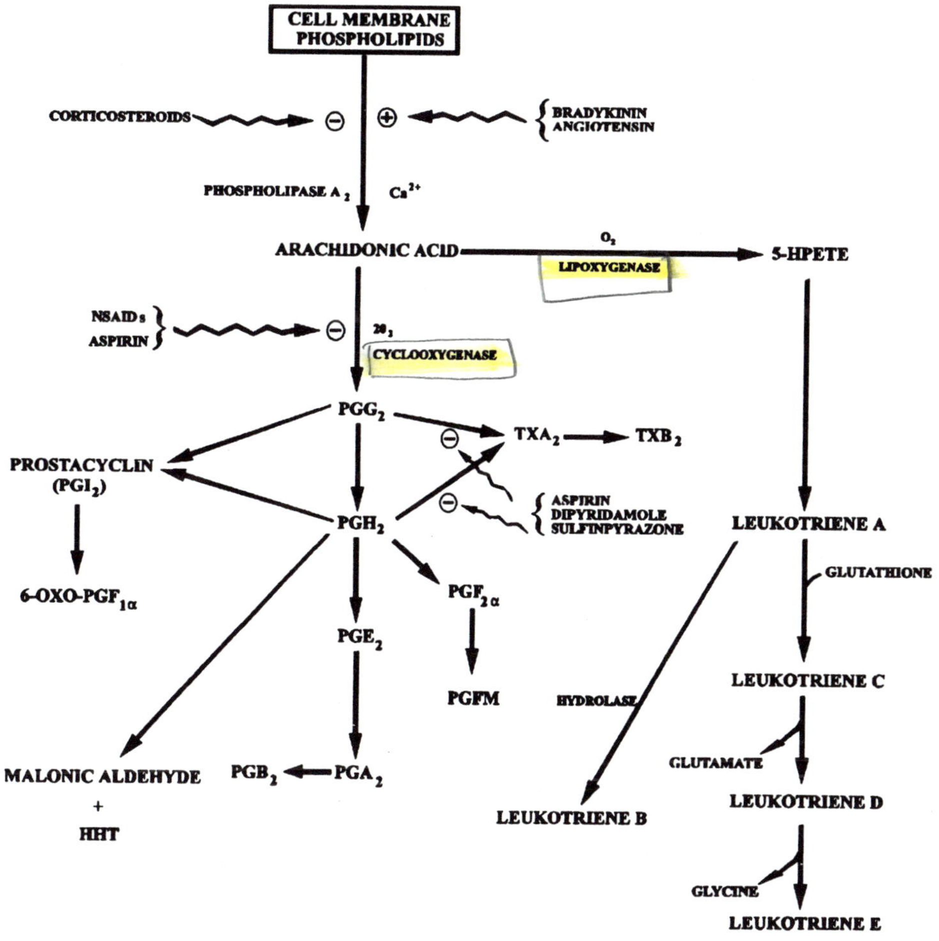

Figure 7.5

Prostaglandins = **PG**, thromboxanes = **TX**, 5-hydroperoxyeicosatetranenoic acid = **5-HPETE**, 1,25-hydroxy-5,8,10-heptadecatrienoic acid = **HHT**

Nonsteroidal anti-inflammatory drugs (NSAIDs) including aspirin inhibit cyclooxygenase and thereby the production of prostaglandins, prostacyclin, and thromboxane. Aspirin is unique in that its inhibition of cyclooxygenase is irreversible. This inhibition of cyclooxygenase by NSAIDs is responsible for the anti-inflammatory, antipyretic, and anticlotting blocking the availability of the precursor molecule arachidonic acid. This effect of the corticosteroids is achieved via induction of lipocortins, which are proteins that inhibit the action of phospholipase A_2. This is most likely the major mechanism by which corticosteroids produce the anti-inflammatory effect.

Ticlopidine inhibits platelet aggregation and clot retraction. Its mechanism of action does not, however, involve effects on eicosanoid metabolism. Instead, it prevents normal functioning of the platelet surface receptor for fibrinogen, thereby destabilizing the platelet plug.

ANSWER AND TUTORIAL ON ITEMS 98

The answer is: **98-C**. **Coronary heart disease** (CHD) is a major cause of death in the US and much of the rest of the industrialized world. The development of CHD is strongly correlated with abnormal levels of cholesterol- and triacylglycerol-containing lipoproteins in the blood. Lipoproteins are synthesized in the liver and intestinal mucosa and occur in four basic classes: high-density lipoprotein (HDL), intermediate-density lipoprotein (IDL), low-density lipoprotein (LDL), and very low-density lipoprotein (VLDL). Increased risk of CHD is associated with depressed levels of HDL and increased levels of IDL, LDL, and VLDL. In addition, increased risk of CHD is associated with elevated triglycerides and chylomicrons in blood.

The levels of lipoproteins, triglycerides, and chylomicrons can be elevated by diet, metabolic problems such as diabetes mellitus, hypothyroidism, biliary cirrhosis, and/or inherited defects in lipoprotein metabolism. Drugs used to treat hyperlipidemias have four basic mechanisms of action:

1) decrease secretion of lipoprotein by tissues

2) increased lipoprotein catabolism

3) inhibition of de novo cholesterol synthesis

4) increased excretion of cholesterol via removal of bile acids.

Figure 7.6 illustrates the basic features of lipoprotein metabolism.

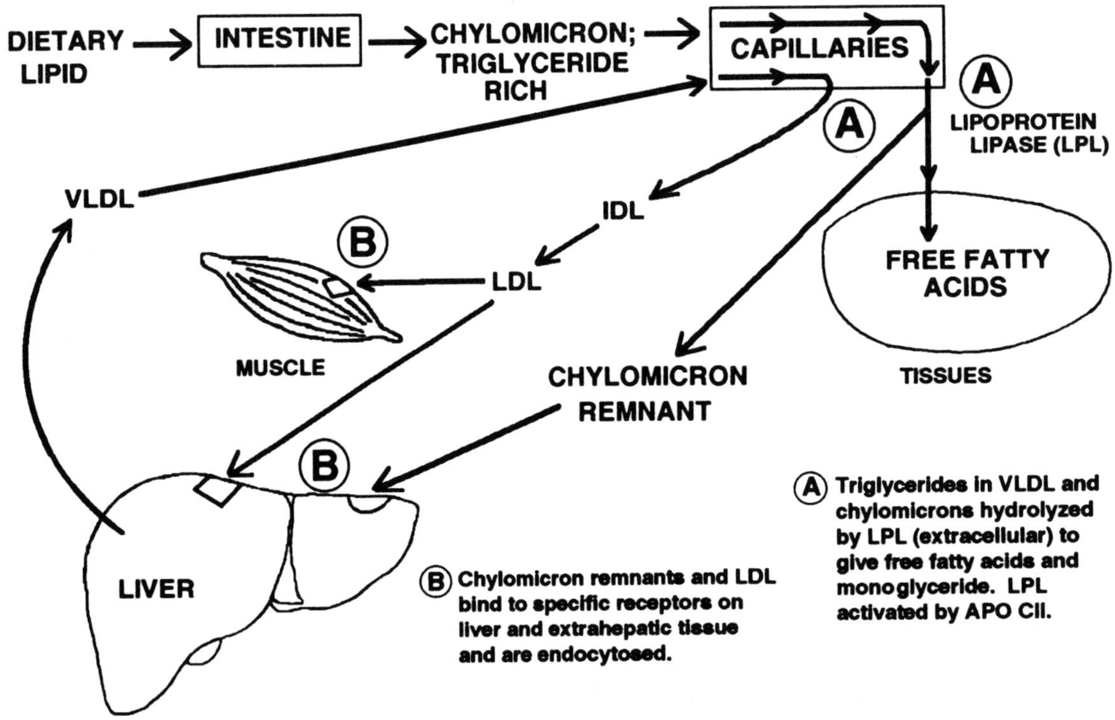

Figure 7.6

There are four major lipoprotein metabolic enzymes relevant to management of hyperlipidemias. Acyl-CoA:cholesterol acyltransferase (CACAT) esterifies cholesterol in the liver, extrahepatic tissues, and chylomicrons. Lecithin:cholesterol acyltransferase (LCAT) is an HDL-associated enzyme which esterifies cholesterol by transferring a fatty acid residue from lecithin to cholesterol. Lipoprotein lipase (LPL) hydrolyses triglycerides to free fatty acids and glycerol. 3-Hydroxy-3-methylglutaryl-CoA (HMG-CoA) reductase catalyses the formation of mevalonate, a key intermediate in cholesterol synthesis.

Primary hyperlipidemias have been divided into several broad classes based on biochemical differences in these disease entities (see below). Secondary hyperlipidemias are associated with other metabolic diseases, eg, hepatic disease, diabetes mellitus, or hypothyroidism.

Type I (familial hyperchylomicronemia) occurs when there is a normal dietary fat intake but fasting levels of chylomicrons, VLDL, and consequently plasma triglycerides are greatly elevated. It is caused by a deficiency in lipoprotein lipase or apoprotein C11. There is no single drug or combination of drugs efficacious in treatment. Low fat diet helps manage this condition.

Type IIA (familial hyperbetalipoproteinemia) manifests with elevated LDL and normal VLDL. It is due to decreased LDL receptors leading to decreased LDL degradation and concomitant elevated cholesterol with normal triglycerides. Xanthoma formation and CHD are serious problems here. This type is treated by low cholesterol and saturated fat diet. Useful medications include cholestyramine/colestipol and/or lovastatin/mevastatin. Probucol and niacin may also be used.

Type IIB [familial combined (mixed) hyperlipidemia] is similar to Type IIA but VLDL is also elevated leading to increased plasma triglycerides and cholesterol. It is treated by reducing intake of cholesterol, saturated fats, and alcohol. Drug treatment is similar to type IIA; however, when VLDL is very high, clofibrate or gemfibrozil may also be used.

Type III (familial dysbetalipoproteinemia) exhibits VLDL remnants, chylomicron remnants, and elevated plasma IDL. Plasma cholesterol and triglycerides are also increased. It is caused by excessive production or lowered utilization of IDL due perhaps to a mutant apoprotein. Here, accelerated xanthoma and atheroma formation is seen by middle age. This type is treated by reduced intake of cholesterol and alcohol and weight reduction. Drugs useful here include clofibrate or gemfibrozil and niacin. Lovastatin or mevastatin may also be used.

Type IV (familial hypertriglyceridemia) presents with very high levels of plasma triglycerides, normal to elevated cholesterol, elevated VLDL but normal or lowered LDL. It is caused by excessive production or decreased removal of VLDL from plasma. CHD is accelerated. Treatment includes restriction of fat, carbohydrate, and alcohol intake and treatment with either niacin, clofibrate, or gemfibrozil.

Type V (familial mixed hypertriglyceridemia) presents with very high triglycerides and an elevation in plasma chylomicrons, VLDL, and cholesterol. LDL is either normal or decreased. It is caused by increased production or decreased clearance of VLDL and chylomicrons. Treatment includes weight reduction and low fat diet, elimination of alcohol, and drug therapy with niacin, clofibrate, and/or gemfibrozil. Lovastatin (or mevastatin) may also be helpful.

Treatment of hyperlipidemias always begins with alteration of diet to reduce intake of cholesterol, total fat (particularly saturated fats), and alcohol. Drug treatments are secondary. All of the drugs described below are administered orally.

Cholestyramine and **colestipol** are anion exchange resins that bind bile acids and ensure their fecal elimination rather than allowing reentry into the enterohepatic circulation. The liver thus diverts cholesterol for bile acid synthesis, reducing the availability of cholesterol for lipoprotein synthesis. The drop in hepatocyte cholesterol levels also induces an increase in high-affinity LDL receptors on the hepatocyte cell surface. The overall effect of these resins is to reduce plasma cholesterol levels. These resins are used mainly in the management of Type IIA and Type IIB hyperlipidemias. GI disturbances are common side effects. Anion exchange resins will also bind vitamins and drugs although this problem can be circumvented by timing the other drugs with resin administration.

Clofibrate stimulates lipoprotein lipase (LPL) activity and thus causes a decrease in plasma VLDL levels. The increased clearance of triglyceride-rich lipoproteins caused by the increased LDL activity results in lower plasma triglycerides. Secondarily, an inhibition of hepatic cholesterol biosynthesis also occurs by an unknown mechanism. It is used primarily in treating Type III hyperlipidemia in which LDL accumulates and may also benefit Type IV and Type V patients. Clofibrate can cause GI disturbances and potentiates anticoagulants.

Gemfibrozil lowers plasma triglycerides (TG) by decreasing hepatic VLDL synthesis and increasing VLDL clearance from plasma. This is achieved by inhibition of hepatic incorporation of free fatty acids into TG thus lowering the availability of TG for VLDL synthesisand by increasing LPL activity. An increase in HDL may also occur. Gemfibrozil is used in treating Types III, IV, and V hyperlipidemias when elevated plasma VLDL and IDL are seen. GI disturbances and rashes may occur when gemfibrozil is used therapeutically and it also potentiates coumarin anticoagulant activity.

Lovastatin and mevastatin are analogs of 3-hydroxy-3-methylglutarate (HMG), a cholesterol precursor. They inhibit HMG-CoA reductase, leading to a decrease in intracellular cholesterol synthesis and an increase in high-affinity cell surface LDL receptors. These receptors bind and endocytose LDL, a major cholesterol carrier. The net result is increased LDL catabolism and decreased cholesterol synthesis, leading to decreased plasma cholesterol and reduced risk of CHD. These drugs are most effective in heterozygotes for familial hypercholesterolemia. Homozygotes lacking the LDL receptors benefit less from these drugs. Type III, IV, and V hyperlipidemic patients may also benefit from use of these drugs. These drugs are lipophilic and therefore poorly absorbed after oral administration. Once removed from blood, they are removed from the portal circulation in the liver and eliminated in bile and feces. Only small doses enter the systemic circulation and thus there are few adverse side effects with short-term treatment. Caution is indicated in patients with liver disease.

Niacin is a potent inhibitor of lipolysis in adipose tissue, the primary source of free fatty acids used by the liver for TG synthesis. Decreased hepatic TG synthesis leads to decreased hepatic VLDL synthesis which in turn leads to a lower plasma LDL level (LDL-cholesterol-rich particles are derived from VLDL in the plasma). The overall effect is lowering of plasma TG (from VLDL) and cholesterol (from VLDL and LDL). Oral niacin is converted into nicotinamide which is incorporated into NAD+ although nicotinamide itself has no lipid lowering effects. Niacin is used to treat Type IIB hyperlipoproteinemia where both VLDL and LDL are elevated. It is often used with other antihyperlipidemic drugs to treat other severe hypercholesterolemias. The most common side effects are cutaneous flushing and pruritus. Aspirin taken prior to niacin will reduce flushing which is probably prostaglandin mediated.

Probucol reduces plasma cholesterol by lowering plasma LDL levels. The exact mechanism is not understood but perhaps it stimulates a low-affinity LDL uptake pathway. It may also reduce CHD risk by a mild antioxidant effect. It also decreases HDL levels. This limits it usefulness because decreased HDL is associated with increased risk of CHD. It is used to treat Type IIA disease not responsive to other drugs. Adverse side effects include GI upset and cardiac arrhythmias.

Answer and Tutorial on Item 99

The answer is: **99-A.** The primary factor underlying the cause and pain of **peptic ulcer** is the enhanced secretion of HCl by gastric parietal cells. Treatment of peptic ulcer can be approached by 1) decreasing stimuli causing HCl secretion; 2) neutralizing acid after release; 3) protecting the gastric mucosa. Recently, ***Helicobacter pylori*** has been implicated as a causative agent in gastritis and peptic ulcer formation and/or recurrence. Thus, treatment of peptic ulcers may include a course of antibiotics along with an antisecretory agent. New treatment regimens are currently being developed.

DRUGS USED IN PEPTIC ULCER TREATMENT

DRUG CLASS	EXAMPLES
Antacids	Sodium bicarbonate Calcium carbonate Aluminum hydroxide Magnesium hydroxide
Antimuscarinic agents	Pirenzepine Telenzepine
H_2-histamine receptor blockers	Cimetidine Famotidine Nizatidine Ranitidine
Mucosal protectants	Colloidal bismuth Sucralfate
Prostaglandins	Misoprostol
Proton pump inhibitors	Omeprazole
Antibiotics	Amoxicillin Metronidazole Tetracycline

Antacids are divided into two groups–systematic and nonsystematic. Systematic antacids (eg, sodium bicarbonate) are very effective; however, they are readily absorbed enterically, leading to metabolic alkalosis and increased gastric HCl secretion. Their use has been discontinued by physicians but they are still widely used in over-the-counter remedies.

Nonsystematic antacids (eg, calcium carbonate, aluminum hydroxide, and magnesium hydroxide) are less soluble and buffer the gastric contents to approximately pH 4.0. They act locally and produce no drastic changes in acid-base chemistry. Furthermore, they do not trigger gastric HCl secretion. $Al(OH)_3$ reacts with HCl to form insoluble $AlCl_3$ which may cause constipation. It also binds to tetracycline, preventing absorption of this antibiotic. $CaCO_3$, in addition to aiding in healing of duodenal ulcers and esophagitis, is also a good source of Ca^{2+} but may lead to hypercalcemia. $Mg(OH)_2$ ("milk of magnesia") forms insoluble salts when it neutralizes HCl, slowing their removal from the stomach and drawing fluid into the GI tract, thus they act as good cathartics. Many antacids combine $Al(OH)_3$ and $Mg(OH)_2$ so they counteract each other's side effects (ie, constipation and diarrhea).

Pirenzepine and telenzepine are cholinergic antagonists used as adjuncts in patients not responding to treatment with H_2histamine receptor blockers alone. Pirenzepine, in contrast to other anticholinergics, shows more specificity for gastric secretory function and less against smooth muscle and salivary glands.

H_2-histamine receptor blockers Briefly, histamine exerts a potent effect on stimulation of HCl secretion by gastric parietal cells. It binds to H_2 receptors on the parietal cells, initiating a cAMP-mediated cascade. Cimetidine and other drugs in this class competitively block the H_2-histamine receptor, decreasing acid secretion and promoting healing of ulcers in 3-4 weeks. They are administered orally, distributed throughout the body, and excreted in the urine.

Colloidal bismuth coats and binds to both gastric and duodenal ulcers, thus protecting them from acid and pepsin. Sucralfate (aluminum sucrose sulfate) selectively binds to ulcerated tissue, forming a barrier to further ulceration. It requires an acidic pH for activation and therefore should not be given with antacids or H_2-histamine blockers.

Misoprostol is a methyl ester analog of prostaglandin E_1. It is superior to cimetidine in lowering mucosal damage caused by the chronic ingestion of NSAIDs. Misoprostol has antisecretory and cytoprotective properties and causes healing and pain relief in both peptic and duodenal ulcers. It is very useful in patients with duodenal ulcers who are not responsive to H_2-histamine receptor blockers.

Omeprazol inhibits the gastric parietal cell membrane H^+/K^+-ATPase proton pump required for the final step of HCl secretion. It does not affect pepsin or gastric intrinsic factor secretion. Omeprazol is used in the treatment of ulcers in patients who do not respond to H_2-histamine receptor blockers. It also offers symptomatic relief in Zollinger-Ellison syndrome. It is effective in a once-daily dose and is safe and well tolerated.

All of these treatments often provide only temporary relief from ulcers. Although there has been strong evidence for involvement of *Helicobacter pylori* in causing some ulcers, the medical community has been slow to respond by treating ulcers with antibiotics. When antimicrobial therapy has been coupled with treatment for excessive HCl secretion in patients with ulcers and *H. pylori* infection, there has been a marked decrease in recurrence of ulcers following eradication of *H. pylori* infection.

Answers and Tutorial on Items 100-101

The answers are: **100-E; 101-E**. There are five major classes of diuretic drugs. The first class is **carbonic anhydrase inhibitors**, the most widely used example of which is **acetazolamide**. This weak diuretic drug acts by inhibiting the exchange of H^+ for Na^+ in the proximal convoluted tubule.

The second class is **loop diuretics**. These potent diuretics include ethacrynic acid, bumetanide, **furosemide**, and muzolimine. These drugs have their effects on the ascending limb of the loop of Henle where they inhibit $Na^+/K^+/Cl^-$ cotransport. Since these ions are retained, water is also retained and urine product increases.

The third class is **thiazide diuretics**. These include **chlorothiazide**, hydrochlorothiazide, chlorthalidone, and metolazone (a thiazide analog). These drugs have their effects on the distal convoluted tubules . They cause retention of ions and consequently water in the distal convoluted tubules.

The fourth class are the **K^+-sparing diuretics** such as **spironolactone**, triamterene, and amiloride. These drugs have their effects on the distal convoluted tubules, specifically inhibiting Na^+ resorption as well as K^+ and H^+, thus their name. They are often used with loop or thiazide diuretics to combat the hypokalemia caused by these drugs.

The fifth class are the **osmotic diuretics** including **mannitol** and urea. They enter the urinary filtrate but are not efficiently resorbed. Thus, they increase the osmotic pressure of the filtrate drawing water into tubular fluid and increasing the rate of urine production.

Antidiuretic hormone (ADH) is secreted by the neurohypophysis. It is an octapeptide hormone which is secreted under conditions of water deficit. ADH and a synthetic analog **desmopressin** (1-deamino-8-D-arginine vasopressin) act on the **collecting tubules** primarily (having secondary effects on the distal convoluted tubules), reducing their water permeability and thus increasing urine concentration and decreasing water loss. They are used pharmacologically in the treatment of ADH-sensitive diabetes insipidus.

Renin is a secretion product of the specialized cells in the wall of the afferent arteriole, a component of the juxtaglomerular apparatus. Renin catalyzes the conversion of angiotensinogen to angiotensin I. A second enzyme, angiotensin converting enzyme (ACE) cleaves angiotensin I to angiotensin II, a potent vasoconstrictor.

Notes

CHAPTER 8

Pathology

DIRECTIONS (Items 1-117): For each of the numbered items that proceed, you must select the single best answer from among the lettered options listed.

Some of the numbered items will pose a question or incomplete sentence that is followed by a list of 4-5 lettered options. In all cases, select the ONE lettered option that best answers the question or completes the sentence given.

Some of the numbered items are preceded by 5-24 lettered options. In these sets, the lettered options will be preceded by a single instruction asking you to match one of the lettered options to each numbered item most closely associated with it. In all matching sets, you may use any of the lettered options once, more than once or not at all, but you should still only select ONE lettered option per numbered item.

If you wish to simulate actual USMLE testing conditions, you should aim to complete all the items in this chapter in 2 hours.

Do NOT look at the answers and tutorials until you have completed all of the items in this chapter.

Good luck!

Items 1-4

1. A 45-year-old man presented with hyperpigmentation of the skin, ascites, and abnormal liver function tests. His serum iron was 210 µg/dl, and the transferrin saturation was 90%. The most likely diagnosis is

   (A) erythropoietic porphyria
   (B) hepatic porphyria
   (C) iron intoxication
   (D) primary hemochromatosis
   (E) secondary hemochromatosis

2. Which of the following organs is LEAST LIKELY to be affected by this disease?

   (A) brain
   (B) heart
   (C) liver
   (D) pancreas
   (E) skin

3. Which of the following clinical manifestations is LEAST LIKELY to occur in this patient?

   (A) congestive heart failure
   (B) diabetes mellitus
   (C) hepatocarcinoma
   (D) photosensitivity dermatitis
   (E) testicular atrophy

4. Secondary hemochromatosis is most likely to occur in patients

   (A) with Addison's disease
   (B) with high dietary iron content
   (C) with malaria
   (D) with porphyria
   (E) requiring multiple blood transfusions

Item 5

A middle-aged homeless man was found unconscious on the street and died shortly after admission to the hospital. The cause of death was acute liver failure. A photomicrograph of the liver at autopsy is shown below in **Figure 8.1**.

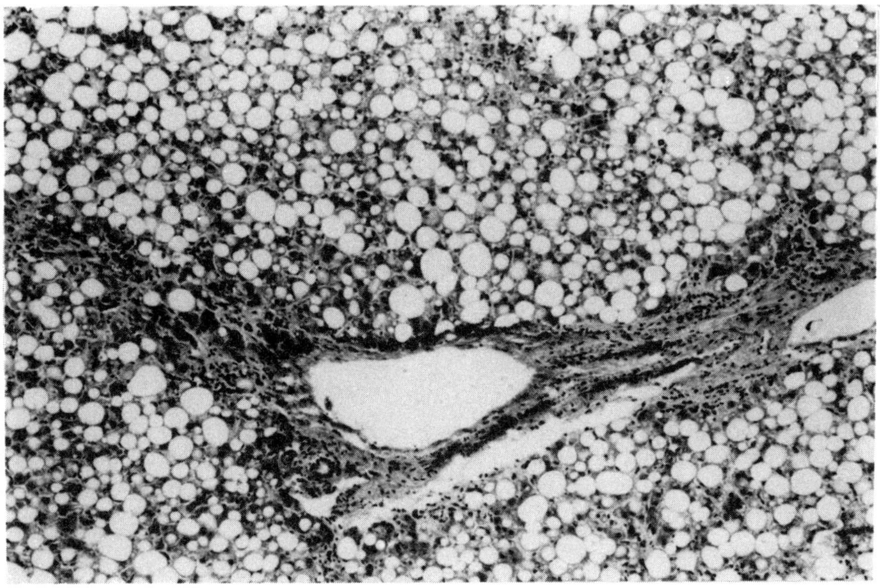

Figure 8.1

5. The most likely pathologic process shown is

   (A) cloudy swelling
   (B) coagulation necrosis
   (C) fatty degeneration
   (D) hydropic degeneration
   (E) inflammation

Items 6-8

A man with poor dentition and oral hygiene developed chills and fever. A chest film revealed a small, round opacity in the RLL. A photomicrograph of the lesion from a segmental resection is shown below in **Figure 8.2.**

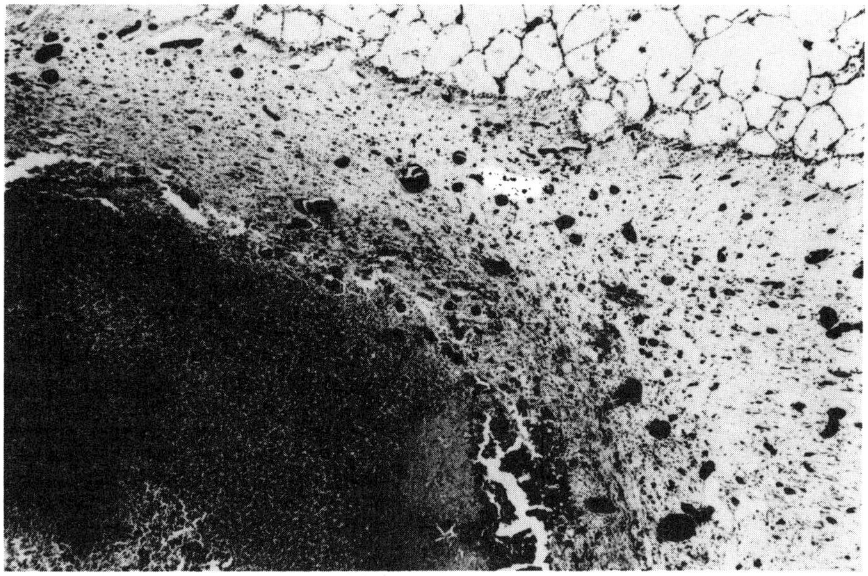

Figure 8.2

6. The most likely diagnosis is

 (A) abscess
 (B) bronchopneumonia
 (C) carcinoma
 (D) infarct
 (E) tuberculosis

7. The type of necrosis in the lesion shown above is

 (A) caseation
 (B) coagulation
 (C) fibrinoid
 (D) hemorrhagic
 (E) liquefaction

8. The cause of the type of necrosis shown above is

 (A) arterial occlusion by an embolus
 (B) bacterial toxins
 (C) cell-mediated immune reaction
 (D) lysosomal enzymes from neutrophils
 (E) outgrowth of blood supply by malignant cells

Items 9-12

Match each type of cancer with the cause known or strongly suspected to be associated with it.

(A) aniline dyes
(B) aflatoxin
(C) Epstein-Barr virus
(D) nitrates
(E) papilloma virus

9. Cervical carcinoma

10. Hepatocarcinoma

11. Burkitt's lymphoma

12. Urinary bladder carcinoma

Items 13-15

13. Following a camping trip, a young man developed a hemorrhagic rash, diagnosed as spotted fever. In spotted fever, the rickettsiae are found within

(A) endothelial cells
(B) epidermal basal cells
(C) Kupffer cells
(D) macrophages
(E) splenic phagocytes

14. On his return from a trip to South America, a 30-year-old man complained of diarrhea as well as tenesmus. *Entamoeba histolytica* was found in his feces. A common complication of amoebic dysentery is

(A) adrenal cortical necrosis
(B) carrier state due to amoebic cholecystitis
(C) liver abscess
(D) perforation of amoebic ulcer in colon
(E) sigmoid colon obstruction due to fibrosis

15. A 60-year-old resident of northern Minnesota who was an inveterate fisherman in nearby lakes became pale and easily fatigued. He was found to have a megaloblastic anemia due to vitamin B_{12} deficiency. Further studies discovered a helminthic infestation. The causative organism is

(A) *Diphyllobothrium latum*
(B) *Echinococcus granulosus*
(C) *Hymenolepis naud*
(D) *Taenia saginata*
(E) *Taenia solium*

Item 16

One month before death, a 65-year-old man suffered sharp costovertebral angle pain and had an episode of hematuria. A photograph of the involved kidney is shown below in **Figure 8.3.**

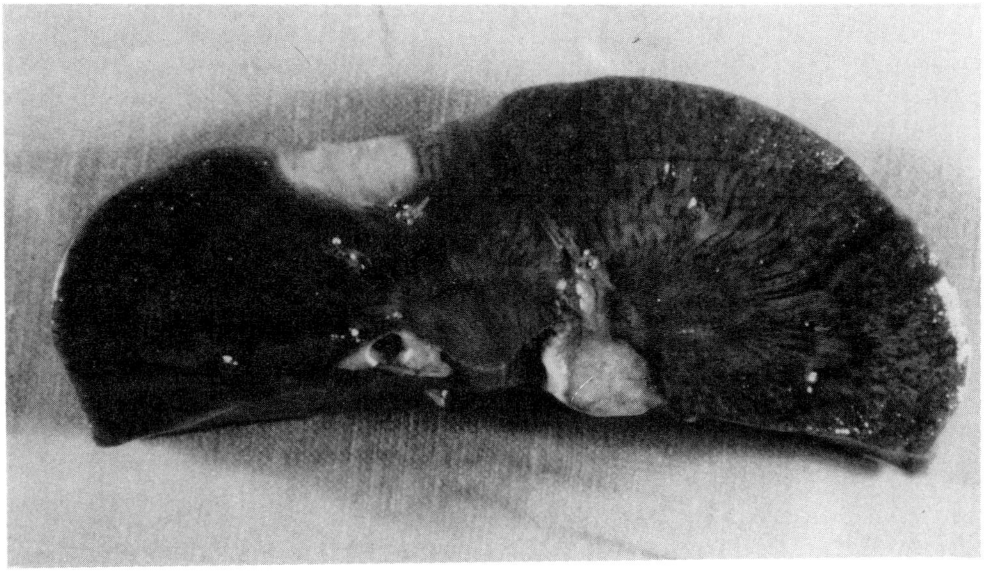

Figure 8.3

16. The likeliest diagnosis in this kidney is

    (A) abscess
    (B) adenoma
    (C) carcinoma
    (D) hematoma
    (E) infarct

Items 17-22

Match each disorder with the type of hemorrhage which typically occurs with it.

(A) Ecchymosis
(B) Epistaxis
(C) Hematemesis
(D) Hemoptysis
(E) Melena
(F) Metrorrhagia
(G) Petechiae

17. Battered child syndrome

18. Duodenal ulcer

19. Fractured nose

20. Portal hypertension

21. Thrombocytopenia

22. Tuberculosis of lung

Items 23-28

Match the change with the vitamin deficiency with which it is most closely related.

(A) Avitaminosis A
(B) Avitaminosis C
(C) Avitaminosis D
(D) Avitaminosis K
(E) Cyanocobalamin deficiency
(F) Riboflavin deficiency
(G) Niacin deficiency
(H) Thiamine deficiency

23. Hemorrhages from prothrombin deficiency

24. Night bindness (nyctalopia)

25. Erythema and hyperpigmentation of skin

26. Bone softening due to formation of osteoid that fails to calcify

27. Delayed callus formation because of deficient cartilage and osteoid formation

28. Dilated cardiomyopathy

Item 29

29. A 30-year-old woman, who had scarlet fever when she was 10 years old, was found to have a cardiac murmur. She was diagnosed as having rheumatic heart disease. The type of valvular lesion most closely related to this disease is

    (A) aortic insufficiency
    (B) aortic stenosis
    (C) mitral stenosis
    (D) pulmonic stenosis
    (E) tricuspid stenosis

Item 30

30. Which of the following would LEAST LIKELY cause myocarditis?

    (A) Coxsackie virus group B infection
    (B) Diphtheria exotoxin
    (C) Chagas' disease
    (D) syphilis
    (E) toxoplasmosis

Item 31

31. A 60-year-old man who had been diagnosed 3 days before as having had an acute myocardial infarct suddenly developed mitral insufficiency. This was most likely due to

    (A) coincidental rheumatic mitral stenosis
    (B) extension of the infarct to a mitral valve leaflet
    (C) rupture of an infarcted interventricular septum
    (D) rupture of an infarcted papillary muscle
    (E) subacute bacterial endocarditis on the mitral valve

Item 32

32. The most common primary neoplasm of the heart is the

    (A) lipoma
    (B) myxoma
    (C) papillary fibroelastoma
    (D) rhabdomyoma
    (E) rhabdomyosarcoma

Items 33-34

33. The presence of HbF in the blood of children and adults is characteristic of

    (A) α-thalassemia
    (B) β-thalassemia
    (C) megaloblastic anemia
    (D) sickle cell anemia
    (E) spherocytic anemia

34. The commonest cause of iron deficiency anemia in adults in the United States is

    (A) chronic blood loss
    (B) chronic renal failure
    (C) inadequate iron intake in diet
    (D) iron loss due to hemolysis
    (E) mucosal block to iron absorption in duodenum

Items 35-37

35. A 60-year-old man complained of bone pain, especially in his spine. X-rays revealed lytic lesions in the vertebrae and skull. He also had anemia and hypercalcemia. The likeliest diagnosis is

    (A) Burkitt's lymphoma
    (B) chronic lymphocytic lymphoma
    (C) heavy chain disease
    (D) multiple myeloma
    (E) Waldenstöm's macroglobulinemia

36. Which of the following findings would LEAST LIKELY be present in this patient?

    (A) Bence-Jones proteinuria
    (B) Decreased resistance to infection
    (C) Infiltration of flat bones by plasma cells
    (D) Macroglobulinemia
    (E) Monoclonal gammopathy

37. A 40-year-old man presented with weight loss and painless lymphadenopathy. A node biopsy showed proliferation of germinal centers in the cortex and medulla. The enlarged centers consisted of poorly differentiated lymphocytes. The likeliest diagnosis is

    (A) acute lymphadenitis
    (B) Burkitt's lymphoma
    (C) diffuse poorly differentiated lymphocytic lympyhoma
    (D) follicular (nodular) lymphocytic lymphoma
    (E) lymphocyte predominance Hodgkin's disease

Items 38-40

A 25-year-old woman had recurrent low grade fever and cervical lymphadenopathy. Photomicrographs of a lymph node biopsy are found in **Figure 8.4** below.

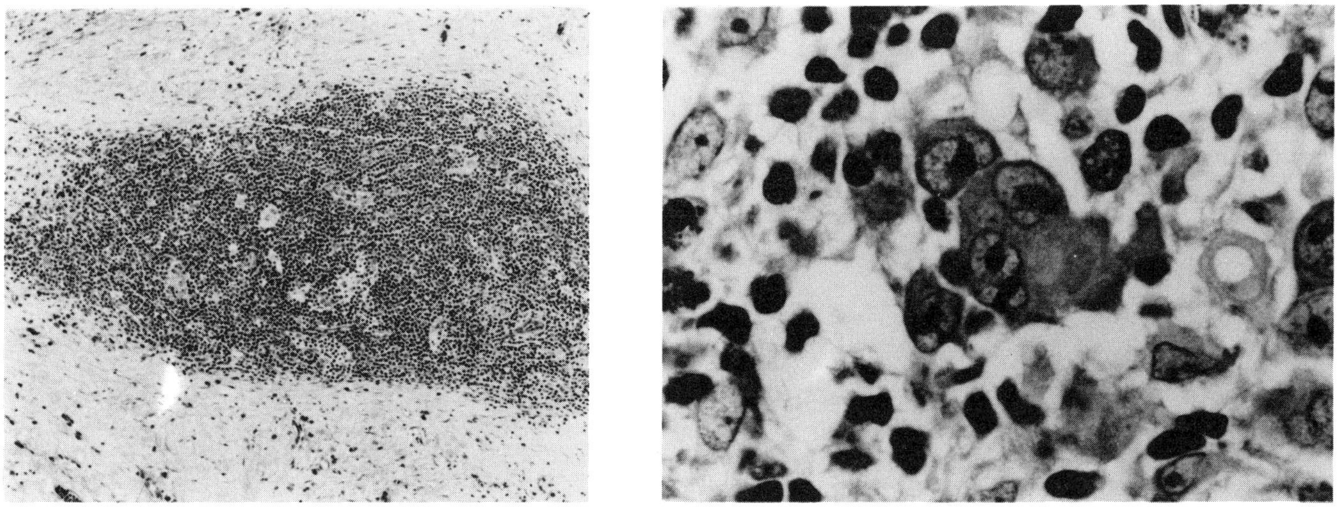

Figure 8.4

38. The most likely diagnosis is

    (A) Burkitt's lymphoma
    (B) chronic lymphadenitis
    (C) histiocytic lymphoma
    (D) Hodgkin's disease
    (E) nodular lymphoma

39. All of the following statements are true concerning Hodgkin's disease EXCEPT

    (A) Burkitt's lymphoma is a variant occurring in Africa
    (B) leukemia and other malignancies have appeared in patients successfully treated for Hodgkin's disease
    (C) lymph nodes and spleen are commonly involved
    (D) nodular sclerosis type is the commonest form
    (E) Reed-Sternberg cells are the most important diagnostic feature

40. The patient was found to have involvement of the cervical and mediastinal lymph nodes and spleen. The extent of the disease was

    (A) Stage IA
    (B) Stage IIB
    (C) Stage IIIA
    (D) Stage IIIB
    (E) Stage IVB

Item 41

41. The most distinctive feature of acute myeloblastic leukemia is the presence of

    (A) Auer bodies (eosinophilic rods) in myeloblasts
    (B) blast crisis
    (C) chloromas
    (D) Philadelphia chromosomes in neutrophils
    (E) virus particles in myeloblasts

Items 42-51

Match the disorder with the type of immune mechanism which is associated with it.

(A) Type I (immediate hypersensitivity)
(B) Type II (antibody dependent hypersensitivity)
(C) Type III (immune complex hypersensitivity)
(D) Type IV (cell-mediated hypersensitivity)

42. Asthma

43. Autoimmune hemolytic anemia

44. Contact dermatitis to poison ivy

45. Erythroblastosis fetalis

46. Goodpasture's syndrome

47. Hay fever

48. Lupus erythematosus

49. Polyarteritis nodosa

50. Post-streptococcal glomerulonephritis

51. Urticaria

Items 52-58

Match the item with the disease with which each is most closely associated.

(A) Amyloidosis
(B) Dermatomyositis
(C) Disseminated lupus erythematosus
(D) Polyarteritis nodosa
(E) Progressive systemic sclerosis (scleroderma)

52. Collagenous thickening of dermis

53. Fibrinoid necrosis of medium-sized arteries

54. Hematoxylin bodies

55. Immunoglobulin light chain deposition in glomeruli

56. Increased incidence of malignant neoplasms

57. Soluble immune complex deposits in glomeruli

58. Sterile vegetations on heart valves

Item 59

59. A striking increase in the incidence of malignant neoplasms occurs in patients with

(A) atopic disorders
(B) disseminated lupus erythematosus
(C) immune deficiency disorders
(D) scleroderma
(E) tuberculosis

Items 60-67

Match each clinical summary with the type of anemia with which it is most closely related.

(A) α-Thalassemia
(B) Anemia due to glucose-6-phosphate dehydrogenase (G6PD) deficiency
(C) Aplastic anemia
(D) Autoimmune hemolytic anemia
(E) β-Thalassemia
(F) Hereditary spherocytic anemia
(G) Iron deficiency anemia
(H) Myelophthisic anemia
(I) Pernicious anemia
(J) Sickle cell anemia
(K) Sideroblastic anemia

60. A 10-year-old boy was found to have mild jaundice, with an elevation mainly of unconjugated bilirubin, and splenomegaly. His erythrocyte count was 4 million/mm^3, and the corrected reticulocyte count was 3%. The serum iron was 120 mg/dL.

61. A 4-year-old African-American child developed pneumonia. While being treated for this he began to have episodes of bone pain. His erythrocyte count was 3 million/mm^3, and the corrected reticulocyte count was 3%. The serum iron was 120 μg/dl.

62. An Italian-American child was noted to be listless, easily fatigued, and pale. His erythrocyte count was 2 million/mm^3, corrected reticulocyte count 5%, and serum iron 100 mg/dL. Numerous target cells were seen on the peripheral blood smear. HbF and HbA2 were present in significant amounts.

63. A 25-year-old woman had menometrorrhagia for several months. She complained of being weak and chronically tired. Her erythrocyte count was 3.5 million/mm^3, corrected reticulocyte count 1%, and serum iron 50 μg/dl with a high total iron binding capacity.

64. A 60-year-old man gave a 6-month history of gradually worsening fatigue and dyspnea on exertion. He had tingling in his feet. His erythrocyte count was 2 million/mm^3. Gastric analysis revealed achlorhydria.

65. A 64-year-old woman with a history of a mastectomy for breast cancer 2 years before suffered collapse of several vertebrae. She was found to have extensive bony metastases. Her erythrocyte count was 3 million/mm^3 and corrected reticulocyte count 1%.

66. A 40-year-old woman developed weakness, pallor, skin hemorrhages, and fever. Her erythrocyte count was 1.5 million/mm^3, leukocyte count 1500/mm^3, and platelet count 40,000/mm^3.

67. A 40-year-old African-American Vietnam War veteran developed episodes of hemolysis on using certain drugs. Numerous Heinz bodies were found in his erythrocytes during these periods.

Items 68-73

Match the antigen with the organ specific autoimmune disease in which it is a principal target.

(A) Addison's disease
(B) Goodpasture's syndrome
(C) Grave's disease (primary hyperthyroidism)
(D) Idiopathic thrombocytopenic purpura
(E) Juvenile diabetes mellitus
(F) Lymphocytic (Hashimoto's) thyroiditis
(G) Myasthenia gravis
(H) Pernicious anemia

68. Acetylcholine receptor

69. Gastric parietal cells

70. Glomerular and lung basement membranes

71. Microsomal antigen

72. Pancreatic islet cells

73. Thyroid stimulating hormone (TSH) receptor

Items 74-75

74. A 50-year-old woman had tuberculosis involving the left upper lobe years ago. It had been treated successfully with isoniazid, but there was considerable residual fibrosis. A carcinoma had developed in the LUL. The type of lung cancer most often associated with pulmonary scars is

(A) adenocarcinoma
(B) anaplastic small cell carcinoma
(C) epidermoid carcinoma
(D) giant cell carcinoma
(E) metastatic carcinoma

75. A 60-year-old man, who had been a heavy smoker for years, noted weight loss, dyspnea, and coughing. Bronchoscopy revealed a mass in the right main bronchus. A photomicrograph of the biopsy is shown below in **Figure 8.5**. The likeliest diagnosis is

(A) anaplastic small cell carcinoma
(B) carcinoid bronchial adenoma
(C) lymphoma
(D) poorly differentiated adenocarcinoma
(E) squamous cell carcinoma

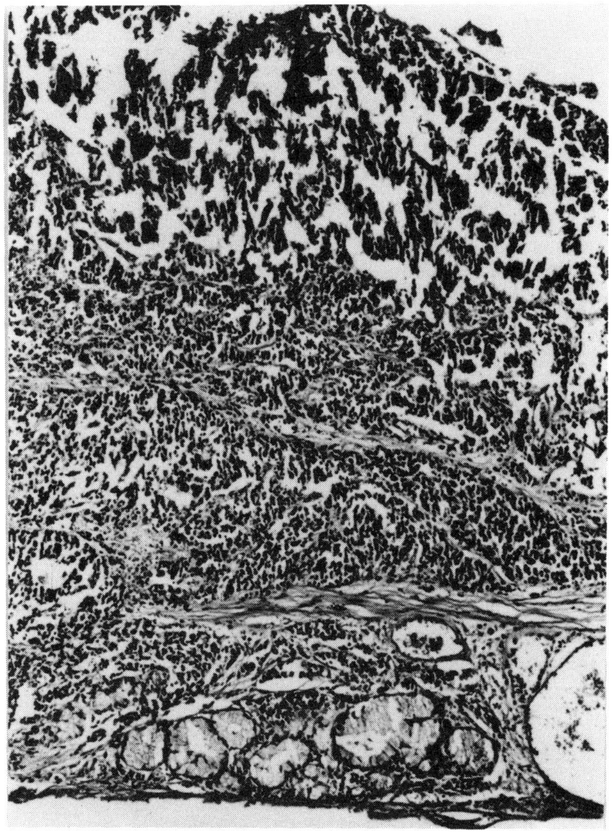

Figure 8.5

Item 76

76. A 50-year-old man who had smoked over a pack of cigarettes daily for many years had a hacking cough productive of mucoid sputum for 2 years. He had scattered rhonchi and wheezing. The likeliest diagnosis is

(A) asthma
(B) bronchiectasis
(C) chronic bronchitis
(D) chronic pneumonitis
(E) diffuse pulmonary fibrosis

Items 77-78

77. Of the following, the lung disorder which is most characteristically associated with the development of pulmonary tuberculosis is

(A) anthracosis
(B) bronchiectasis
(C) centrilobular emphysema
(D) lipid pneumonia
(E) silicosis

78. The cause of farmer's lung is

(A) hypersensitivity to actinomycetes in moldy hay
(B) hypersensitivity to actinomycetes in bagasse
(C) hypersensitivity to antigen in bird droppings
(D) hypersensitivity to antigen in wheat weevil
(E) nitrogen dioxide in silage

Item 79

79. A 50-year-old man attended a banquet where he had several drinks and a heavy meal. A few hours later he had severe upper abdominal pain and vomiting. He went into shock. The most likely diagnosis is

(A) acute cholecystitis
(B) acute gastroenteritis
(C) acute pancreatitis
(D) intussusception
(E) perforated duodenal ulcer

Items 80-81

80. Adenoma of the liver occurs in increased incidence in patients taking

(A) chlorpromazine
(B) cimetidine
(C) erythromycin
(D) oral contraceptives
(E) reserpine

81. The most common malignant neoplasm of the liver in the United States is

(A) cardinoid
(B) cholangiocarcinoma
(C) hepatocarcinoma
(D) Kaposi's sarcoma
(E) metastatic carcinoma

Item 82

82. Several weeks after surgery during which he received a blood transfusion, a 45-year-old man developed jaundice, fever, nausea, and vomiting. Hepatitis was diagnosed. The virus most commonly transmitted during blood transfusion is

(A) hepatitis A
(B) hepatitis B
(C) hepatitis C
(D) hepatitis D (delta)
(E) human immunodeficiency virus (HIV)

Item 83

83. The commonest complication of diverticulosis of the colon is

(A) development of carcinoma
(B) diverticulitis
(C) hemorrhage
(D) obstruction
(E) perforation

Items 84-87

84. A 10-year-old boy developed a pharyngitis due to B-hemolytic streptococci. It subsided after a few days of penicillin therapy. Two weeks later his eyelids became puffy, and he had a fever, elevated blood pressure and gross hematuria. The likeliest diagnosis is

(A) acute proliferative glomerulonephritis
(B) antiglomerular basement membrane disease
(C) membranous glomerulonephropathy
(D) minimal change disease
(E) rapidly progressive glomerulonephritis

85. A 35-year-old man developed hematuria, proteinuria, mounting azotemia, and hypertension. A renal biopsy confirmed the diagnosis of rapidly progressive glomerulonephritis. The most characteristic microscopic finding in this condition is

(A) epithelial crescents within glomeruli
(B) hyalinization of numerous glomeruli
(C) hyalinization of walls of afferent arterioles
(D) proliferation of glomerular tuft and mesangial cells
(E) uniform thickening of glomerular basement membranes

86. A 25-year-old man developed hematuria and hemoptysis. Immunofluorescent studies on a renal biopsy demonstrated linear immune globulin deposits along glomerular basement membranes. The most likely diagnosis is

(A) acute proliferative glomerulonephritis
(B) diabetic glomerulosclerosis
(C) Goodpasture's syndrome
(D) lupus nephritis
(E) membranous glomerulonephropathy

87. An 8-year-old girl was found to have nephrotic syndrome. The commonest cause of this disorder in children is

(A) acute proliferative glomerulonephritis
(B) membranous glomerulonephropathy
(C) minimal change glomerulonephropathy
(D) nephroblastoma (Wilms' tumor)
(E) rapidly progressive glomerulonephritis

Items 88-90

88. The typical microscopic feature of toxic nephrosis is

(A) degeneration of proximal convoluted tubular epithelium
(B) degeneration of distal convoluted tubular epithelium
(C) interstitial edema and lymphocytic infiltration
(D) necrotizing papillitis
(E) tubulorrhexis (focal rupture of tubular basement membranes)

89. The most characteristic feature in a patient with acute tubular necrosis is

(A) hematuria
(B) hyposthenuria
(C) oliguria
(D) proteinuria
(E) pyuria

90. The drug which causes renal papillary necrosis is

(A) acetophenetidin
(B) gentamicin
(C) gold
(D) methicillin
(E) methoxyflurane

Item 91

91. A 35-year-old mother of six children with a history of hypertension died of renal failure. At autopsy the kidneys were atrophic and unequal in size (right 80 gm, left 100 gm), had wide U-shaped scars on their surfaces, and slightly dilated pleves and calyces with scarring of their walls. The cut surfaces were grossly fibrotic. The likeliest diagnosis is

(A) arteriolonephrosclerosis
(B) chronic glomerulonephritis
(C) chronic pyelonephritis
(D) hereditary nephritis
(E) stenosis of one renal artery

Item 92

A 50-year-old man developed hematuria. He was found to have a large neoplasm in his right kidney, which was surgically removed. A photograph of the gross specimen is shown below in **Figure 8-6**.

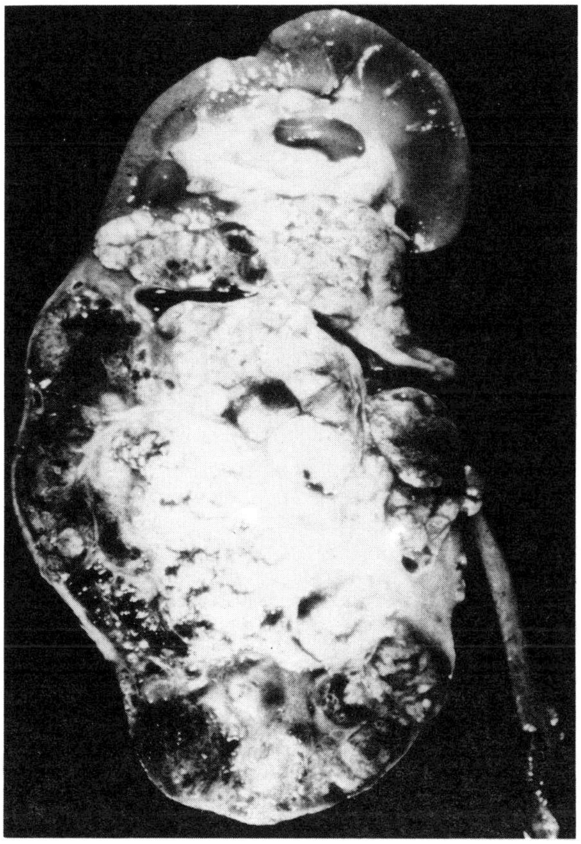

Figure 8.6

92. The neoplasm shown in the photograph arises from

 (A) adrenal cortical rests
 (B) glomerular epithelium
 (C) metanephrogenic blastema
 (D) proximal convoluted tubular epithelium
 (E) collecting tubular epithelium

Items 93-95

93. A 30-year-old male prostitute developed severe constipation and passed only cigarette-sized fecal masses. The most likely cause is

 (A) AIDS
 (B) carcinoma of the rectum
 (C) granuloma inguinale
 (D) lymphopathia venereum
 (E) syphilis

94. A 60-year-old man developed urinary frequency and retained residual urine. Digital rectal examination revealed a nodular prostate which was neither hard nor fixed. His serum prostate specific antigen (PSA) level was 1.5 units. The likeliest diagnosis is

 (A) acute prostatitis
 (B) adenocarcinoma of prostate
 (C) hyperplasia of prostate
 (D) chronic prostatitis
 (E) tuberculous prostatitis

95. After puberty the most frequent complication of cryptorchidism is

 (A) atrophy of the undescended testis
 (B) development of a neoplasm in the undescended testis
 (C) gynecomastia
 (D) femoral hernia
 (E) varicocele

Items 96-98

96. Of the following, the pathologic change in a 20-year-old woman which has been significantly associated with intrauterine exposure to diethylstilbestrol is

 (A) adenocarcinoma of endometrium
 (B) clear cell adenocarcinoma of vagina
 (C) endometriosis
 (D) leiomyomata of uterus
 (E) serous cystadenoma of ovary

97. The usual cause of death in fatal cases of cervical carcinoma is

(A) hepatic failure due to liver metastases
(B) hypercalcemia due to bone metastases
(C) intestinal obstruction
(D) pulmonary embolism
(E) uremia due to urinary obstruction and infection

98. During an infertility work-up a 30-year-old woman was found to have enlarged ovaries with "chocolate cysts." The most likely diagnosis is

(A) corpora hemorrhagica
(B) endometriosis
(C) hemorrhage into serous cystadenomas
(D) dermoid cysts
(E) metastatic melanoma

Item 99

A 25-year-old woman felt a rubbery, movable 2 cm mass in her right breast. It was removed surgically. A photomicrograph of the lesion pictured in **Figure 8.7**.

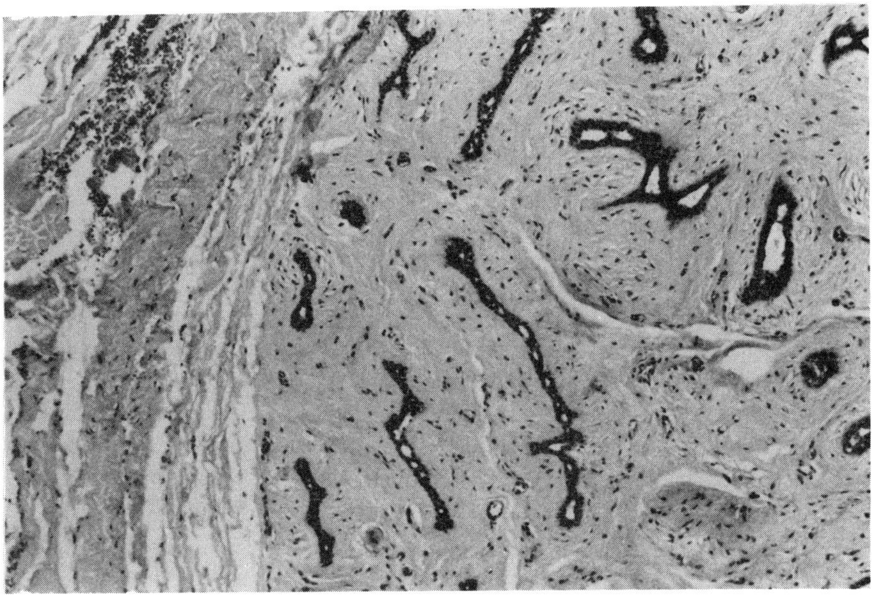

Figure 8.7

99. This is most likely a diagnosis of

(A) fibroadenoma
(B) fibrocystic mastopathy
(C) carcinoma
(D) periductal mastitis
(E) sclerosing adenosis

Items 100-102

100. By the age of 16, a young man had grown to a height of 7 feet. Skull films showed an enlargement of the sella turcica. The most likely causative lesion is

   (A) acidophil adenoma of pituitary
   (B) basophil adenoma of pituitary
   (C) craniopharyngioma
   (D) pinealoma
   (E) pituitary adenocarcinoma

101. A 30-year-old man developed bilateral homonymous hemianopsia. He also had moderate enlargement of his lower jaw and hands. Of the following the likeliest cause is

   (A) adamantinoma
   (B) basophil adenoma of pituitary
   (C) chromophobe adenoma of pituitary
   (D) craniopharyngioma
   (E) glioma of optic chiasm

102. During labor, a 25-year-old grava 3 para 2 had a premature placental separation and lost 500 ml. of blood. Postpartum she developed panhypopituitarism. The cause of the hypopituitarism in Sheehan's syndrome is

   (A) chromophobe adenoma of pituitary
   (B) craniopharyngioma
   (C) hemorrhage into sella turcica
   (D) idiopathic atrophy of pituitary
   (E) infarction of pituitary

Item 103

103. A 40-year-old Caucasian male became weak and easily fatigued. His skin and gingiva were tan, and his blood pressure was 110/60. Addison's disease was diagnosed. In chronic adrenal cortical insufficiency, the commonest adrenal lesion is

   (A) amyloidosis
   (B) histoplasmosis
   (C) idiopathic atrophy
   (D) metastatic carcinoma
   (E) tuberculosis

Item 104

A 30-year-old woman became hyperactive and irritable. There was a mass in her neck, and her eyes protruded. A subtotal thyroidectomy was performed. A photograph of the thyroid is shown in **Figure 8.8** below.

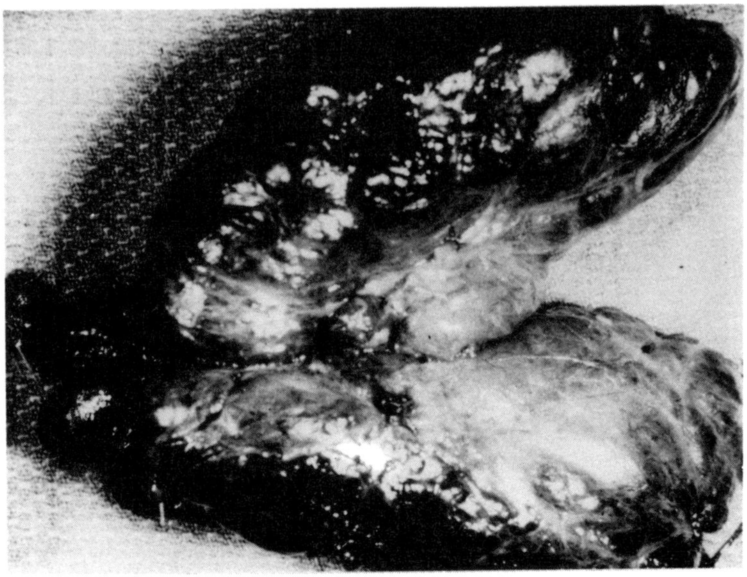

Figure 8.8

104. The likeliest diagnosis is

(A) diffuse primary hyperplasia
(B) follicular carcinoma
(C) lymphocytic thyroiditis
(D) medullary carcinoma
(E) nodular goiter

Item 105

105. An 80-year-old man suffered a cerebrovascular accident with left hemiplegia. The cause was a cerebral hemorrhage. Such bleeding frequently originates in the

(A) basal ganglia and internal capsule
(B) frontal lobe
(C) midbrain
(D) occipital lobe
(E) temporal lobe

Item 106

106. Several years after a case of measles, a 10-year-old girl began to have signs of CNS degeneration. She had most likely developed

(A) herpes zoster
(B) multiple sclerosis
(C) post-infectious encephalomyelitis
(D) progressive multifocal leukoencephalopathy
(E) subacute sclerosing panencephalitis (SSPE)

Item 107

107. Neuronal loss without inflammation in the anterior horns of the spinal cord is characteristic of

(A) amyotrophic lateral sclerosis
(B) cerebral infarction involving the internal capsule
(C) multiple sclerosis
(D) myasthenia gravis
(E) poliomyelitis

Item 108

108. The most common malignant neoplasm of bone is

(A) chondrosarcoma
(B) giant cell tumor
(C) metastatic carcinoma
(D) multiple myeloma
(E) osteogenic sarcoma

Item 109

109. A premature infant was treated with increased oxygen concentrations because of respiratory distress. A few months later it was noted that the child was blind. The ocular lesion induced by oxygen therapy is

(A) congenital cataracts
(B) congenital glaucoma
(C) granulomatous endophthalmitis
(D) interstitial keratitis
(E) retrolental fibroplasia

Items 110-117

Match each item with the dermatitis or dermatosis with which it is most closely related.

(A) Acne vulgaris
(B) Acute dermatitis due to poison ivy
(C) Dermatitis herpetiformis
(D) Erythema multiforme
(E) Lichen planus
(F) Pemphigus vulgaris
(G) Pityriasis rosea
(H) Psoriasis
(I) Seborrheic keratosis
(J) Urticaria pigmentosa

110. Delayed hypersensitivity reaction

111. Dense dermal infiltration by mast cells

112. Herald patch

113. IgA deposits along basal layer of epidermis

114. Large bullae on skin and oral mucosa

115. Papules and pustules on skin of face

116. Sprue-like pattern in jejunum

117. Violaceous papules on forearms and wrists

STOP.

YOU HAVE COMPLETED THIS SECTION.

Notes

Pathology

Answers and Tutorials

Answers and Tutorial on Items 1-4

The answers are: **1-D; 2-A; 3-D; 4-E. Primary** (endogenous) **hemochromatosis** is a rare disturbance of iron pigment metabolism, usually occurring in middle-aged males. It is inherited as an autosomal recessive, with incomplete expression. An association with HLA-A3 and HLA-B14 antigens has been noted. The hemochromatosis gene is on chromosome 6, tightly linked to the HLA region. There appears to be an inborn defect in the duodenal mucosa; absorption of a greatly increased amount of iron results. The total body iron may reach 50 gm. The principal clinical features are bronzing of the skin and signs of diabetes mellitus and pigmentary cirrhosis of the liver. The so-called bronze diabetes is usually mild. In the skin, hemosiderin deposits occur in the dermis about sweat glands, and there is also an increase in melanin deposition in the epidermis. The pancreas is usually slightly enlarged, firm, and deeply pigmented. The liver is usually enlarged, rusty red or ochre in color, and nodular. The lobules are separated by dense fibrous tissue (pigmentary cirrhosis). Hemosiderin is found mainly in the hepatic parenchymal cells. In about 7% of the cases of pigmentary cirrhosis, a hepatocarcinoma develops. Significant amounts of hemosiderin are deposited in the myocardial fibers and may contribute to the development of cardiac failure.

Secondary (exogenous) **hemochromatosis** occurs in cases of chronic refractory anemia, especially in those receiving multiple blood transfusions and prolonged intravenous or oral iron therapy. This rare form of hemochromatosis occurs at any age and in males and females about equally. Diabetes mellitus and full-blown hepatic cirrhosis are rare. In contrast to primary hemochromatosis, in the secondary form hemosiderin pigment is deposited mainly in reticuloendothelial cells, with a lesser involvement of epithelial cells. In patients on hemodialysis for chronic renal disease, heavy iron deposits may be present in the liver and spleen even when the bone marrow is iron depleted.

Answer and Tutorial on Item 1

The answers is: **5-C. Figure 8.1** Show a grossly enlarged, yellow liver. These changes are characteristic of **fatty degeneration**. The lipid in hepatocytes in fatty change is mainly in the form of triglycerides. The commonest cause is ethyl alcohol poisoning. Continued excessive use of alcohol commonly leads to hepatic cirrhosis.

Cloudy swelling is due to failure of the cellular sodium pump. This allows excess sodium to enter cells and eventually increases cellular water. Hydropic degeneration is a severe form of cloudy swelling. It occurs with hypokalemia due to vomiting or diarrhea. Potassium is drawn from cells and replaced by sodium and water in large amounts.

When the cells of an organ are affected diffusely by an adverse circumstance, as by bacterial toxins or by inadequate oxygen supply, the affected organ is increased in size and weight. The tissues lose their normal glistening translucency and resemble boiled meat. This is cloudy swelling caused by an increase in intracellular water due to injury to the plasma membrane and mitochondria. The mitochondrial damage leads to decreased oxidative phosphorylation and ATP production. Sodium enters the cells in increased amounts and draws in water. Chiefly affected are certain highly specialized cells such as the epithelial cells of the convoluted tubules of the kidneys and hepatocytes. The kidneys and liver are somewhat enlarged and pallid. Affected cells are swollen, and fine granules and vacuoles can be seen in the cytoplasm. Nuclei are usually not affected. Electron microscopy shows swelling of mitochondria and dilation of the endoplasmic reticulum and Golgi due to accumulation of water. The cell surface becomes "blebby."

Hydropic (vacuolar) degeneration results from a more severe degree of water imbibition into the cell cytoplasm. It occurs in some severe bacterial infections with high fever, certain types of poisoning, and hypokalemia. In its most striking form, hydropic degeneration involves the renal tubular epithelium, but small vacuoles may develop in hepatocytes and myocardial fibrils. Translucent intracytoplasmic vacuoles, which may be so large as to push the nucleus against the plasma membrane, appear in the proximal convoluted tubular cells. The vacuoles represent great accumulations of water in the endoplasmic reticulum, Golgi, and mitochondria and, in some cases, lysosomes.

Functional manifestations of cloudy swelling and hydropic degeneration are usually minimal. If the patient recovers from the underlying condition, the changes in the parenchymal cells usually disappear, and their functional capacity returns to normal.

Fatty degeneration (fatty metamorphosis, fatty change, steatosis) is the abnormal appearance of fat within parenchymal cells. Fat vacuoles may accumulate in liver cells under either physiologic or pathologic conditions. The physiologic type of fatty liver may occur after a fatty meal. The pathologic type of fatty liver may occur as a result of poisoning by hepatotoxic agents such as ethyl alcohol, chloroform, or carbon tetrachloride, during severe infections, in prolonged anemia, and in toxemia of pregnancy. The defect in the pathologic type of fatty liver may be a reduction in the capability of the liver cells to synthesize the phospholipid or protein moiety of lipoprotein; decreased lipoprotein release from hepatocytes; or increased triglyceride production. As a consequence, lipid accumulates in the liver cells mainly in the form of triglycerides.

When the liver is affected by severe fatty degeneration as in a patient with severe alcoholism, the organ is enlarged, soft, flabby and friable. The edges are rounded as a result of enlargement, and the surface is yellow and greasy. Usually the degree of dysfunction is relatively mild, but occasionally there may be total hepatic failure, with jaundice, coma, increased serum ammonia level and portal hypertension.

Answers and Tutorial on Items 6-8

The answers are: **6-A; 7-E; 8-D**. The photomicrograph in **Figure 8.2** shows a focus of lung tissue destruction due to **liquefaction necrosis**. This is caused by release of lytic lysosomal enzymes from dead neutrophils in the lung abscess. The abscess is walled off by a collagenous membrane. Lung abscess due to anaerobic bacteria from the mouth is associated with poor dentition and oral hygiene due to inhalation. An abscess is a localized collection of pus in a tissue. It is filled with viable and dead phagocytes and bacteria.

The local reaction of tissues to an injurious agent is **inflammation**. When the injurious agent is particularly irritating, the reaction is quick and violent, and the inflammation is said to be acute. Illnesses characterized by acute inflammation generally last hours or days, constitutional symptoms such as fever are prominent, and the patient can usually recall exactly the time and manner of onset. Illnesses characterized by chronic inflammation are usually less severe and more protracted. The process may last weeks or months, constitutional symptoms are usually minimal, and the patient often cannot recall the precise time or manner of onset. In most instances, factors inherent in the injurious agents account for the differences in the reaction of the host. In some instances, the differences are due to factors inherent in the host. Thus, a first exposure to a particular agent may be characterized by a mild or chronic reaction, while subsequent contacts result in an acute response because of prior sensitization.

When a tissue is inoculated with a small quantity of living culture of virulent bacteria, a series of vascular changes takes place, sometimes beginning with a transient constriction of blood vessels. Soon the arterioles dilate, causing a speeding of blood flow. Next, venules and then capillaries dilate, resulting in hyperemia, with stagnation of the circulation. As the vessels dilate and the flow of blood slows, the vessel walls become more permeable. Leukocytes and plasma move out of vessels into the connective tissues, forming the inflammatory exudate. Subsequent developments depend chiefly upon the amount of tissue destroyed. If tissue destruction is minimal, the dead cells are removed, hyperemia subsides, and the tissues return almost to normal, leaving no scar. If there is extensive destruction of tissue, great numbers of leukocytes come into the area and release their lytic enzymes. The central portion of the affected tissues liquefies, forming an abscess, or, if at a surface, an ulcer. If bacterial multiplication gets ahead of the host's response, the infection may spread to adjacent parts, and the process may end with the death of the host due to systemic effects of the infection.

The vascular response in acute inflammation is **biphasic**. The early phase lasting a few minutes is mediated by histamine released locally from tissue mast cells. Vasodilation and increased endothelial permeability are produced by histamine. This reaction can be blocked by the prompt administration of antihistaminic drugs. The delayed and sustained phase, which becomes maximal in 3-4 hours, is mediated mainly by kinins. In this system, an activator (Hageman factor) is released which reacts with an inactive precursor substance (kallikreinogen) in blood, releasing an enzyme (kallikrein). This in turn reacts with plasma kininogens to release the active substances, kinins. Following tissue injury, kinins incite vascular dilatation, increased vascular permeability, and emigration of leukocytes. **Bradykinin** is a nine amino acid peptide which, when injected locally, causes severe pain and tissue changes which closely simulate those occurring naturally in an acute inflammation. **Prostaglandins PGE** and **PGI_2** cause vasodilation and pain synergistically with bradykinin in foci of inflammation. These actions are inhibited by aspirin and other nonsteroidal anti-inflammatory agents. **Leukotrienes** C, D and E (slow reacting substance, SRS) are chemically related to prostaglandins. They cause a short-lived vasoconstriction, especially of arterioles, followed by increased vascular permeability. Acetyl glyceryl ether phosphorylcholine (AGEPC) (platelet-activating factor), released from basophils and mast cells, also produces vasoconstriction and both transient and prolonged increased vascular permeability.

In the focus of acute inflammation leukocytes escape from the bloodstream into the affected tissues. First the cells move out of the axial stream and adhere to the vascular lining (margination). Divalent cations, especially Ca^{2+}, play a key role in mediating leukocyte sticking. As the venules dilate, endothelial cells lining these vessels are pulled apart, exposing the underlying basement membrane to the leukocytes. These cells then emigrate into the perivascular connective tissues, passing between endothelial cells and through the basement membrane. Cells are attracted to the area of tissue injury by a positive force known as chemotaxis. Chemo-attractants include C5a complement fragment, leukotriene B4, and bacterial soluble products.

As the leukocytes move into the area of tissue injury, they provide an additional source of kinins. Plasma always seeps out of the vessels along with leukocytes. This exudation of leukocytes and plasma separates the fixed tissues of the affected part and leads to swelling (inflammatory edema). Plasma brings with it its various ingredients such as the plasma proteins, including in some instances, specific antibodies capable of acting against the infectious agents or neutralizing its toxins.

The **polymorphonuclear leukocyte** (PMN) or neutrophil is particularly important in acute inflammation. The PMNs contain lysosomes. These granules contain several potent lytic enzymes which make it possible for these cells to destroy many types of bacteria and to liquefy the cell fragments resulting from tissue injury. The formation of hydrogen peroxide within neutrophils contributes to the bactericidal effect of these cells, as does the presence of superoxide, myeloperoxidase, halide ions, especially Cl^- and I^-.

Meanwhile other changes have occurred in the area of injury. The blood in the small vessels, already stagnant from vasodilatation, has become more viscous. **Thrombosis** of small vessels commonly occurs. Strands of fibrin also form in tissue interstices as the result of the interaction of the coagulation-prompting factors present in the exudate. The fibrin web tends to block the movement of tissue fluids, thereby localizing the bacterial agent in the case of staphylococcal infections. In streptococcal infections, fibrinolytic enzymes are active in the exudate, and there is less tendency for the infection to remain localized. A spreading infection (cellulitis) is common.

Abscess formation or ulceration followed by healing is a common end result of inflammation. Bacteria multiply within a localized area walled off by a fibrin barrier, the pyogenic membrane; fixed tissue cells of the host are destroyed by bacterial toxins; leukocytes are attracted in large numbers; and leukocytic enzymes liquefy fibrin and dead tissue cells (liquefaction necrosis). If the area of injury is deep in the tissues, a cavity is formed, filled with pus. This abscess must be drained surgically before healing can occur. If the area of the injury involves the skin or a mucosal surface, an ulcer is formed. In either event, healing is slow and imperfect, and is followed by scar formation.

The gross features are important, because they provide the visible evidence that leads the physician to recognize the nature of the process. The cardinal signs of inflammation have been known for centuries. **Calor** (heat) and **rubor** (redness) are manifestations of the active hyperemia in the affected part. **Tumor** (swelling) is due chiefly to the accumulation of the inflammatory exudate but also to hyperemia. **Dolor** (pain) and functio laesa (disturbed function) are due to a combination of factors including the stimulation of sensory nerve endings as the exudate stretches the tissues, and the direct effect of kinins. Fever is due to resetting of the hypothalamic thermoregulator by endogenous pyrogens (interleukin-1 and prostaglandins) released from macrophages and neutrophils. Leukocytosis results from the release of colony stimulating factory from macrophages.

In **chronic inflammation**, the injurious agent acts over a longer period of time but is less damaging than in the examples of acute inflammation. In such cases, tissue destruction, hyperemia, and exudation may be minimal or nonexistent, lymphocytes and macrophages predominate in the exudate, and fibrous tissue proliferation may be marked.

A special form of chronic inflammation is seen in response to tissue invasion by **Mycobacterium tuberculosis**. Macrophages and multinucleated giant cells accumulate about the organisms, and fibrous tissue forms about these small focal lesions or tubercles. This combination of macrophages and fibrosis is known as granulomatous inflammation. These lesions may heal by scarring and become calcified, or they may undergo a distinctive form of necrosis known as caseation, whose characteristic cheesy yellow appearance is due to the waxy material from the capsule of the organisms. Similar focal collections of macrophages without caseation may be seen in certain other disease (fungus infections, leprosy, syphilis, sarcoid, brucellosis); these focal lesions are often spoken of as tuberculoid granulomas. Beryllium, when inhaled into the lung or deposited in a wound, may incite a similar granulomatous inflammation.

Another form of chronic inflammation is seen as a reaction to foreign material in the tissues. Usually the material is organic matter, such as vegetable fibers or hair, but a similar reaction occurs with suture material. Macrophages are attracted to the area, and a number of them, perhaps a dozen or even as many as 50, fuse resulting in a multinucleated giant cell. These cells engulf the foreign matter. Lymphocytes and fibrous tissue formation are always seen in conjunction with the giant cells.

The special role of leukocytes is emphasized by the peculiar susceptibility to infection of those individuals whose leukocytes are reduced in number or impaired in quality. Patients with marked leukopenia are very susceptible to infections. Patients who receive cancer chemotherapy may show a leukocyte count of 1,000 or less per mm^3 as a result of the cytotoxic effect of the drug on leukocyte precursors in the bone marrow. These patients often develop opportunistic infections–bacterial, fungal, or viral–to which they succumb. In such cases, the inflammatory exudate may contain fewer leukocytes than in usual with the organism in question making microscopic diagnosis difficult.

There are many instances in which leukocytes are present in normal numbers but are somehow impaired in quality. Since leukocyte dysfunctions are usually caused by hereditary disorders, the effects are manifest in infancy or early childhood as an unusual susceptibility to infection. These dysfunctions include defective **chemotaxis** and migration related to deficiency or inhibition of complement components; failure of recognition related to absence of opsonization of bacteria as a result of a lack of activation of C′3; a disorder of degranulation caused by the absence of NADPH oxidase and failure of peroxidation (formation of hydrogen peroxidase), which usually occurs as an X-chromosome-linked chronic granulomatous disease of young males.

Chédiak-Higashi syndrome is inherited as an autosomal recessive trait. The disease appears to be a generalized abnormality of unit membrane-bound organelles, such as lysosomes.

The syndrome becomes clinically apparent at from 1-8 years of age with partial albinism, photophobia, lymphadenopathy, hepatosplenomegaly, and decreased resistance to infections. The last is caused by decreased bactericidal activity of neutrophils. This is due to decreased chemotactic responsiveness and phagocytic activity. Death typically occurs by the age of 10 years due to infection or development of a malignant lymphoma. Large cytoplasmic granules are present in leukocytes. In the skin, hair, and uvea melanin pigment is present in clumps of large granules.

Job's syndrome occurs in light-skinned, red-haired girls. There is defective neutrophilic chemotactic response. The patients have repeated suppurative lymphadenitis and staphylococcal abscesses without signs of inflammation. Serum levels of immunoglobulin E (IgE) are markedly elevated. In the lazy leukocyte syndrome, there is defective chemotaxis, leukocytes showing random movement in response to inflammatory stimuli.

Inflammation and healing should be looked upon as two parts of a single vital function, the physiologic response to tissue injury, the objective of which is restoration of normal structure and function. Perfect restoration of function is dependent upon the replacement of lost cells by like cells (regeneration), and the orderly arrangement of these new cells in relation to preexisting cells so that intercellular functions are restored. This is not possible in all human tissues. Repair, ie, filling in of a wound or tissue defect, may restore lost tissue mass, but this is not the same as regeneration. Certain cell strains (epidermis, intestinal epithelium, and hematopoietic tissues) continue to undergo cell division throughout life (intermitotic cells), whereas others (fixed postmitotic cells, such as neurons, skeletal muscle, and cardiac muscle) do not. This difference in reproductive capability is apparently due to the presence or absence of intermitotic cells in adult tissues. Tissues which have them are able to regenerate after injury; tissues which lack them cannot. Intermediate between these two extremes are reverting postmitotic cells, such as hepatocytes, renal tubular epithelial cells, and connective tissues in general. Tissues composed of these cells normally contain few intermitotic cells, but when tissue is lost, surviving cells are capable of a rapid increase in the rate of cell division.

All wounds heal in roughly the same way: new cells are formed from preexisting cells and fill in the area of tissue loss, receiving support and nourishment from connective tissue and blood vessels as they grow. Small wounds heal quickly, large wounds slowly. A clean, dry surgical wound heals rapidly and readily by primary union. By contrast, a gaping wound must fill in by a process known as granulation before the surface epithelium can cover it over. Healing is then said to have occurred by secondary union.

Collagen is the chief constituent of **scar tissue**. Tropocollagen is synthesized by the myofibroblast and extruded into the extracellular space, where it polymerizes to form the banded collagen fibrils. These fibrils then arrange themselves parallel to each other to form an orderly sheet. As collagen ages, the bonds between fibrils continue to grow stronger. Thus, the healed wound continues to gain tensile strength.

The following systemic factors promote wound healing; (1) youth (wound healing is a slower process in the elderly person), (2) warmth, (3) ultra-violet light, and (4) good nutrition, particularly adequate reserves of protein. The following systemic factors delay or prevent wound healing: (1) vitamin C or zinc deficiency, (2) protein starvation, (3) prolonged therapy with steroids (by suppressing the vascular phase of inflammation), and (4) ionizing radiation. Local factors which inhibit wound healing include presence of foreign matter, poor blood supply, and persistence of infection. Vitamin C enhances conversion of proline and lysine to hydroxyproline and hydroxylysine, which are important in collage formation.

Answers and Tutorial on Items 9-12

The answers are: **9-E; 10-B; 11-C; 12-A**. A **neoplasm** is a focal autonomous new growth of cells which has no useful function. Neoplasia is the process of development of neoplasms (tumors).

Benign neoplasms do not invade adjacent tissue, do not spread to distant sites, and are the cause of localized effects. In contrast, malignant tumors invade normal tissue, spread elsewhere in the body, and cause death by local and disseminated effects. Benign tumors are much more common than malignant tumors and they tend to arise at an earlier age and to enlarge at a slower rate. Benign tumors are cured by total excision, whereas malignant tumors are often incurable because of spread outside the resectable region.

Grossly, benign neoplasms are characterized by sharply circumscribed margins that are often encapsulated, by central portions that tend to remain solid and viable, and by a texture that is uniformly soft or resilient. The microscopic feature is the resemblance of benign tumor cells to normal cells so that while the tissue pattern is altered and ordinarily easily distinguished from normal, the individual cells are often not.

Malignant neoplasms (cancers) are characterized grossly by serrated margins due to irregular invasion of adjacent tissues, by foci of necrosis in their centers, and sometimes by a hard consistency. Microscopically, they are characterized by a pronounced distortion of cell pattern. The most conspicuous changes are variations in cell size and shape; increase in nuclear size and nucleocytoplasmic ratio; increased nuclear staining (hyperchromatism); and increased numbers of mitotic figures, some of which are abnormal. Malignancy often involves appearance of discrete tumor nodules in parts of the body separated from the primary site. This phenomenon, called metastasis, is due to the detachment of tumor cell clusters from the site of origin and their transport in the lymph or blood streams to other tissues, especially the liver and lungs. While this phenomenon is proof of malignancy, the absence of metastasis does not establish benign behavior.

Certain biochemical changes are also utilized for the diagnosis of cancer. Galactosyl transferase isoenzyme (GT-II) is found in the serum of about 80% of patients with cancer. Choriocarcinoma is accompanied by high concentration of chorionic gonadotrophin in the serum, and the decline of this substance in the blood after the removal of the uterus is indicative of cure, while persistence of an elevated blood level is suggestive of metastatic disease. Normal cells and malignant epithelial tumors of the prostate produce the enzyme acid phosphatase which usually escapes in the pathway of secretions of the gland, ie, through the urethra. With cancerous invasion of parapsoriatic tissue, and especially with metastasis to bone, the circulating level undergoes a sharp rise and is accordingly useful in the diagnosis of metastatic disease from this site. **Prostate specific antigen** (PSA) is a more specific screening test, being elevated in prostatic carcinoma. Additional examples are the presence of significant amounts of **5-hydroxytryptamine** (serotonin) in the blood in cases of metastatic carcinoid, **calcitonin** in medullary thyroid carcinoma, **α-fetoprotein** in hepatocarcinoma, and **carcinoembryonic antigen** (CEA) in colon carcinoma.

Some neoplasms produce potent clinical manifestations by excessive secretion of hormones. **Islet cell adenoma** or carcinoma may cause severe **hypoglycemia** by insulin secretion, and hypertension may result from release of large amounts of catecholamines from a pheochromocytoma of the adrenal medulla. A paraneoplastic syndrome occurs when neoplastic cells produce a hormone not normally secreted by the cells of origin. Anaplastic bronchogenic carcinoma sometimes elaborates significant amounts of adrenocorticotrophic hormone, antidiuretic hormone, or parathormone with resultant endocrine effects.

The ultimate cause of malignant transformation in a cell or group of cells is unknown. It appears to be an alteration in nuclear DNA which produces a modification of gene expression, either as the result of a random mutation or the effect of a carcinogenic agent. Once induced, malignant transformation is a hereditably transmissible cellular change characterized by escape from normal growth controls; increased capacity for growth; cell membrane alterations and decreased adherence between cells which lead to a loosening of intercellular bonds; loss of contact inhibition between adjacent cells; development of new antigens on cell surfaces, such as the **tumor specific antigens** (TSA) in neoplasms produced by viruses; and the appearance of a great variety of karyotypic abnormalities in the nucleus. In vitro, neoplastic cells show decreased contact inhibition, growth on soft agar, and continuous proliferation, being potentially immortal. The loss of cell cohesiveness is associated with a decrease in calcium ion concentration and an increase of negative electric charges at the cell borders. Cell membrane alterations may be fundamental to the ability of malignant cells to escape normal control mechanisms in cell societies and to invade adjacent tissues and metastasize. Most cancers arise by malignant transformation of a single cell (clonal origin); some derive from a group of altered cells (field cancerization). Malignant teratomas, in which tissues from more than one germ layer are present, arise from multipotential embryonic cells.

The known causes of cancer include hereditary defects, ionizing radiation, chemical carcinogens, and living agents. Hereditary defects are presumably due to randomly acquired mutations. Three conditions associated with malignant tumor formation are clearly inherited, two as dominant genes. These are some cases of retinoblastoma of the eye, familial polyposis of the colon, and xeroderma pigmentosum of the skin; all are uncommon.

A number of neoplasms are associated with specific chromosomal defects in malignant cells. In about 95% of cases of chronic myelocytic leukemia, the **Philadelphia chromosome**, in which a portion of a chromosome 22 is translocated on number 9, is present. Various translocations are found in some cases of acute myeloblastic and lymphoblastic leukemia and in non-Hodgkin's lymphomas. In cases of **retinoblastoma**, there is often a deletion in the long arm of a chromosome 13, and children with birth defects associated with **Wilms' tumor** of the kidney have deletion in the short arm of a chromosome 11. Patients with **Down syndrome**, in which there is a defect in the 21 chromosomes in body cells, have an increased incidence of acute leukemia in childhood.

Ionizing radiation causes cancer. The mechanism is not entirely clear, but it is probably an alteration in cellular DNA. A relatively high dose and a relatively long time are required for the process to take place. When these conditions exist, a wide variety of malignant tumors may arise, the kind depending especially on the tissue exposed, the intensity of the ionization, and the duration of the exposure. Ultraviolet radiation in sunlight causes skin cancer after prolonged and excessive exposure.

Numerous **chemical agents** cause cancer. Carcinogenic materials in coal tar include benzpyrene, methylcholanthrene, and derivatives of anthracene. The aromatic amines are known to be carcinogenic, and naphthylamines selectively cause cancer of the urinary bladder. Occupational exposure is a risk of the aniline dye industry. Vinyl chloride has been implicated in the causation of angiosarcoma of the liver. Arsenic induces papillomas and carcinomas of the skin, and asbestos causes mesothelioma of the pleura and peritoneum, as well as bronchogenic carcinoma.

A number of the cancer chemotherapeutic drugs, especially the alkylating agents and antibiotics, have proved to be carcinogenic. Children and immunosuppressed patients are especially susceptible to the development of a second malignant neoplasm following the use of anticancer drugs.

The mechanism of **chemical carcinogenesis** is not completely known. It is considered to be at least a two-stage process. Some chemical carcinogens act as initiators, producing discrete, irreversible, additive, and transmissible dose-dependent effects on cell DNA. Other chemicals, such as croton oil, act as promoters, probably by stimulating cell division. Phorbol esters, one of which is the active principle in croton oil, are potent tumor promoting agents. Chemical agents most likely induce malignant transformation in cells by binding to and altering cell DNA.

Extensive epidemiologic evidence implicates **diet and nutritional** status in the incidence of certain forms of cancer, especially carcinoma of the breast, stomach, and colon. The exact relationship of diet and nutrition to cancer is unclear. Breast, prostate, and colon carcinoma are especially common in populations with a high fat and caloric intake. Colon carcinoma is positively related to low fiber content in the diet. Stomach carcinoma is especially common where large amounts of nitrate preservatives and small amounts of vitamin C are ingested. The vitamin C inhibits the conversion of nitrites to carcinogenic nitrosamines.

With respect to living agents, **viruses** have the principal role in carcinogenesis. Many oncogenic (tumor producing) viruses have been identified in lower animals. Viruses strongly suspected as causes of human cancers are human papilloma virus (cervical carcinoma); hepatitis B virus (hepatocarcinoma); Epstein-Barr virus (Burkitt's lymphoma, nasopharyngeal carcinoma); and human T cell leukemia virus (HLTV-1) (hairy cell leukemia). Oncogenic DNA viruses include papilloma, polyoma, herpes, and adenoviruses. DNA oncoviruses induce an abortive infection in cells of a foreign host. Viral DNA is incorporated in the host cell genome, modifying it and causing malignant transformation of the cell. Oncogenic RNA viruses (oncornaviruses) produce leukemia and sarcomas in many species of animals and mammary cancer in mice. RNA These viruses replicate in infected host cells by synthesizing a DNA copy of viral RNA by means of an RNA-directed DNA polymerase (reverse transcriptase). The DNA copy is then inserted into the host cell DNA.

Oncogenes, when expressed, are involved in the transformation of normal to malignant cells. They were first detected in oncogenic RNA viruses, and have been found in chemically-induced neoplasms in animals and in human cancer cells. Oncogenes are also present in the DNA of normal cells as potential transforming genes. Normally they are controlled within cell DNA by regulator genes. Loss of such control and activation of an oncogene appears to be one step in the multi step process of cell transformation.

Other living agents are associated with tumor formation although a direct causal relationship is not established. Bacterial infections, especially when associated with chronic draining sinuses, may be complicated by tumor formation in the living cells of the sinus tract. Certain parasitic ova are also associated with cancer–**Schistosoma haematobium** with carcinoma of the urinary bladder, *S. mansoni* with cancer of the colon. Aflatoxin, a metabolic product of the fungus *Aspergillus flavus*, has been found to be a potent hepatocarcinogen.

Immune responses play an important role in the body's reaction to a malignant neoplasm. Most cancerous cells have tumor specific surface antigens. Tumors produced by a virus cross-react with others caused by the same virus. Those produced by chemical and physical agents usually have unique antigens on their cell surfaces. Both humoral and cell-mediated immune responses to tumor cells have been identified. Patients in whom a striking lymphocytic infiltration is found about and within neoplastic tissue generally have a better prognosis than those with a few stromal lymphocytes. In cases of primary immune deficiency diseases, the likelihood of development of a malignant neoplasm is ten thousand times greater than in age-matched controls. Cancer also occurs significantly more frequently in patients under immunosuppression by drugs than the expected rate. It is possible that the development of a malignant neoplasm depends on a failure of the body's immune surveillance to detect the presence of cells with foreign antigens. This failure may be due to coating of the surface antigens by blocking antibodies from the circulation. T and Tn antigens have been found on the cells of most carcinomas but not on mesenchymal neoplasms or normal cells.

Natural killer (NK) **cells** are lymphocytes which are capable of destroying neoplastic cells, especially those of early leukemias and lymphomas. Suppressor T-lymphocytes may inhibit the activity of NK cells. Suppressor cells may interfere with other types of immune response and thus enhance neoplastic cell growth. Activated macrophages have been shown to be cytotoxic for malignant neoplastic cells. However, decreased macrophage chemotactic responsiveness to malignant tumor cells, especially in neoplasms with a poor prognosis, has been found in about 60% of cancers.

Answers and Tutorial on Items 13-15

The answers are: **13-A; 14-C; 15-A**. **Spotted fever** is caused by **Rickettsia rickettsii**. Rickettsiae are Gram-negative, bacterium-like, obligate intracellular parasites. Most are transmitted by ticks or mites. The gross changes are not distinctive and consists mainly of petechiae or ecchymoses. The typical microscopic change in rickettsial infections is a mononuclear cell inflammatory reaction (lymphocytes, plasmocytes and macrophages) about small blood vessels. The rickettsiae enter the bloodstream via the bites and are carried to the capillary beds throughout the body. They enter and proliferate in the endothelial cells lining arterioles, venules and capillaries in many parts of the body.

The rash in spotted fever usually appears on the third day, beginning on the extremities and face and later extending to the trunk. The rash is hemorrhagic, with numerous petechiae and ecchymoses, because of vascular necrosis.

The gross and microscopic changes in spotted fever occur in the skin and viscera. The rickettsiae are found in the endothelial and smooth muscle cells of small blood vessels. In the brain, there are proliferation of glial tissue to form nodules, sometimes around small blood vessels; perivascular infiltration of lymphocytes, with endothelial swelling; and necrosis and thrombosis of arterioles, with small infarcts of the brain.

Rubella (German measles) is caused by a spherical togavirus of the Rubivirus genus. Rubella virus contains single-stranded RNA. Transmission is by direct contact, droplet infection, and transplacentally. The incubation period is 14-21 days. Clinically rubella is a mild childhood exanthem, the rash being maculopapular and purplish red. Numerous congenital anomalies are related to the incidence of rubella in women during the first trimester of pregnancy. Rubella virus has been isolated from defective newborns. The most common anomalies are those of the heart, deaf-mutism, microcephaly, and lenticular cataracts. The pathologic changes in childhood rubella are little known. There is a lymphocytic dermal infiltrate in the skin macules and papules.

Rubeola (measles) is caused by paramyxovirus. Transmission of the virus is by direct contact and droplet infection from secretion of the nose, mouth, and eyes. The incubation period is usually 10-12 days. There is a period of invasion lasting 2-3 days with fever, malaise, lacrimation, photophobia, conjunctival injection, and signs of a respiratory infection. The earliest characteristic sign is the Koplik spot. The period of eruption usually begins about 145 days after exposure, and the maculopapular rash lasts 4-7 days. It begins on the forehead and neck and gradually involves the entire body. Subacute sclerosing panencephalitis develops rarely years after clinical rubeola as a slow virus infection.

The **Koplik spot** is a small, grayish yellow focus with a red halo on the buccal mucosa opposite the first molar. Microscopically, there is an infiltration of polymorphonuclear leukocytes, with capillary dilatation and small hemorrhages. In the skin, lesions the dermis is edematous and infiltrated by lymphocytes and macrophages. Small hemorrhages may occur. The formation of multinucleated giant cells is the most specific change in rubeola. Reticuloendothelial (Warthin-Finkeldey) giant cells, with up to 100 closely packed nuclei, are found in the tonsils, lymph nodes, spleen and lymphatic tissue of the intestines and appendix. Epithelial giant cells have been found in the tracheobronchial mucosa and in nasal and bronchial secretions.

Mumps is caused by paramyxovirus. Transmission is by droplet infection and direct contact. Clinically most cases of mumps occur in children, but adult infections are not rare and may be severe. The incubation period is about 3 weeks, and the first symptom is usually pain below the ear. Soon parotid enlargement is noted, along with fever, malaise, and headache. In about 70% of the cases, there is bilateral parotid involvement.

Mumps is a systemic disease with localization in the parotid glands, testes or ovaries, pancreas, and meningis. The parotid glands are enlarged and pink, the edematous interstitial tissue being infiltrated by mononuclear cells. Similar changes are found in the testes. The orchitis is usually unilateral and patchy and is rarely followed by sterility. In acute meningoencephalitis, the meningis are infiltrated by lymphocytes, up to 200 per cubic millimeter appearing in the cerebrospinal fluid. The brain is edematous and shows perivascular lymphocytic cuffing.

Infectious mononucleosis is a mildly contagious disease affecting adolescents and young adults. It is caused by the herpesvirus Epstein-Barr (EB) virus. The disease is usually manifest clinically by sore throat, fever, swelling of the cervical lymph nodes, and sometimes splenomegaly. The blood leukocytes usually number 10,000 to 20,000 mm^3, and many immature large lymphocytes with foamy basophilic cytoplasm and indented nuclei (Downey cells) are noted in the blood smear; similar cells are also seen in the sinuses of the lymph nodes. In up to 90% of cases of mononucleosis, a heterophil antibody appears in the serum, capable of agglutinating sheep's red blood cells. The disease is usually mild, terminating spontaneously after a few weeks, but in some instances it is quite severe, even fatal. Hepatitis is an important complication. Massive intraperitoneal hemorrhage due to spontaneous rupture of the spleen has occurred occasionally. The spleen may show a rather characteristic lesion microscopically, consisting of infiltration of the capsule and trabeculae by the immature lymphocytes.

Acquired immunodeficiency syndrome (AIDS) occurs in male homosexuals, drug addicts, and boys with hemophilia (due to transmission via blood transfusions). It also develops in female sexual partners and children of patients in high risk groups. The cause of AIDS is a retrovirus, HIV1. Patients, after a usually prolonged latent period, become immunodeficient due to infection of CD4-helper T lymphocytes. This leads to their depletion, making patients susceptible to opportunistic infections and the development of cancers. Opportunistic infections include pneumonitis due to *Pneumocystis carinii* (often in association with the cytomegalovirus), ulcerative perianal Herpes simplex infections, atypical tuberculosis due to *Mycobacterium avium-intracellulare*, oral and esophageal candidiasis, cryptococcal infections, toxoplasmosis, and profuse diarrhea due to the intestinal protozoan, *Cryptosporidium*. Malignancies in AIDS patients include Karposi's sarcoma (a usually rare form of blood vessel cancer) and Burkitt's, immunoblastic and primary central nervous system lymphomas. The mortality rate in AIDS is 75% within one year of onset.

Amebiasis is caused by *Entamoeba histolytica*, a protozoan found in feces as trophozites, precystic forms, and cysts. The trophozoite, the only form found in tissues, moves by pseudopodia. Its cytoplasm may contain erythrocytes and vacuoles. Usually transmission occurs by ingestion of food or water contaminated with human feces containing cysts of *E. histolytica*. Food is contaminated by flies and soiled fingers of food handlers. Cysts are ingested and pass into the small intestine where they encyst, each releasing four amebulae. These travel to the colon and develop into trophozoites which invade the mucosa and multiply in colonies and the submucosa. Amebic dysentery is characterized by the formation of deep, ragged ulcers with undermined edges in the colon and rectum. Because of the undermining, amebic lesions are called flask-shaped or water-bottle ulcers. Microscopically, the margins and floor show little inflammatory reaction, with only a few macrophages and lymphocytes. Hordes of amoebae are found in the submucosa. Complications of amebic dysentery include liver abscess. This is common due to infiltration of the portal venules. The abscesses are due to liquefactive necrosis of the liver cells by the proteolytic enzymes of the amoebae. Brown "anchovy sauce" material fills the cavity. The wall consists of necrotic liver cells infiltrated with lymphocytes and plasm cells. There are many amoebae in the abscess.

Diphyllobothrium latum (fish tapeworm) infestation is common in northern Michigan and Minnesota. There is usually a single worm, which grows to be 10 meters long. Larvae are ingested in raw fish. In about 1% of cases, the tapeworm ingests large enough amounts of vitamin B_{12} to cause a megaloblastic anemia in the host.

Answer and Tutorial on Item 16

The answer is: **16-E**. Formation of a coagulum of blood in a vessel during life is **thrombosis**, and the coagulum is a thrombus. The process is often initiated by contact of platelets with subendothelial collagen. Platelets release ADP which causes platelet aggregation. The coagulation mechanism is triggered and thrombosis results.

The photograph in **Figure 8.3** shows a roughly wedge-shaped pale subcapsular focus of old **infarction** in the kidney. It may have resulted from thrombosis in or embolism to a renal arterial branch supplying the infarcted zone. This infarct is pale (anemic). Hemorrhagic infarcts usually occur in soft organs, such as the lungs or intestine. Infarcts due to venous occlusion are often hemorrhagic.

Splenic arterial embolism cannot be due to a thrombus from an abdominal aortic aneurysm because this vessel is distal to the splenic circulation.

Slowing or eddying of the blood in an auricular appendage, such as in auricular fibrillation, often leads to thrombosis. Such a thrombus as well as a mural one may become pedunculated and act as a ball-valve thrombus. Thrombosis may also occur in an aneurysmal sac due to eddying within the bulged-out portion of the vessel. Thrombosis occurring without a precedent alteration in a vein wall is phlebothrombosis and is usually due to slowing or stasis of the blood within the vein. Such thrombosis usually originates in the pockets behind valve cusps in lower extremity veins. Pressure of a space-occupying mass or of a pregnant uterus on veins produces slowing of the venous flow distally, and thrombosis sometimes follows. The general circulatory slowing in congestive heart failure, together with the inactivity of the cardiac patient, is accompanied by a tendency to venous thrombosis.

Increased coagulability of the blood is caused by the release of tissue thromboplastin or other procoagulants in **disseminated intravascular coagulation**. A tendency to thrombosis may also be present in conditions characterized by increased blood viscosity due to a striking increase in the number of cells. These include chronic leukemia and polycythemia. A migratory phlebothrombosis complicates some cases of malignant neoplasm, especially pancreatic carcinoma, due to increased coagulability of the blood.

Occlusion of a vein may produce stasis in the area drained, causing passive hyperemia or even necrosis of the involved tissues. Occlusion of an artery causes ischemia of the tissue supplied. Unless collateral circulation is present and adequate, infarction will follow. If the thrombus becomes detached and free in the circulation, it is an embolus. Some thrombi are removed by lysis. If a thrombus remains attached and the patient survives, it becomes organized from the lining of the vessel. Capillaries bud into the thrombotic mass, fibroblasts proliferate, and gradually the thrombus is replaced. New vascular channels develop through it (recanalization), or the mass becomes fibrous.

Embolism is the lodging of an embolus in a blood vessel at a point beyond which it cannot pass. An embolus is a foreign substance such as a thrombus or fragments of a thrombus, tissue cells, clumps of bacteria, parasites, bone marrow, amniotic fluid, globules of fat, or bubbles of gas carried in the bloodstream. Fragments of or entire thrombi are by far the most common type of emboli. Venous emboli originate in the peripheral veins and almost always lodge in a pulmonary artery, producing infarction of a lung, or sudden death in cases of massive embolism.

Pulmonary embolism is a fairly common sequela of congestive heart failure, surgery, and obstetric delivery. In over 90% of the cases, pulmonary emboli arise in veins of the lower extremities, especially the deep calf veins. Small or large thrombi break off from a site of phlebothrombosis and are carried in the venous bloodstream up the inferior vena cava and though the right side of the heart into the pulmonary arterial circulation, where they impact. When a large embolus is suddenly jammed into the main pulmonary artery or is impacted astride the bifurcation to block both great pulmonary trunks (saddle embolus), the pulmonary circulation is completely obstructed and an enormous strain is immediately placed on the right ventricle. There is a rapid rise in the pulmonary arterial pressure proximal to the block, and the right ventricle and atrium become dilated (acute cor pulmonale). Death usually ensures within a few minutes due to the failure of venous return to the left side of the heart. A shower of small emboli which lodge in numerous pulmonary arterial branches may produce similar results.

Arterial emboli originate from the left side of the heart, an aneurysmal sac, an atheromatous plaque on a large arterial trunk, or rarely, the pulmonary veins. The effects of arterial emboli depend on the size and nature of the embolus, the organ involved, and the state of collateral circulation. If collateral circulation is absent or deficient, an embolus of any size will produce infarction in the heart, brain, spleen, intestine, kidney, or an extremity.

Paradoxical embolism results when a venous embolus enters the arterial circulation through a patent foramen ovale or other cardiac septal defect.

Septic embolism is the lodgement of infected foreign material in a blood vessel. Masses of bacteria, usually within a septic embolus, are carried in the bloodstream. Septic infarcts or abscesses are produced where the emboli lodge. In some cases, necrosis of the artery in which the infected embolus lodges leads to thinning and outpouching of the wall (mycotic aneurysm). Septic embolism commonly originates in acute bacterial endocarditis.

Neutral fats from injured tissue or the bone marrow, or injected fats and oils, may act as fat emboli, obstructing capillaries in the lungs, brain, and elsewhere. Most cases follow fractures or other trauma to fat. Fat embolism also occurs in cases of fatty liver in acute and chronic alcoholism, carbon tetrachloride poisoning, diabetes mellitus, and decompression sickness.

Talc, cellulose, and cornstarch embolism in the pulmonary circulation occurs in addicts who inject oral drug preparations intravenously. The starch and talc are used as fillers for drugs, such as amphetamines and barbiturates, or as adulterants with heroin. In persons who inject drugs, foreign-body granulomas that consist of filler granules, macrophages, and epithelioid and multinucleated giant cells develop in and around the walls of small pulmonary arteries. Thrombi develop within the lamina of these vessels. Extensive occlusion of the pulmonary arterial tree may occur with resultant pulmonary hypertension and cor pulmonale (thickening of the right ventricle secondary to increased pulmonary blood pressure).

Air embolism results when air is drawn or forced into the circulation as into the jugular vein during neck surgery, uterine veins during abortion, and during pneumothorax. The air tends to lodge in the right ventricle, mixing with blood and producing a frothy mass which obstructs blood flow.

Aeroembolism refers to the presence of tiny bubbles of gas, especially nitrogen, in the bloodstream. The nitrogen is released by sudden lowering of the air pressure such as may occur in the raising of divers (bends) or the decompressing of workers in tunnels (caisson disease). The gas comes out of solution in the blood and lodges in the capillaries of the heart, lung, muscles, and bones, producing severe pain.

Infarction is the production of an infarct, a local focus of necrosis resulting from vascular obstruction. When an artery is occluded suddenly, cell death occurs in the tissues supplied by it. The vessels and capillaries deprived of blood later dilate and fill with blood from surrounding anastomoses. A fresh infarct is therefore dark and congested. In soft organs, such as the lungs and intestines, hemorrhagic infarcts occur. In a firm organ, such as the kidney, swelling of parenchymal cells presses the blood out of small vessels so that a pale (anemic) infarct occurs. This area is surrounded by a hemorrhagic zone.

Infarction of the lung results from occlusion of a branch of the pulmonary artery from embolism. However, a large embolus occluding the main pulmonary artery or lodged in the right or left pulmonary artery usually causes almost immediate death without infarction. Clinically, pulmonary infarction is characterized by a sudden, sharp chest pain which later localizes over the infarct and is worsened by deep inspiration, a pleural friction rub due to fibrin, hemoptysis, fever, tachycardia, and dyspnea.

Answers and Tutorial on Items 17-22

The answers are: **17-A; 18-E; 19-B; 20-C; 21-G; 22-D**. Hemorrhage is the escape of blood from a vessel incident to a mechanical defect in the vascular or cardiac wall. Definitions relating to hemorrhage

Ecchymosis— blotchy, purplish hemorrhage into the subcutaneous tissues due to leakage from venules; a bruise. Typically due to blunt trauma.

Epistaxis— A hemorrhage from the nose.

Hematemesis— The presence of a significant amount of blood in vomitus, due to a ruptured esophageal varix secondary to portal hypertension.

Hematoma— A localized mass of blood, usually clotted, within a tissue.

Hemoptysis— The presence of blood in the sputum. Common causes are bronchiectasis and pulmonary tuberculosis.

Hemostasis— The stopping of blood flow from the vascular tree.

Melena— The presence of dark, digested blood in the feces. A bleeding duodenal ulcer is a common cause.

Menorrhagia— Excessive endometrial bleeding during a menstrual period.

Metrorrhagia— Irregular endometrial bleeding between menstrual periods.

Petechia— A tiny hemorrhage due to leakage from a capillary or venule. It is often associated with thrombocytopenia.

The causes of hemorrhage include injury, infection, or ulceration of a blood vessel wall; atherosclerosis, in which the arterial wall becomes brittle; rupture of an aneurysm (a bulge in a vessel wall); purpuras (bleeding diseases in which small hemorrhages occur in the skin and mucosa); leukemia, because of the suppression of platelet formation; avitaminosis K, because of the deficiency of prothrombin formation; scurvy (avitaminosis C), because of fragility of the vessel walls; certain poisons and bacterial toxins; and hypoxia.

When even a large amount of blood is lost over a long period of time, as in chronically bleeding hemorrhoids, the body is able to compensate by increasing the activity of the bone marrow to replace the shed erythrocytes. When blood loss outstrips replacement, anemia ensues.

When a large amount of blood is lost suddenly, a decrease in both blood pressure and blood volume flow develops. The body reacts quickly to counter-act the loss. Reduced blood pressure or flow stimulates the carotid sinus reflex. This produces increased cardiac action and selective vasoconstriction. If the blood pressure cannot be maintained, the decreased capillary blood pressure results in the movement of fluid from the tissue into the blood vessels. Thus the blood volume is partly restored by hemodilution. Eventually the erythrocyte loss produces tissue hypoxia, which leads to increased capillary and venular permeability and dilatation. The outcome of this is hypovolemic shock. While there is some individual variability, the sudden loss of 30% or more of the blood volume is usually fatal.

Hemorrhage into the gastrointestinal tract, abdominal cavity, or retroperitoneal region has the same effect as external hemorrhage. Pleural or pericardial hemorrhage may compress the lungs or heart (cardiac tamponade). Cerebral hemorrhage infiltrates the adjacent brain substance and destroys it.

Answers and Tutorial on Items 23-28

The answers are: **23-D; 24-A; 25-G; 26-C; 27-B; 28-H.** **Vitamin K** is essential for synthesis of prothrombin in the liver; **vitamin A** is necessary for the synthesis of rhodopsin (a light sensitive pigment in the retina); niacin prevents the development of pellagra with its rough skin, diarrhea, and mental changes; **vitamin D** prevents rickets in children by its effect on calcification of osteoid in bones; **vitamin C** is essential for the development of intercellular substances including cartilaginous and bone matrix; thiamine prevents beriberi heart disease in which there is cardiac enlargement, due to dilatation, and heart failure.

Answer and Tutorial on Item 29

The answer is: **29-C**. Weeks before the development of **rheumatic fever**, the related streptococcal infection has cleared, so there would be no positive throat culture. Poststreptococcal **glomerulonephritis** does not develop concomitantly with rheumatic fever often, although they share a remote causative factor. While the **Aschoff body** is due to an immunologic reaction, there are no eosinophiles in it. Both rheumatic heart disease and floppy valve syndrome most often affect the **mitral valve**. Myxomatous degeneration is responsible for the floppiness of the floppy valve. Calcific aortic stenosis is characterized by an aortic systolic murmur and heart block due to compression of the conduction bundle.

Alpha-hemolytic streptococci cause the less virulent subacute bacterial endocarditis (SBE), β-hemolytic streptococci (among others), acute bacterial endocarditis (ABE). Both result from a bacteremia. ABE develops on normal valves and causes fenestration (perforation) of valve cusps and septic embolism and infarction, because the causative organisms are highly virulent. Embolism and infarction in SBE are usually bland. Focal ("embolic") glomerulonephritis occurs in SBE, probably on an immunologic basis.

Answer and Tutorial on Item 30

The answer is: **30-D**. **Myocarditis** signifies inflammation of the myocardium. **Rheumatic myocarditis** is the most common type and occurs during the course of acute rheumatic fever. Interstitial myocarditis, characterized by focal collections of lymphocytes and macrophages about small vessels, may be seen in fatal cases of many infectious diseases, including varicella, diphtheria, scarlet fever, typhoid fever and group B Coxsackie viral infections. Myocarditis also occurs in toxoplasmosis and **Chagas' disease** (due to *Trypanosoma cruzii*). **Fiedler's myocarditis** is idiopathic and is characterized by cardiomegaly and the presence of granulomas in the myocardium. **Hypersensitivity myocarditis** due to drugs such as methyldopa, sulfonamides, ampicillin, and furosemide, is characterized by an infiltration of eosinophils, macrophages, and predominantly T lymphocytes.

Acute pericarditis usually follows infection of some other organ. Suppurative pericarditis is usually a complication of bacteremia or spread from an adjacent pleuritis. Tuberculous pericarditis is usually due to spread to the pericardial sac from adjacent tuberculous lymph nodes. Rheumatic pericarditis may occur along with rheumatic endocarditis and myocarditis. Pericarditis occurs in uremia, myocardial infarction, and viral infections, especially Coxsackie B.

In acute pericarditis due to pyogenic bacteria, the fluid is frankly purulent. In nonspecific pericarditis and in pericarditis due to rheumatic fever, the fluid is sterile, usually slightly cloudy, and contains fibrin. In tuberculous pericarditis, there may be frank caseation necrosis of the involved tissues and a thick layer of fibrin may collect, or there may be a blood-tinged effusion. In pericarditis due to myocardial infarction, fibrin is commonly deposited over the necrotic area of the myocardium. In uremic pericarditis, a dry fibrinous exudate is usual.

Adhesions of minor degree are often encountered between the two layers of the pericardium. When pericardial adhesions are thick, and particularly when they are associated with mediastinal, pleural, and chest wall adhesions, they may produce heart failure. Sometimes adhesions may be so dense that retraction of the chest wall is noted with each systole (Broadbent's sign). Constrictive pericarditis (Pick's disease) is a crippling disease, sometimes a sequel of mediastinal tuberculosis. Dense scar tissue, often with a heavy layer of calcium frosting, may surround the ventricles, atria, or great vessels as an unyielding band. As a result the heart chambers may be unable to dilate to receive blood during diastole. Clinically dyspnea, ankle edema, and especially abdominal swelling due to peritoneal effusion are the chief symptoms. Distention of the cervical veins, hepatomegaly, high venous pressure, and a reduction of cardiac output are the chief signs.

A cardiomyopathy is a noninflammatory disorder in which the involvement is primarily in the myocardium. It may be classified as idiopathic, infiltrative or endomyocardial in type. The idiopathic form is divided into dilated and nondilated (hypertrophic) types. In the latter, the hypertrophy may be symmetric or asymmetric.

Dilated (congestive) cardiomyopathy occurs in men more often than in women and is frequently associated with chronic alcoholism (possibly due to an associated thiamine deficiency). Cobalt formerly added to beer was a causative factor. It may also be related to nutritional deficiency in pregnancy and the post partum period. Doxorubicin therapy and viral myocarditis have also been indicated. The average heart weight is 600 gm. The left ventricular wall is usually less than 1.5 cm thick. The myocardium is flabby. All four cardiac chambers are dilated. Recent and old thrombi are often present in the ventricles and atrial appendages, and embolism is common. Death is usually due to congestive heart failure.

In symmetric hypertrophic cardiomyopathy the heart is enlarged, averaging over 600 gm and the left ventricular myocardium is more than 1.5 cm thick. The interventricular septum is similar in thickness to the ventricular free wall, and ventricular outflow obstruction does not occur. Asymmetric hypertrophic cardiomyopathy is more common than the symmetric type and is usually associated with ventricular outlet obstruction (idiopathic hypertrophic subaortic stenosis, IHSS). It is transmitted as an autosomal dominant. In IHSS, the septal myocardium is thicker than the free wall. The ventricular cavities are small (muscle bound heart), and the atria are dilated. There is thickening of the mitral valve, and a plaque forms on the septal endocardium where it is slapped by the anterior leaflet of the mitral valve. Microscopically, the myocardial fibers of the septum are disoriented, running in all directions rather than parallel to each other. Hypertrophic cardiomyopathy often occurs in young adults and may lead to sudden death during athletic activity or strenuous exercise.

Infiltrative (restrictive) cardiomyopathy may occur in amyloidosis, sarcoidosis, hemochromatosis (iron deposition), glycogen storage disease types II, III and IV, and Fabry's disease (glycolipid deposition). Endomyocardial disease with eosinophilia (Loeffler's endocarditis) is an idiopathic cardiomyopathy which occurs in men more often than in women. The heart is enlarged, the average weight being about 475 gm. There is marked fibrous thickening of the left ventricular endocardium at the inflow tract. Thrombosis is common over the fibrous foci. The myocardium shows interstitial fibrosis and infiltration by eosinophils. Peripheral eosinophilia may be over 20%. Endomyocardial fibrosis without significant eosinophilia occurs in Africa among children and young adults. It may be related to eating large amounts of fruits rich in serotonin.

Answer and Tutorial on Item 31

The answer is: **31-D**. **Atheroma** is the generic name for both types of plaque. The fatty streak occurs in children and disappears later in life. The fibrous plaque is formed by accumulation of cholesterol and other lipids and collagen laid down by myointimal cells which have entered the intima from the media. Calcium deposits in the intima, cholesterol, ulceration of the endothelial surface, and thrombosis all occur in a complicated plaque. Calcification of the media occurs in Mönckberg's sclerosis and is not related to atherosclerosis. As to complications of atherosclerosis, although myointimal cells participate in formation of plaque, they do not produce smooth muscle tumors.

Of the risk factors for **coronary** (and other) **atherosclerosis**, obesity alone is probably not a primary cause. However, it is frequently associated with other risk factors. **Rupture of an infarcted papillary muscle** allows a mitral cusp to fly free and produce mitral insufficiency. The infarct in the photomicrograph shows the degree of coagulation necrosis and leukocyte infiltration found in one about 3 days old. No or little change is apparent in the first day, and by a week granulation tissue would be present. In about two thirds of cases of acute MI, a thrombus is found in the atherosclerotic artery supplying the infarcted zone.

Answer and Tutorial on Item 32

The answer is: **32-B**. Many forms of **syphilis** of the cardiovascular system have their beginnings in syphilitic aortitis. The interval between the appearance of the chancre and clinical evidence of syphilitic aortitis is usually 5-15 years. The spirochete has an affinity for the ascending and transverse limbs of the aortic arch. Grossly, the affected portion of the aorta is somewhat dilated. Syphilitic fibrosis of the media, with destruction of muscularis and elastica, results in puckered stellate depressions of the intima, separated by wrinkled areas. The aorta is greatly weakened. Microscopically, the media shows scattered foci of necrosis and fibrous scarring. The adventitia and outer portion of media show perivascular infiltration by plasma cells and lymphocytes. The vasa vasorum show luminal narrowing due to endarteritis obliterans.

Insufficiency of the aortic valve results when the syphilitic fibrosis of the aortic media spreads to the commissure of the aortic valve, separating one cusp from another, and causing thickening, shortening, and rolling of the cusp edges. Left ventricular dilatation and hypertrophy develop and often become extreme. Coronary insufficiency is an important although uncommon complication of syphilitic aortitis. When the inflammatory fibrosis of the aortic wall happens to surround one or both coronary ostia, the scarring may narrow the lumen sufficiently to cause symptoms. Sudden death is common in such cases.

Any localized dilatation of the lumen of a blood vessel is a true **aneurysm**. A false aneurysm is a localized external widening of a vessel without dilatation of the lumen often due to a hematoma between its layers.

Most aneurysms occur in the aorta or its major branches, often at a localized area of weakening in the vessel wall. Atherosclerosis and medial dissection are the major causes. All aneurysms are more common in males. When rupture occurs, it may cause exsanguinating hemorrhage, or the accumulation of blood may so compress vital structures such as the heart due to intrapericardial hemorrhage (cardiac tamponade) as to cause death. When an aneurysm of an intracranial artery ruptures, it usually causes death by increased intracranial pressure due to subarachnoid hemorrhage.

Atherosclerosis is the most frequent cause of aortic aneurysm. In most instances, the affected patients are males in the seventh or eighth decade. The abdominal aorta, generally below the renal arteries, is the most common site. The iliac arteries are the next most frequent sites of atherosclerotic aneurysm development.

Atheromatous lesions weaken the affected vessels and, when combined with loss of elastica in the media, result in dilatation. An unruptured arteriosclerotic aneurysm of the abdominal aorta often causes no symptoms. When rupture occurs, it is usually into the retroperitoneal tissues, where a mass appears and enlarges over a period of a few hours. Exsanguination is the usual end result, but many patients are saved by surgical excision of the aneurysm and replacement with a graft or prosthesis.

A **dissecting aneurysm** (dissecting hematoma) is a form of false aneurysm in which there is a splitting of the media of the aorta, usually at the juncture of the inner two thirds and outer third. Blood enters the split and extends it, resulting in an elongated hematoma in the wall. Most patients with dissecting aneurysm have a long history of severe hypertension. Some patients with dissecting aneurysm show evidence of Marfan's syndrome.

Severe chest pain, usually substernal or in the back, and described as ripping or tearing, commonly marks the onset of dissecting aneurysm. The pain extends with the dissection.

"Congenital" (berry) aneurysm occurs on or near the **circle of Willis**, especially the anterior communicating artery, the middle or anterior cerebral arteries, or the basilar artery, usually at or near a point of bifurcation, where the media is thin normally. About 30% develop on the anterior, middle and posterior cerebral arteries respectively and 10% on the basilar and vertebral arteries. "Congenital" aneurysms are saccular in form and vary from 0.1 to 3 cm in diameter. The wall of the aneurysm is composed of a greatly thickened intima, with complete absence of the media and internal elastic lamina. With rupture or leakage of the aneurysm, subarachnoid hemorrhage develops. Bright red blood floods the subarachnoid space. Clinically leakage or rupture of the aneurysm often occurs in young individuals. Marked dizziness and violent headache suddenly develop. If the hemorrhage is severe, coma follows quickly. The neck is rigid on flexion, and the deep tendon reflexes are hyperactive. The cerebrospinal fluid is under greatly increased pressure and is grossly bloody.

Cor pulmonale signifies right ventricular strain. As the term is generally used it implies a chronic disorder, associated with right ventricular hypertrophy. Acute cor pulmonale is the term for the sudden right ventricular strain that is a sequel to massive pulmonary embolism.

Primary obstruction to pulmonary blood flow may be due to (1) stenosis of the pulmonic valve; (2) conditions which block blood flow in major pulmonary arteries (recurring pulmonary embolism), or in pulmonary arterioles (idiopathic pulmonary hypertension; left-to-right-shunts due to septal defects or persistent ductus arteriosus); or (3) stenosis of the mitral valve orifice.

Primary difficulty in ventilation may result from **emphysema** (about 80 percent of cases), pulmonary fibrosis, or diseases restricting thoracic mobility (kyphoscoliosis, extreme obesity). Patients with these conditions show cyanosis and dyspnea, and examination reveals thoracic deformity and expiratory wheezes. Cor pulmonale results from pulmonary vasoconstriction due to hypoxia and respiratory acidosis and from the development of bronchopulmonary vascular shunts.

Primary neoplasms of the heart are rare and are usually benign. **Myxoma** is the most common primary neoplasm. It is a soft mass, consisting of edematous connective tissue irregularly covered by thrombus, commonly attached to the endocardium by a pedicle, and hanging free into a cavity, usually the left atrium. It may block the mitral orifice, producing a murmur like that of mitral stenosis. Embolism from the surface of the neoplasm or an overlying thrombus is common. The papillary fibroelastoma is very rare and occurs on heart valves. Rhabdomyoma (which is associated with tuberous sclerosis) and rhabdomyosarcoma are extremely rare neoplasms arising in cardiac muscles cells in children. Metastatic neoplasms of the heart, especially in the pericardium, are widespread. The neoplasms commonly giving rise to cardiac metastases are those primary to the breasts and lungs, as well as lymphomas and melanomas.

Answers and Tutorial on Items 33-34

The answers are: **33-B; 34-A**. **Thalassemia** (Mediterranean or Cooley's anemia) is a hemoglobinopathic anemia in children of Italian and Greek heritage due to partial or complete failure of formation of a globin chain in their erythrocytes. In α-thalassemia there is a gene deletion on chromosome 16, and in β-thalassemia there is a defect on chromosome 11. Children in whom the train is homozygous develop a severe anemia (thalassemia major). Those who are heterozygous have a mild anemia (thalassemia minor). In β-thalassemia, beta chain formation is defective. HbA production is decreased, and there is increased formation of HbF (fetal hemoglobin) and HbA2, which do not contain β-chains. The hemoglobin in erythrocytes contains an excess of α chains, which may be responsible for the hemolysis in β-thalassemia.

Iron deficiency anemia results from a chronic blood loss, an inadequate iron intake, or to interference with iron absorption in the intestine. The anemia is hypochromic and microcytic. In the bone marrow there is no stainable iron. Plummer-Vinson syndrome is iron deficiency anemia in middle-aged women together with atrophic glossitis, difficulty in swallowing due to an esophageal web, and spoon-shaped nails.

Answers and Tutorial on Items 35-37

The answers are: **35-D; 36-D; 37-D**. In Item 36, the age, bone pain, lytic lesions in flat bones, hypercalcemia, and anemia are indicative of **multiple myeloma** (MM). Macroglobulinemia is not typical of MM.

Lymphomas occur in increased incidence in autoimmune disorders such as rheumatoid arthritis and lupus erythematosus; chromosome defects, such as t 18q+; 14q- in follicular lymphoma; both congenital and acquired immunodeficiencies, such as AIDS; and exposure to certain viruses, such as Epstein-Barr in Burkitt's lymphoma.

In Item 38, the overgrowth of poorly differentiated lymphocytes throughout the lymph nodes in a pattern mimicking germinal centers in typical of **nodular lymphoma.**

Answers and Tutorial on Items 38-40

The answers are: **38-D; 39-A; 40-D.** In Item 38, the age, sex, recurrent fever and lymphadenopathy, sclerosis, lacunar cells, the Reed-Sternberg cell, and eosinophils are characteristic of the nodular sclerosis type of **Hodgkin's disease**. Involvement of lymph nodes and spleen (on both sides of the diaphragm) and the presence of symptoms would place this case in Stage III B.

Answer and Tutorial on Item 41

The answer is: 41-A. The sudden onset with a severe infection, markedly elevated white cell count, and very immature myeloid cells (myeloblasts) in the peripheral blood are indicative of **acute myeloblastic leukemia**. **Auer rods** in the cytoplasm of myeloblasts are a distinctive feature in AML.

Answers and Tutorial on Items 42-51

The answers are: **42-A; 43-B; 44-D; 45-B; 46-B; 47-A; 48-C; 49-C; 50-C; 51-A**. Asthma, hay fever, and urticaria are due to Type I hypersensitivity; autoimmune hemolytic anemia, erythroblastosis fetalis, and Goodpasture's syndrome, to Type II; lupus erythematosus, polyarteritis nodosa, and post-streptococcal glomerulonephritis, Type III; and contact dermatitis, Type IV.

Answers and Tutorial on Items 52-58

The answers are: **52-E; 53-D; 54-C; 55-A; 56-B; 57-C; 58-C**. Collagenous dermal thickening is typical of scleroderma; fibrinoid vascular necrosis of polyarteritis; hematoxylin bodies (complexes of nucleoprotein-antinucleoprotein) of DLE; an increased incidence of cancer of dermatomyositis; and glomerular immune complex deposits and valvular vegetations of DLE.

Answer and Tutorial on Item 59

The answer is: **59-C**. Patients with either inherited, acquired, or induced forms of immune deficiencies, as well as those with autoimmune disease show an increased incidence of lymphoma and other forms of malignant neoplasia. This may be due to inadequacy of immune surveillance over the emergence of forbidden clones or the expression of viral oncogenes in malignant cells.

Answers and Tutorial on Items 60-67

The answers are: **60-F; 61-J; 62-E; 63-G; 64-I; 65-H;66-C; 67-B**. In Item 60, hemolysis, splenomegaly, and increased osmotic fragility of erythrocytes point to congenital **spherocytic anemia.**

In Item 61, the triggering of a crisis by pneumonia and the bone pain in an African-American child are indicative of **sickle cell anemia**.

In Item 62, severe anemia with target cells and HbF and HbA2 in this child is indicative of **β-thalassemia**.

In Item 63, chronic blood loss has led to iron depletion and anemia, which is corroborated by the low serum iron and high iron binding capacity.

In Item 64, the tingling of the feet, achlorhydria, and severe anemia are characteristic of **pernicious anemia**.

In Item 65, extensive bony metastases lead to a diagnosis of **myelopathic anemia**.

In Item 66, the presence of anemia, leukopenia, and thrombocytopenia are indicative of **aplastic anemia**.

In Item 67, hemolysis on use of an antimalarial drug and Heinz bodies occur with **G-6-PD deficiency** in erythrocytes.

Answers and Tutorial on Items 68-73

The answers are: **68-G; 69-H; 70-B; 71-F; 72-E; 73-C**. These items are targets in organ-specific autoimmune disease. Antiacetylcholine receptor antibodies, acting at the myoneural junction, cause the muscle weakness in **myasthenia gravis**. In **pernicious anemia** an atrophic gastritis and failure to produce intrinsic factor necessary for vitamin B_{12} absorption is caused by antiparietal cell antibodies. Anti-glomerular and -lung basement membrane antibodies cause pulmonary hemorrhages and glomerulonephritis in **Goodpasture's syndrome**. Anti-microsomal (and antithyroglobulin) antibodies are responsible for the development of **lymphocytic thyroiditis**. In **juvenile diabetes** islet β-cells are destroyed by antibodies against them. In **Graves' disease** anti-TSH receptor antibodies stimulate TSH and cause excessive thyroid hormone production.

Answers and Tutorial on Items 74-75

The answers are: **74-A; 75-A**. In 74, **scar carcinoma** is usually an **adenocarcinoma**. Adenocarcinoma arises from epithelial cells of the bronchial surface or glands. This tumor comprises about 30% of all lung carcinomas and affects both sexes about equally. It is generally located more peripherally in the bronchial tree than the other types. Microscopically it is composed of gland-forming mucin-secreting epithelial cells. Its spread is chiefly by the blood stream.

Anaplastic small cell (oat cell) **carcinoma Figure 8.5** may arise from pulmonary endocrine cells especially of the main stem bronchi, and comprises about 20% of all bronchogenic carcinomas. It is more common in men than women. Microscopically this neoplasm is composed of small cells resembling lymphocytes, with scanty cytoplasm and darkly staining nuclei. Distant hematogenous spread is common.

Answer and Tutorial on Item 76

The answer is: **77-C**. Chronic bronchitis is one of the most common respiratory diseases due to cigarette smoking. While bacteria are sometimes present in foci of chronic bronchitis they are not a primary causative factor. Chronic bronchitis is one of the chronic obstructive lung diseases, the others being asthma, emphysema, and diffuse bronchiectasis.

The smoking history and productive hacking cough for at least 2 years is indicative of chronic bronchitis.

Answers and Tutorial on Items 77-78

The answers are: **77-E; 78-A**. **Coal worker's pneumoconiosis** (CWP, black lung disease), is characterized by the formation of interstitial nodules of anthracotic pigment with associated fibrosis. It may lead to massive fibrosis of the lungs. Silicosis is associated with an increased incidence of tuberculosis (miner's phthisis) as well as of bronchogenic carcinoma.

The lungs are the site of a host of immunologic diseases due to inhaled or circulating allergens. The offending agent in farmer's lung is thermophilic actinomycete, *Micropolyspora faeni*. This is also the cause of extrinsic hypersensitivity alveolitis. Actinomycetes (*M. vulgaris*) also cause bagassosis, due to inhalation of sugar cane residue dust. Nitrogen dioxide from nitrates in corn causes silo-filler's lung.

Answer and Tutorial on Item 79

The answer is: **79-C**. **Acute pancreatitis** is seen chiefly in males after age 40 and often associated with obesity and alcoholism. In about 50% of the cases, gallstones are also present. Pancreatitis occurs in about 10% of cases of hyperparathyroidism. In some cases, calculi resulting from the hypercalcemia of hyperparathyroidism develop in pancreatic ducts and lead to obstruction and inflammation. A few cases of pancreatitis have occurred in patients taking chlorothiazide diuretics.

Answers and Tutorial on Items 80-81

The answers are: **80-D; 81-E**. **Primary neoplasms** of the **liver** are uncommon in the United States, although **metastatic tumors** to the liver are very frequent. Adenoma is a circumscribed, liver-colored mass consisting of well-differentiated hepatocytes without lobular organization. A number of cases of this rare neoplasm have developed in women taking oral contraceptives. Such adenomas tend to be large and undergo hemorrhage spontaneously or after mild trauma. Adenomas occasionally develop in children and adults on androgen therapy.

Answer and Tutorial on Item 82

The answer is: **82-B**. **Viral hepatitis** is caused by hepatitis viruses A, B, C, and D (delta). Hepatitis C (formerly non-A, non-B) is responsible for most cases transmitted via blood transfusions. Hepatitis virus A is transmitted by ingestion of fecally contaminated water or food. Hepatitis B virus is transmitted by plasma and blood transfusion, vaccines containing human serum, injections with contaminated needles and tattoo needles. Some cases of B virus hepatitis are transmitted by fecal contamination and by sexual contact. The delta agent can replicate only in the presence of hepatitis B surface antigen. The virus D can produce marked damage to hepatocytes.

Answer and Tutorial on Item 83

The answer is: **83-B**. A **diverticulum of the intestine** is a mural outpouching whose mucosal lining is continuous with that of the intestine. If multiple diverticula are present, as is common in the acquired form, the condition is diverticulosis. If one or more diverticula become inflamed, the process is diverticulitis. Acquired diverticula are usually multiple. They are most common in elderly persons, especially those subject to constipation. A low residue diet which leads to excessive segmental colonic contraction has been implicated as the cause. Diverticula are most common in the sigmoid colon where they bulge between the longitudinal muscle bands.

Answers and Tutorial on Items 84-87

The answers are: **84-A; 85-A; 86-C; 87-C**. Item 85 gives a classical history for the development of **acute poststreptococcal glomerulonephritis**. Epithelial crescents are the typical microscopic feature of rapidly progressive glomerulonephritis.

The combination of hematuria and hemoptysis in Item 87 in a young man is characteristic of Goodpasture's syndrome in which autoantibodies develop against the glomerular and pulmonary capillary basement membranes.

The **nephrotic syndrome** occurs most often in minimal change disease in children and in membranous glomerulonephropathy in adults.

Acute proliferative (postinfectious) **glomerulonephritis** is a generalized inflammation of the glomeruli with secondary tubular, interstitial, and vascular changes. In about 90 percent of patients with acute glomerulonephritis, there is an associated Group A, type 12 β-hemolytic streptococcal infection, but occasional cases are associated with types 4, 1, 25, and 49. Usually the preceding infection is in the form of streptococcal pharyngitis or tonsillitis. Acute proliferative glomerulonephritis typically follows the antecedent infection after an interval of about 2 weeks. Most cases occur in the 5 to 20 age group. There is no correlation between the occurrence of acute rheumatic carditis and poststreptococcal glomerulonephritis.

In **acute glomerulonephritis** the kidneys are swollen, red, and smooth, with tense capsules which strip easily. The glomeruli are enlarged, and there is marked endothelial and mesangial cell proliferation. Many PMNs are present intra- and extravascularly. RBCs may be found in Bowman's spaces. Immunofluorescence reveals the presence of immune globulin G (IgG) and complement along the glomerular basement membranes in a lumpy, bumpy pattern characteristic of immune complex glomerulonephritis.

Proliferative glomerulonephritis with crescents (rapidly progressive glomerulonephritis) is usually idiopathic but may occur in poststreptococcal GN, Goodpasture's syndrome, lupus erythematosus, or Henoch-Schönlein purpura. The kidneys are large, pale and soft with widespread glomerular epithelial crescent formation due to proliferation of Bowman's capsular epithelium. The epithelial cells become fusiform. Collagen may be laid down in the crescents. The escape of fibrinogen through the damaged glomerular basement membrane with the formation of fibrin in the glomerular space is the stimulus for epithelial crescent formation.

Goodpasture's syndrome is an autoimmune disorder in which antiglomerular basement membrane antibodies are formed. This results in the deposition of immune globulin G and complement in a uniform linear pattern along the glomerular basement membranes. IgG and complement are also deposited along alveolar septa in the lungs, because the anti-GBM antibodies cross-react with alveolar basement membranes. In Goodpasture's syndrome, the lungs are heavy, often weighing up to 2000 gm together. There is an acute necrotizing alveolitis with hemorrhage into the alveolar spaces. Early kidneys show an acute proliferative glomerulonephritis, which changes into rapidly progressive glomerulonephritis with epithelial crescent formation in glomeruli.

Minimal change glomerulonephropathy, which occurs in males more often than in females, is the commonest cause of nephrotic syndrome in children. The nephrotic syndrome consists of massive proteinuria; hypoalbuminemia due to the urinary loss; widespread edema due to decreased plasma osmotic pressure; and hyperlipidemia, probably due to increased hepatic lipoprotein synthesis. The cause of minimal change disease is unknown. The kidneys are slightly enlarged and pale or yellow due to tubular lipids. The glomeruli have diffuse obliteration of the epithelial foot processes.

Answers and Tutorial on Items 88-90

The answers are: **88-A; 89-C; 90-A**. **Acute tubular necrosis** includes all damage to renal tubules whether it is caused directly by chemical or drugs (toxic nephrosis) or indirectly by a reduction in blood supply or precipitation of hemoglobin or myoglobin (hypoxic nephrosis). Oliguria or anuria is the most common clinical feature of all types of acute tubular necrosis. Degeneration of **proximal convoluted tubules** are involved. Shock and hemolytic reactions are the basis for most cases of hypoxic nephrosis.

Renal papillary necrosis due to acetophenetidin is a gradual process with slow loss of renal function.

Answer and Tutorial on Item 91

The answer is: **91-C**. It is often difficult to determine the underlying cause of chronically scarred kidneys. In arteriolonephrosclerosis and chronic glomerulonephritis, both kidneys are affected equally and so are symmetrically scarred. In **chronic pyelonephritis**, involvement is often uneven, and the pelves and calyces show signs of infection. In renal artery stenosis, the ipsilateral kidney is atrophic while the contralateral one is compensatorily large.

Answer and Tutorial on Item 92

The answer is: **92-D**. **Adenocarcinoma of the kidney (Figure 8.6)** arises from **proximal convoluted tubular epithelium**, and the nephroblastoma from the metanephrogenic blastema. Wilms' tumor is sometimes part of a multiple developmental defect complex.

Answers and Tutorial on Items 93-95

The answers are: **93-D; 94-C; 95-A**. The lymphogranuloma (lymphopathia) venereum is caused by *Chlamydia trachomatis*. Transmission is by sexual contact, especially in conditions of uncleanliness. The primary lesion is transient and disappears after a few days. Within 2-8 weeks inguinal lymph nodes enlarge to form buboes. In homosexual men, anorectal infection may occur. Early there is procitis with a mucopurulent discharge, shallow ulcers of the mucosa, and the formation of polypoid masses on the mucosa. Rectal stricture follows the procitis and is usually within 6 cm of the anus. The rectal wall is thick, fibrous, and rigid, and the lumen is greatly narrowed.

Prostatic hyperplasia is the commonest cause of urinary obstruction in men over age 50. The normal PSA rules out prostatic carcinoma in Item 95. An elevated PSA points to carcinoma, which is not related to sexual promiscuity.

Cryptorchidism is the failure of one or both testes to descend into the scrotal sac. The involved testis may have stopped in its downward descent anywhere along its path from the coelomic cavity to the inguinal canal. The cause is not always apparent. Cryptorchidism occurs in about 1 percent of males. Until puberty the undescended testis remains normal, but after puberty a gradually progressive atrophy with hyaline thickening of the tubular basement membranes, loss of germinal cells, and interstitial fibrosis occurs. thus bilateral cryptorchidism in the adolescent or the young adult produces sterility. The undescended testis is roughly 15 times as likely to develop a neoplasm as is the normal scrotal testis.

Answers and Tutorial on Items 96-98

The answers are: **96-B; 97-E; 98-B**. **Gonorrheal complications** in females may be by spread to vulval glands and internal genitalia or joints hematogenously. During birth, gonococci may infect the newborn's eyes causing keratoconjunctivitis.

Acute salpingitis does not lead to rectal stricture, which is a complication of lymphopathia venereum.

The uterine leiomyoma occurs in about a third of all women, being the most common internal neoplasm.

Cervical cancer is more common in women who begin sexual activity early in their teens and have multiple partners and pregnancies. Stage 4 carcinoma extends to surround the **ureters** and causes bilateral urinary obstruction and failure. Endometrial carcinoma on the other hand occurs in older women who have had no or few children.

In **endometriosis externa**, the ectopic glands respond to hormonal activity and bleed at menstrual periods, causing hemorrhagic cysts in the ovaries.

Dermoid cysts are made up mainly of tissues derived from ectoderm or endoderm. They contain no placental villi. Granulosa-theca cell tumors secrete estrogens and can produce isosexual precocious pseudopuberty in girls.

Answer and Tutorial on Item 99

The answer is: **99-A**. **Fibroadenoma (Figure 8.7)** is a very common, slowly growing, estrogen-induced, fibroepithelial neoplasm, usually occurring in women between 25 and 35 years of age. Growth is rapid during pregnancy and lactation and usually ceases at the menopause. The skin over the fibroadenoma is unchanged, and it is movable under the skin. Grossly, the tumor feels rubbery and is smooth or lobulated, sharply outline, encapsulated, and 0.5 to 3.5 cm in diameter. The color is pearly-gray or pink. The cut surface is delicately fissured by ducts and feels moist or sticky. Old tumors may show hyalinization or calcification.

Answers and Tutorial on Items 100-102

The answers are: **100-A; 101-C; 102-E**. **Gigantism** is due to excessive secretion of growth hormone by a neoplasm of the adenohypophysis before epiphyses are closed. This hormone is normally produced by acidophil cells, but is also secreted by some chromophobe adenomas. In adults, excessive growth hormone causes acromegaly with enlarged bones and viscera. Pituitary adenomas are histologically benign but may grow out of the sella turcica to compress the optic chiasm and produce bilateral homonymous hemianopsia.

Cushing's syndrome may be caused by ACTH-producing neoplasms of the pituitary or certain malignant tumors such as small cell bronchogenic carcinoma or by autonomous over-production of corticosteroids by an adrenal neoplasm or hyperplasia. It is also an iatrogenic disorder due to long term adrenocorticosteroids therapy. Crooke's hyaline change in basophils is a retrogressive change due to high levels of corticosteroids from an adrenal neoplasm or hyperplasia.

In Cushing's syndrome there is an over-production of the adrenal glucocorticoids. The syndrome is more common in females than in males. The usual manifestations are: (1) obesity, chiefly of the trunk and face; (2) skin disorders such as acne and purplish striae of the thighs and abdomen; (3) diminished sexual function (amenorrhea in females; impotency in males); (4) hypertension; (5) hirsutism in females; (6) diabetes mellitus, ore more often a diabetic type of glucose tolerance curve; and (7) osteoporosis.

Primary hyperaldosteronism (Conn's syndrome) consists of hypertension, polyuria, hypokalemia, and severe muscle weakness, simulating paralysis. In most instances, it is associated with an adrenal cortical adenoma, occasionally with an adrenal carcinoma or adrenal hyperplasia. The adenomas consist almost entirely of zona glomerulosa cells or of a mixture of glomerulosa–and fasciculata-type cells.

Increased production of the two hormones–epinephrine and mainly norepinephrine–of the adrenal is usually due to tumor of the chromaffin cells of the medulla (pheochromocytoma), but may be due to tumor of the related chromaffin bodies of the sympathetic nervous system. The characteristic manifestations are a result of paroxysmal hypertension. Increased levels of catecholamines appear in the urine.

Hyperfunction of the acidophil cells is usually a result of an eosinophilic adenoma. The hyperfunction is usually manifest by increased bone growth. When the condition arises before epiphyseal closure has occurred, it results in abnormal tallness or gigantism. When the hyperfunction has its onset after age 20, there is little opportunity for increase in height because the epiphyses of the long bones are already closed. Instead the bone growth is manifest by a general increase in bone mass, the condition being known as acromegaly. This is especially evident in the lower jaw (prognathism). The fingers broaden and the hands become spade-like. The viscera are also enlarged. Some patients develop diabetes mellitus due to insulin resistance.

Simmond's disease (hypophyseal cachexia) is due to extreme hypofunction of the adenohypophysis. It is usually a result of a destructive process, either vascular or neoplastic. Vascular causes include infarction of the pituitary gland, usually due to prolonged circulatory failure following severe intrapartum or postpartum hemorrhage (Sheehan's syndrome). Neoplasms causing Simmond's disease may be primary, either in the pituitary gland or in adjacent structures or they may be metastatic, as from breast cancer. Chromophobe adenoma is the commonest cause. Congenital hypopituitarism occurs in boys twice as frequently as in girls. The child develops into a well-proportioned but short person (Lorain-Levi type). Hypopituitarism in children is usually due to a craniopharyngioma, a squamous neoplasm which destroys the pituitary by compression.

Pituitary adenomas vary in size from microscopic to 10 cm in diameter. These may greatly enlarge the sella turcica and may compress nearby brain structures. After a certain size is reached, the neoplasm breaks through the diaphragma sellaa. Many structures may be compressed by the growing neoplasm, particularly the optic chiasm, nerves and tracts, and the non-neoplastic cells of the gland. In most instances, pituitary neoplasms are encapsulated and are benign. Over half of these neoplasms are chromophobe adenomas, and most of the remainder are eosinophilic adenomas or mixed in cellular types. Basophilic adenomas are uncommon.

Pheochromocytomas of the adrenal medulla are variable in size, ranging from 1 gm to over 1 kg. Most are encapsulated, and on section they are pink and soft. Microscopically, they are composed of nests of polyhedral cells, usually constant in size and morphology. A fine network of fibers usually separates the cell nests. About 1 percent are malignant, and in about 10 percent of cases pheochromocytomas are bilateral.

Chronic adrenal cortical insufficiency (Addison's disease) occurs chiefly in middle life. In crisis, circulatory collapse may be profound. More than 90% of adrenal cortical cells must be lost before hypofunction becomes manifest. Tuberculosis of the adrenal glands is a common cause of Addison's disease. In such cases, both glands are almost totally destroyed. In recent years, idiopathic cortical atrophy of the glands has become the most important cause. It may be due to an autoimmune reaction. Anti-adrenal antibodies are found in the sera of over half the cases. The atrophic glands are reduced to as little as 2.5 gm combined weight (normal 8 gm.). Occasionally Addison's disease is a result of histoplasmosis, bilateral adrenal metastases, especially from bronchogenic carcinoma, or of amyloid disease of the adrenal glands.

Answer and Tutorial on Item 103

The answer is: **103-C.** Chronic adrenal cortical insufficiency (**Addison's disease**) occurs chiefly in middle life. In crisis, circulatory collapse may be profound. More than 90% of adrenal cortical cells must be lost before hypofunction becomes manifest. Tuberculosis of the adrenal glands is a common cause of Addison's disease. In such cases, both glands are almost totally destroyed. In recent years, idiopathic cortical atrophy of the glands has become the most important cause. It may be due to an autoimmune reaction. Anti-adrenal antibodies are found in the sera of over half the cases. The atrophic glands are reduced to as little as 2.5 gm combined weight (normal 8 gm). Occasionally Addison's disease is a result of histoplasmosis, bilateral adrenal metastases, especially from bronchogenic carcinoma, or of amyloid disease of the adrenal glands.

Answer and Tutorial on Item 104

The answer is **104-A**. The commonest cause of hyperthyroidism is diffuse hyperplasia (**Figure 8.8**) (**Graves' disease**). The hyperplasia is due to the development of autoantibodies to thyroid stimulating hormone (TSH) receptors on the follicular cells. these antibodies cause thyroid hyperplasia and hypersecretion of thyroid hormones. In Graves' disease, the thyroid gland is diffusely and symmetrically enlarged, vascular, and beefy. Microscopically, the amount of colloid is somewhat reduced, and the colloid is scalloped around the edges of the follicles. The cells lining the follicles are enlarged. Papillary projections into the follicles are frequent. Collections of lymphocytes, some having germinal centers, are commonly noted.

Answer and Tutorial on Item 105

The answer is: **105-A**. Most **cerebral emboli** enter the middle cerebral artery, apparently because it is the straightest course. The commonest site of cerebral hemorrhage is the **basal ganglia** and **internal capsule** due to bleeding from a lenticulostriate artery. These small branches come off the middle cerebral artery and under high pressure at a right angle. Cerebrovascular accidents (CVA's) result from embolism, thrombosis, or hemorrhage. Bleeding into a neoplasm is not a CVA.

Answer and Tutorial on Item 106

The answer is: **106-E**. **Slow virus infections** of the central nervous system are progressive, degenerative and usually lethal. Progressive multifocal leukoencephalopathy is caused by a papovavirus. This demyelinating disease occurs in patients whose immune response has been impaired by immunosuppression or by a disease such a leukemia or

Hodgkin's disease. Intranuclear viral particles are found in oligodendrocytes, the cells which produce and maintain the myelin sheaths. Multiple demyelinated patches are found in the cerebral white matter. The cause of **subacute sclerosing panencephalitis** (Dawson's encephalitis) has been shown to be measles (rubeola) virus. This disease may occur more than 10 years after the clinical attack of measles. The brain lesions are possibly due to development of an autoimmune reaction. Intranuclear and intracytoplasmic viral particles are found in neurons, astrocytes, and oligodendrocytes. The changes in the brain are similar to those in other types of viral encephalitis plus scattered foci of demyelinization. Kuru and Creutzfeldt-Jakob disease are human subacute spongiform encephalopathies which have been transmitted to experimental animals, although no virus has been identified in brain tissue. Prions have been proposed as the cause. These are proteinaceous infectious particles smaller than viruses. Both diseases are characterized by spongy vacuolation (status spongiosus) of the cerebral and cerebellar gray matter.

Answer and Tutorial on Item 107

The answer is: **107-A**. Degeneration of posterior columns and posterior nerve roots is characteristic of **tabes dorsalis**, the spinal form of CNS tertiary syphilis. Quiet degeneration of anterior horn occurs in amyotrophic lateral sclerosis (Lou Gehrig's disease). A tubular cavity in the cervical segment of the spinal cord develops in syringomyelia.

Amyotrophic lateral sclerosis (ALS) is a chronic, progressive, idiopathic disease with degeneration of the lower and upper motor neurons and marked muscular atrophy. It is more common in males by 4:1 and usually appears in the fourth and fifth decades. A marked loss of anterior horn cells in ALS leads to atrophy of the anterior horns. Many cells disappear, and the remaining ones show all degrees of degeneration. The pyramidal tracts degenerate, and there is a corresponding involvement of the Betz cells of the motor cortex. The motor nuclei of the pons and medulla degenerate late in the course.

Answer and Tutorial on Item 108

The answer is: **108-C**. **Metastatic tumors of bone** are much more common than primary tumors, especially after middle age. Carcinomas of the prostate often metastasize to the bones of the pelvis and lower spine. Carcinomas of the lungs, breasts, thyroid gland, and kidneys also metastasize to bone.

Answer and Tutorial on Item 109

The answer is: **109-E**. **Retrolental fibroplasia** is an oxygen-induced degeneration in the premature infant in whom the peripheral retina is not completely vascularized. In such an infant, an increased oxygen tension causes immediate but transient closing down of terminal arterioles and the arterial side of the capillary bed. With continued increased oxygen levels an irreversible vaso-obliteration occurs. The involved vessels degenerate, and vasoproliferation from adjacent vessels begins. Newly formed capillaries invade the retina, penetrate the internal limiting membrane, and grow into the vitreous. Retinal detachment may be caused by organization of vitreous hemorrhages and exudates and the formation of a preretinal membrane. In severe cases, a completely detached retina and organized vitreous form an opaque retrolental mass giving a white cat's-eye reflex (leukocoria).

Answers and Tutorial on Items 110-117

The answers are: **110-B; 111-J; 112-G; 113-C; 114-F; 115-A; 116-C; 117-E**. **Psoriasis** is a common chronic, recurrent skin disease which is sometimes associated with arthritis. It may be a disorder of epidermal cell replication. The number of basal cells is increased, and the time of cell passage from basal layer to stratum corneum is only 3 days (normal 27 days). The extensor surfaces of the elbows and knees are most commonly affected, but the entire skin may be involved.

Acute dermatitis occurs in the contact reaction due to poison ivy and to other agents. It is a delayed hypersensitivity reaction. there is intense itching and even burning. The affected skin areas are swollen, reddened, and vesiculated. the vesicles are intra-epidermal, with cellular necrosis. The superficial dermis has edema, capillary dilation, and perivascular infiltration with neutrophils, eosinophils, and lymphocytes.

Dermatitis herpetiformis is chronic, recurrent, and characterized by itching. It is often associated with persons with HLA-B8. Deposits of IgA are found along the basal layer in skin adjacent to the lesions. there is a symmetrical distribution of groups of papules, vesicles, and, rarely, bullae surrounded by zones of erythema. These lesions occur most commonly on the shoulders, extensor surfaces of the extremities, and the buttocks. Microscopically, the epidermis is only slightly affected, but there is subepidermal vesicle formation with a marked neutrophilic and eosinophilic infiltrate of these lesions and the surrounding dermis. Some patients with dermatitis herpetiformis have a sprue-like pattern in the jejunum, and DH appears to be due to a gluten hypersensitivity.

Pemphigus vulgaris is a severe bullous dermatitis characterized by itching and burning. It occurs most often in the fifth through the seventh decade of like. The skin of the axilla and groin in particularly affected, however, any part of the skin may be involved. Oral lesions often appear first. The bullae are soft and break easily, releasing fluid with an offensive odor. Degenerated squamous cells (Tzanck cells) are found singly and in clusters within bullae. In pemphigus vulgaris IgG autoantibodies against an antigen in intercellular spaces and circulating autoantibodies are found.

Erythema multiforme is an acute dermatosis which is part of a self-limited systemic disease with fever and sore throat. It is most commonly idiopathic, but may be drug-induced or following herpes simplex. The skin lesions are pleomorphic with macules, papules (the commonest manifestations), vesicles, and bullae. The papules often enlarge peripherally and clear centrally to form the typical iris lesions. The vesicles and bullae form by complete separation of the epidermis from the dermis.

Acne vulgaris is persistently chronic disorder which usually appears during adolescence, involving the face and upper chest and back. Sebaceous gland ducts become blocked, and sebum accumulates. When sebaceous follicles rupture, keratin in the comedos stimulates foreign body reactions. Lipolytic enzymes elaborated by bacteria act on lipids in sebum to release free fatty acids, which mediate papule and pustule (pimple) formation. The papules show a lymphocytic and plasmacytic infiltrate, with occasional foreign body giant cells about pilosebaceous glands which contain inspissated sebum. Bacterial infection, often by *Corynebacterium acnes* or Staphylococcus epidermidis, causes pustulation and subcutaneous abscesses. In the later stages, dermal fibrous scarring develops in some of the lesions.

Pityriasis rosea is probably due to a virus and usually lasts 4-6 weeks. the disease occurs most often in the spring and summer in children and young adults. It begins with a patch on the trunk, followed by the appearance of numerous round, pinkish buff patches on the trunk. thin scales overlie the lesions. There are occasional small vesicles in the epidermis.

Lichen planus is idiopathic, persists for months or years, and usually causes severe pruritus. The flexor surfaces of the wrists, forearms and legs often have small, angulated, plateau-like violaceous papules. A heavy lymphocytic infiltrate is present in the upper dermis and crowds up against the epidermis.

Notes

CHAPTER 9

Behavioral Science

DIRECTIONS (Items 1-81): For each of the numbered items that proceed, you must select the single best answer from among the lettered options listed.

Some of the numbered items will pose a question or incomplete sentence that is followed by a list of 4-5 lettered options. In all cases, select the ONE lettered option that best answers the question or completes the sentence given.

Some of the numbered items are preceded by 5-24 lettered options. In these sets, the lettered options will be preceded by a single instruction asking you to match one of the lettered options to each numbered item most closely associated with it. In all matching sets, you may use any of the lettered options once, more than once or not at all, but you should still only select 1 lettered option per numbered item.

If you wish to simulate actual USMLE testing conditions, you should aim to complete all the items in this chapter in one hour and 20 minutes.

Do NOT look at the answers and tutorials until you have completed all of the items in this chapter.

Good luck!

Item 1

1. A 16-year-old boy is brought to the doctor after apparently trying to take off his clothes during the showing of a filmstrip. He describes having started to see wavy lines on the screen, then experiencing a brief period of mental blankness, followed by fatigue and headache. The most probable diagnosis of this patient is

   (A) grand mal epilepsy
   (B) migraine behavioral syndrome
   (C) partial complex seizure
   (D) exhibitionism

Items 2-4

A 55-year-old man with a history of heavy alcohol use comes to the ED for treatment of an infected gash in his hand. He is not currently intoxicated. His clothes fit loosely, and he mentions that he thinks he has lost weight since becoming homeless "sometime this year." In preparation for giving him antibiotics, he gets an intravenous infusion of D5 glucose. Two hours later, he is confused, agitated, and ataxic, with bilateral 6th nerve palsies (intranuclear ophthalmoplegia) and nystagmus.

2. This patient is most likely exhibiting

   (A) alcoholic ketoacidosis
   (B) Wernicke's encephalopathy
   (C) Friedreich's ataxia
   (D) sepsis

3. Immediate treatment should include

   (A) 100 mg of thiamine in each bag of IV fluid
   (B) insulin, glucose, potassium and saline
   (C) vitamin B_{12} IM and oral folic acid for 3 days
   (D) intravenous lorazepam 2 mg every 4 hours until agitation subsides

4. The patient is treated and admitted to the hospital. In 3 days, his wound is healing, and he no longer shows signs of neuropathy. However, his mental status is remarkable for mild confusion, even though he seems awake and alert. He is socially appropriate and denies hallucinations, delusions or ideas of reference. He is oriented to place but not date, able to give his correct date of birth, do simple calculations, and provide the correct address of the house where he lived for 10 years. However, he cannot recall even one of three objects at 5 minutes. He seems unable to remember what he ate at his most recent meal. When asked by the examiner if he remembers the two of them having met and enjoyed an evening together, he cheerfully says he does, though in fact this never occurred. Vital signs are BP 110/60; P 82 and regular. Liver function tests, serum electrolytes and BUN/creatinine are all within normal limits, except for slight elevation of alkaline phosphatase to 652 u/mL (upper limit of normal = 600 u/mL) and SGPT to 50 u/mL (upper limit of normal = 35). CBC shows a hemoglobin of 11.3 gm/100mL (nl 12-15 gm/ml); HCT of 37% (nl 40-50%) MCV 101 fL for femtoliter = a very tiny volume (nl = 82-92). Having recovered from his presenting illness, this patient is now exhibiting

(A) malingering
(B) multi–infarct dementia
(C) alcohol amnestic syndrome (Korsakoff's syndrome)
(D) Wernicke's encephalopathy

Items 5-6

5. A 60-year-old woman comes to the physician's office complaining of unsteadiness and a burning sensation in her feet. She reports that she is under a lot of stress, because her husband is threatening divorce. On closer questioning, she admits the issue is that he thinks she drinks too much. Her neurological exam reveals apparent loss of position and vibratory sense in stocking distribution in both lower extremities with intact reflexes, muscle strength, cerebellar functions and cranial nerves. On mental status exam she seems mildly anxious, and some of her answers are rambling. She is oriented to place, year and day of the week but not date. She claims she can't do serial subtractions because she is not good in math. She remembers two of three objects at 5 minutes, can recall five digits forward and three in reverse. She then refuses the rest of the mental status exam. The most likely diagnosis is

(A) conversion disorder
(B) dementia secondary to alcohol induced hypocalcemia
(C) alcohol induced anxiety disorder
(D) folate deficiency

6. Immediately available laboratory screening will show

(A) normal CBC, elevated sedimentation rate
(B) Hgb 10.3 gm/100 mL (nl = 12-16 gm/100 mL); HCT 32% (nl 37-47%); MCV 79 fL (nl = 82-92); MCHC 30% (nl = 32-36%) (microcytic anemia)
(C) Hgb 10.3 gm/mL (nl = 12-16 gm/ml); HCT 34% (nl = 37-47%); MCV 101 fL (nl = 82-92); MCHC = 33% (nl = 32-36%) (macrocytic anemia)
(D) Na^+ 139 mEq/L (nl 135-145) K^+ 3.4 mEq/l (nl = 3.5-5.5) Cl^- 99 mEq/l (nl = 98-106); HCO_3^- 18 mEq/l (nl = 26-28); anion gap = 25 (nl < 15)

Items 7-13

Choose from the following list the answer that best fits the description given. The same answer may be used more than once or not at all.

(A) Somatization disorder
(B) Panic disorder with agoraphobia
(C) Generalized anxiety disorder
(D) Somatoform disorder
(E) Post-traumatic stress disorder
(F) Social phobia
(G) Brief psychotic disorder
(H) Borderline personality disorder
(I) Panic disorder without agoraphobia
(J) Acute stress disorder

7. Intense anxiety stimulated by feelings of abandonment or mistreatment by important people.

8. Fears of dying, going crazy or losing control, associated with signs of autonomic arousal and avoidance of situations from which escape might be difficult or help unavailable during an episode.

9. Uncontrollable, excessive worry about a variety of events or activities, occurring more days than not for at least 6 months. Associated symptoms of muscle tension, sleep disturbance, and decreased concentration.

10. Three months of intrusive thoughts of an event that evoked intense fear and horror in the face of threatened severe injury or death. Avoidance of stimuli that bring the event to mind, emotional detachment, sleep disorder, poor concentration, and exaggerated startle response.

11. Many physical complaints, including pain, sexual dysfunction, gastrointestinal distress, and inexplicable neurological symptoms.

12. History of sexual or physical abuse in childhood. Difficulty with dysphoria, anxiety and anger, self-mutilation to relieve painful numbness and emptiness.

13. Intense anxiety or panic in situations where a person fears acting or showing symptoms in a way that will be humiliating or embarrassing. Predisposing condition for alcohol abuse.

Items 14-17

Match the symptom pattern with the drug groups listed that are generally used to treat it.

(A) Thioridazine, alprazolam, propranolol
(B) SSRIs, MAOIs, desipramine, alprazolam/clonazepam
(C) SSRIs, clomipramine
(D) Alprazolam, buspirone, propranolol
(E) Buspirone, benzodiazepines, imipramine
(F) Clomipramine, thioridazine, propranolol
(G) Propranolol/atenolol

14. Panic attacks

15. Generalized anxiety

16. Performance anxiety

17. Obsessions/compulsions

Item 18

18. In the treatment of anxiety, all the following have a delayed onset of action; and, indeed, may increase anxiety initially, EXCEPT

(A) fluoxetine
(B) phenelzine
(C) desipramine
(D) lorazepam
(E) sertraline

Items 19-21

19. A 27-year-old female graduate student seeks treatment at the university health service for dizziness, palpitations, and pressure in her chest. During these spells, which last for 5 - 10 minutes at a time, she fears she will faint or even die. She takes a circuitous route to school to avoid crossing large streets, where previous episodes have occurred, because she fears being run over if she faints. She avoids classes where she might be called upon to speak. She finds that staying up late to finish papers makes attacks more frequent, and she is having trouble completing assignments. She once took her pulse during an episode and reports it was 110 BPM. The most likely diagnosis is

(A) somatization disorder
(B) panic disorder with agoraphobia
(C) paroxysmal atrial tachycardia
(D) hypoglycemia
(E) specific phobia

20. After a normal physical exam, further medical evaluation of her symptoms

(A) is unwarranted
(B) should include a glucose tolerance test
(C) should include CBC, serum electrolytes, fasting glucose, thyroid function tests, and urine toxicology
(D) should include Holter monitor and an echocardiogram for mitral valve prolapse
(E) should include TRH stimulation test and dexamethasone suppression test

21. Treatment may involve all the following EXCEPT

(A) psychoeducation
(B) cognitive exercises to change her catastrophic appraisal of her symptoms
(C) encouragement to expose herself to the situations she is avoiding
(D) buspirone/propranolol
(E) SSRI, alprazolam

Items 22-28

Match the neurotransmitters with the subcortical cluster of cell bodies that produce the enzymes necessary for the synthesis of these transmitters in the axon terminals of the cell.

(A) Substantia nigra, ventral tegmentum
(B) Raphe (midline and dorsal) of brainstem
(C) Locus ceruleus
(D) Nucleus basalis of Mynert

22. Serotonin (5–HT)

23. Acetylcholine (ACh)

24. Norepinephrine (NE)

25. Dopamine (DA)

26. The disease process most clearly linked to degeneration of ACh neurons and loss of ACh function in the brain is

    (A) dementia of the Alzheimers type
    (B) dementia syndrome of depression
    (C) dementia secondary to Parkinson's disease
    (D) deficit state of schizophrenia
    (E) Huntington's disease

27. The characteristic pathological changes of the condition in Item 26 include all the following EXCEPT

    (A) cell loss
    (B) amyloid deposition
    (C) neurofibrillary tangles
    (D) granulovascular degeneration of neurons
    (E) dendritic proliferation

28. Parkinson's disease and the extrapyramidal side effects of dopamine blocking, antipsychotic drugs, are specifically related to decreased activity in the

    (A) nigrostriatal pathway
    (B) mesolimbic pathway
    (C) mesocortical pathway
    (D) tuboinfundibular tract

Items 29-33

Certain personality traits cause patients to violate the expectations of the sick role and elicit corrective or punitive responses from caretakers, especially in medical settings. Match the personality trait below with the statement about sick role behavior that best matches it. Answers may be used once or not at all.

(A) Dependent strivings
(B) Antisociality
(C) Narcissism
(D) Borderline traits
(E) Compulsiveness
(F) Schizotypy
(G) Suspiciousness/mistrust (non-psychotic paranoia)
(F) Passivity
(H) Histrionicity

29. Patients exaggerate their complaints but present them so vaguely, that physicians doubt they are real.

30. Patients are reluctant to seek medical care and may have trouble forming an appropriately dependent relationship with a physician or complying with recommendations.

31. Patients are reluctant to resume normal responsibilities and detach from the role of recipient of care.

32. Patients have difficulty acknowledging signs of illness in themselves.

33. Hospital staff often find themselves disagreeing with one another over the legitimacy of the patient's distress; patients may alternate between angry rejection of offered help and undue passivity or neediness.

Items 34-35

Match the DSM–IV axis to the best description of its domain from the following list.

(A) Psychiatric disorders related to underlying neurologic dysfunction
(B) Psychiatric syndromes related to underlying neurologic or medical conditions
(C) Clinical disorders, conditions that may be the focus of psychiatric attention
(D) Physical or medical conditions causally related to primary psychiatric disorder
(E) Any physical or medical condition (causative of, resulting from or unrelated to primary psychiatric disorder)
(F) Personality disorders/habitual psychological defenses/mental retardation
(H) Psychosexual developmental stage
(I) Psychosocial/environmental problems that contribute to the development of the primary psychiatric disorder or may exacerbate it
(J) Severity of recent personal events (current and in past year)
(K) Global assessment of function
(L) Rating of severity of disorder on a scale of 1-5

34. Axis II

35. Axis IV

Items 36-39

Each of the following mental status exams points to a particular psychiatric syndrome. Match the number of the case to the most appropriate description from the following list

(A) Delirium
(B) Amnestic disorder (Korsakoff's psychosis)
(C) Dementia
(D) Generalized anxiety
(E) Depression
(F) Mania
(G) Schizophreniform psychosis
(D) Delusional disorder

36. Case I: A disheveled, 52-year-old woman with excess makeup, tight fitting clothes, and elaborate manicure, with some broken nails.

Level of consciousness: alert
Mood: euphoric, irritable
Affect: cheerful, inappropriate at times (giggles describing loss)
Speech: pressured, emphatic
Thought form: flight of ideas without loose associations; circumstantiality
Thought content: grandiose plans to start her own business, take over the hospital; content is quite fluid and she rationalizes extensively when challenged; some assaultive thoughts but not homicidal or suicidal. No hallucinations admitted. Fleeting paranoid ideas that she does not cling to. No ideas of reference.
Formal testing: oriented X 2.5 (off by 1 day on date); 3/3 objects at 5 minutes, remote memory apparently intact except some confusion in sequencing; can name presidents backwards to Carter (omitting Ford); serial sevens done rapidly with three errors; digit span six forward, four backward.
Continuous performance testing: no errors; Proverbs: abstract, personalized. Formal judgment: would mail a stamped letter, knows why criminals are locked up, but history suggests personal judgment impaired (spent $600 on winter clothes in July; keeps calling her ex-husband, despite restraining order).

37. Case II: An unshaven young man in tattered clothing.

Level of consciousness: alert
Mood: mildly depressed
Affect: flat
Speech: long latency in response to questions, laconic
Thought form: circumstantial, tangential, some odd associations
Thought content: delusional, believes that world is color-coded and that he has to figure out who is safe and who is evil based on what they wear; ideas of reference: gets special messages from the television and from what he reads, is sure people are talking about him when around strangers; auditory hallucinations of voices commenting on his behavior; No admitted SI; some desire to mutilate self.
Formal testing: oriented X 3; recalls 3/3 objects at 5 minutes; remote memory grossly intact; categories concrete; proverbs, concrete ("The glass will break.") Serial sevens done slowly with one error. Seven digits forward, five in reverse. Calculations: Knows there are 20 nickels in a dollar and 60 nickels equal $3.
Formal judgment: would leave a letter in the street; knows why criminals are locked up. By history, impaired judgment (acts are based on his delusions).

38. Case III: A 45-year-old woman, neatly dressed, looks sad, inexpressive.

Level of consciousness: alert
Mood: depressed, subdued
Affect: sad, overtly tearful at times
Speech: normal though some hesitancy around painful topics
Thought form: unremarkable
Thought content: themes of inadequacy, hopelessness, worry, including worry about her health. Passive SI without plan or intent; no hallucinations or delusions or ideas of reference
Formal testing: oriented x 3, 3/3 objects at 5 minutes, 7 digits forward, 5 in reverse, proverbs and categories abstract, serial sevens done slowly with no errors; gives up reciting presidents after Reagan; calculations, normal: Formal judgment: normal, personal judgment: has some insight into own condition.

39. Case IV: A 60-year-old man dressed in hospital pajamas

Level of consciousness: alert
Mood: euthymic = Joyfulness
Affect: cheerful
Speech: fluent, some syntactical errors (possibly consistent with level of education); regional accent
Thought form: circumstantial, loses the thread of questions
Thought content: wants to go home, live independently; no insight into problems that caused family to bring him in to hospital (poor self care, including nutrition); no hallucinations, delusions or ideas of reference; not homicidal or suicidal.
Formal testing: oriented to name, place but not date. 3/3 objects immediately; O/3 objects at 5 minutes, can't recall what he had for breakfast. Unable to do digit span. Spells world forward but not backward. Loses the task of serial sevens after two steps. Simple calculations normal. Long term memory grossly normal—knows his birthday, where he lived growing up, dates of military service, names of family members; categories—concrete; proverbs: refuses. Formal judgement: normal, (would mail a letter, know why criminals are locked up).

Items 40-43

40. From the following, choose the most accurate rank ordering of suicide risk factors (highest to lowest).

    (A) Prior suicide attempts; loss of physical health; age greater than 45 (men), 55 (women); alcohol dependence; recent loss or separation; single, widowed or divorced
    (B) Recent loss or separation; single, widowed or divorced; alcohol dependence; loss of physical health; age over 45 (men), 55 (women); prior suicide attempts
    (C) Age over 45 (men), 55 (women); alcohol dependence; prior suicide attempts; recent loss or separation; loss of physical health; single, widowed or divorced
    (D) Alcohol dependence; age over 45 (men), 55 (women); prior suicide attempts; loss of physical health; recent loss or separation; single, widowed or divorced
    (E) Loss of physical health; recent loss or separation; alcohol dependence; age greater than 45 (men), 55 (women); prior suicide attempts; single, widowed or divorced.

41. Among medical specialties, the one with the highest suicide rate is

    (A) general practice
    (B) anesthesiology
    (C) ophthalmology
    (D) psychiatry
    (E) internal medicine

42. A person with a history of several prior failed suicide attempts or gestures

    (A) is at less risk for suicide than people who have never attempted suicide
    (B) has suicide risk equal to people who have never attempted suicide
    (C) has a greater risk of suicide than people who have never attempted suicide
    (D) has a greater risk of suicide than people who have never attempted suicide only if a prior attempt failed accidentally

43. Across diagnostic categories, the biological marker most clearly associated with completed suicide by violent means is

    (A) decreased norepinephrine in the locus ceruleus
    (B) decreased serotonin metabolite (5-HIAA) in the cerebrospinal fluid
    (C) increased dopamine metabolites (HVA, MHPG) in urine
    (D) decreased dopamine metabolites (HVA, MHPG) in urine

Items 44-46

Match the appropriate intervention to the case. Given interventions may be used once, more than once, or not at all.

(A) Admit to hospital voluntarily
(B) Offer voluntary hospitalization, but commit to hospital if patient refuses
(C) Comfort and reassure; send home with instructions to avoid drugs and alcohol
(D) Reassure the patient and send home after arranging for someone trustworthy to provide supervision until the first outpatient mental health visit
(E) Admit to hospital if no reliable person can be found to stay with patient until outpatient treatment can be arranged.
(F) Refer to a physician who will countenance assisted suicide.

44. A 24-year-old woman who has just broken up with her boyfriend is brought to the ED by her roommate after taking an overdose of sleeping pills and alcohol. The door was unlocked and the patient was found lying in the living room. She reports, and her roommate confirms, that she is normally a social drinker. She admits to having made an overdose attempt under similar circumstances in high school. She says she "just didn't care about ever waking up" when she took the pills. She now feels embarrassed and says she was overreacting and won't try again.

45. A 60-year-old widow, mother of three grown children, with a history of hypertension and a prior left hemisphere stroke with residual weakness of the right leg, comes to the ED with a superficial cut on her wrist. She does not recall deciding she wanted to kill herself. "I had the knife in my hand to slice onions, and suddenly I cut on my wrist." The patient admits to feeling more sad recently, as she often feels around the anniversary of her husband's death. She also reports that she has been depressed since her stroke, with fragmented sleep, irritability, tearfulness and poor appetite. She does not drink and her only medication is clonidine for her blood pressure. In general, she cooperates with medical treatment, and she is glad to be told that her depression might be treatable.

46. A 43-year-old, twice-divorced man with a 5-year cocaine habit comes in asking for treatment. He has had intense suicidal ideation for the past 2 weeks, with a plan to jump from a local traffic bridge. He also describes such depressive symptoms as fatigue, weight gain, sluggishness and self-loathing. He has abstained from cocaine for 2 weeks. When using cocaine, he drank about six beers per day. He has cut down to one per day, but he did drink himself into a state of unconsciousness over the prior weekend, after standing at the edge of the bridge for an hour, trying to decide whether or not to jump. His friends are all drug users and he is in danger of losing his job because of absenteeism. He cannot contract for safety if he goes home.

Items 47-50

After each vignette, chose the appropriate form of psychotherapy

47. 75-year-old woman whose husband died 4 years ago still has disturbed sleep, partial loss of pleasure and interest, crying spells and trouble maintaining her weight. She complains of multiple aches and pains and constipation and worries that the breast cancer she had treated at age 60 may be recurring. She denies alcohol or drug use and says that although she would welcome death, she would never try to hurt herself. Which one of the following is the most appropriate form of psychotherapy for this patient?

    (A) psychoanalytic psychotherapy
    (B) behavior therapy
    (C) brief interpersonal therapy
    (D) emotions Anonymous
    (E) rational emotive therapy

48. 24-year-old graduate student experiences disabling anxiety symptoms when he must speak in class or in front of group. The patient also describes anxiety in informal social interactions—he rarely goes to parties or places where he might have to enter into conversations with strangers. He says he "feels stupid" and thinks others are irritated by his difficulty making conversation. His grades are suffering because of his inhibitions, and he is considering giving up his program to find a less stressful kind of job. Which one of the following is the most appropriate form of psychotherapy for this patient?

    (A) emotions Anonymous
    (B) psychoanalytic psychotherapy
    (C) network therapy
    (D) cognitive behavioral therapy
    (E) vocational counselling

49. 35-year-old, divorced man gives a history of moderately heavy drinking for 10 years. In the 2 years since his divorce, he has been depressed, with disrupted sleep, irritability, fatigue and cynicism. He admits that he typically drinks more than he intends to—on weekends, he can consume a case of beer in 2 days. Recently, he has begun drinking in the morning before work to relieve a persistent hangover. Which one of the following is the most appropriate form of psychotherapy for this patient?

    (A) cognitive behavioral therapy
    (B) self-help (AA or Rational Recovery)
    (C) structural family therapy
    (D) psychoanalytic psychotherapy
    (E) interpersonal psychotherapy

50. 25-year-old woman comes in confused and anxious about her relationships. She describes a pattern of being self-effacing in intimate relationships. She gets involved with men who initially seem charming and protective, only to find that they become dominating and verbally abusive as the relationship proceeds. Her current boyfriend has twice coerced her into sexual activity over her strong objections. The patient mentions that her parents' relationship was overtly abusive. After her parents divorced when she was 8 years old, she lived with her mother, who did not remarry for 10 years. During this time, the patient's mother had three or four boyfriends who were critical and demeaning, both of her mother and of her. At the same time, she discounts her feelings about this as "probably overreacting or something." She presents a cheerful, competent facade to the world but feels she "blocks out" a lot of her most painful feelings and memories as she has done at least since early adolescence. Which one of the following is the most appropriate form of psychotherapy for this patient?

    (A) psychoanalytically oriented psychotherapy, brief or long-term
    (B) emotions anonymous
    (C) assertiveness training
    (D) sex and love addicts anonymous
    (E) family therapy with her mother and stepfather

Item 51

51. The most common delusions in mania are

    (A) bizarre delusions
    (B) grandiose delusions
    (C) belief that people have been replaced by impostors (delusions of Capgras)
    (D) delusions of external control
    (E) delusions of time acceleration

Items 52-56

Match a diagnosis from the following list to the descriptions given below

(A) Delusional disorder
(B) Schizotypal disorder
(C) Schizophreniform disorder
(D) Schizophrenia, paranoid type
(E) Schizophrenia, catatonic type
(F) Schizophrenia, disorganized type
(G) Schizophrenia, undifferentiated type
(H) Bipolar, manic, with mood congruent psychotic features
(I) Substance induced psychosis
(J) Schizoaffective disorder
(K) Brief reactive psychosis

52. A 22-year-old woman is brought in by her parents, for reasons she can't explain. On questioning, she does admit to hearing derogatory voices commenting on her every move for about the past week. She says she first felt not entirely herself about 3 months ago, just after graduating from college. She can't quite say how she felt unwell; things "just seemed different, somehow." She was planning to get a job, but has been staying at her parents' house, often sleeping much of the day and wandering at night. Her speech is a bit odd, with tangential answers to some questions. She has no relevant medical history. She has not smoked marijuana for 2 years and never used other drugs. She drinks only rarely on big social occasions.

53. A 49-year-old woman complains to her primary care physician that she is under intolerable stress at work. Her manager seems to be trying to make her fail, and her coworkers treat her badly. She wonders whether they may be acting under the instructions of the FBI, who have reams of files about her since she worked for the Social Security Administration 10 years ago. She has few friends, but she is close to her family and active in a hiking club. She feels discouraged and unhappy, though she enjoys her time away from work; vegetative symptoms are limited to disrupted sleep on Mondays before work and some fatigue. She is overtalkative and circumstantial in trying to prove she is the target of investigation, but otherwise logical and coherent. She denies drug or alcohol use on the grounds that "You never know what someone might put into your drink."

54. A 50-year-old man is brought in by his wife because "He's going off again." She reports that he is not sleeping much, talk incessantly about plans to increase his business, and has run up unusual credit card debt from impulsive purchases. He is a social drinker, but lately he has been opening beers and leaving them around the house after only a few sips. He seems to be hearing voices, though he refuses to answers questions about this. His behavior includes starting tasks and not finishing them, eating furtively at odd times, rummaging in storage areas, and making lists. His wife reports his presentation is similar to an episode 5 years before. She thinks he has been hearing the voices for months, but his sleep changed only 1 week ago and he was acting fairly normally until 3 weeks ago.

55. A 30-year-old man who works as a custodian, though he has a college degree, presents to your office. He lives alone and has never had an intimate relationship. His chief complaint is that "I was told to come here." He says that he hears voices that tell him what is safe or not and what he should do. He admits to funny shock-like sensations in his body and says that "they" have planted electrical wires that cause him to have an orgasm or to experience pain anytime "they" want to. He smokes a joint of marijuana perhaps once every 2 months and drinks a few beers roughly as often. He presents himself in a stilted, robotic way, as though he were responding to military commands. He says he has had the shocks and heard the voices "for a long time" and was hospitalized when he told his family about them 2 years ago.

56. A 17-year-old high school student who has been in and out of psychiatric treatment for 5 years presents to your office. He was an isolated, quiet child. In adolescence, he gradually developed a thought disorder, keeping a detailed diary that is almost incoherent, filled with references to superheros and sports stars. His answers to questions are tangential, at times frankly illogical. He admits to auditory hallucinations. He smiles inappropriately and seems detached from his surroundings. He seems to lack awareness that anything is wrong. He also lacks initiative, though he will generally accede to requests that he bathe, or put something away, or take his medicine.

Item 57

57. The relevant neuroanatomical finding shown by the CT scans of a normal (A) and a schizophrenic (B) brain found in **Figure 9.1** below is

(A) presence of narrowed lateral ventricles in the schizophrenic brain
(B) presence of enlarged lateral ventricles in the schizophrenic brain
(C) signs of diffuse microcalcification in the schizophrenic brain
(D) absence of any significant abnormality in either brain
(E) narrowing of sulci in the schizophrenic brain

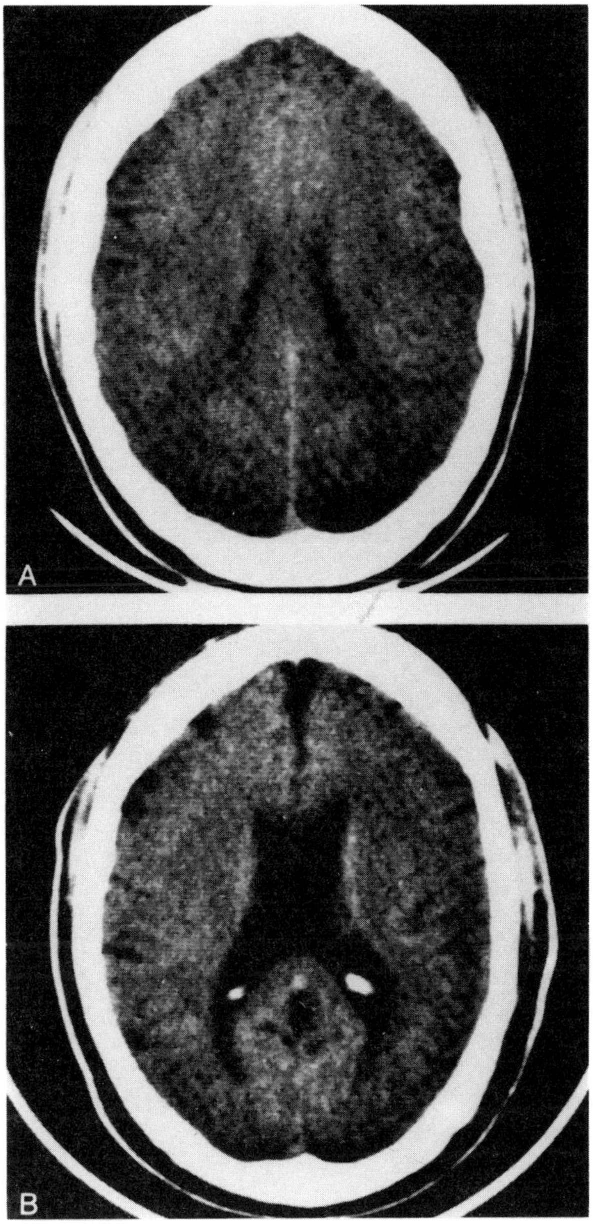

Figure 9.1

Items 58-61

Match the conditions on the following list to the descriptions below

(A) Major depressive episode
(B) Dysthymic disorder
(C) Major depressive episode with mood-congruent psychotic features
(D) Major depressive episode with mood-incongruent psychotic features
(E) Schizoaffective, depressed
(F) Bipolar disorder, most recent episode depressed
(G) Major depressive episode, melancholic
(H) Major depressive episode with atypical features
(I) Substance induced mood disorder
(J) Adjustment disorder with depressed mood
(K) Normal bereavement

58. 50-year-old woman who is admitted to the hospital for the sixth time. She is withdrawn, irritable, fearful and restless. She reports feeling depressed for about 6 weeks, with difficulty falling and staying asleep and a 15-lb weight loss due to loss of appetite. She has suicidal ideation with a plan to take an overdose, which she has done in the past under the influence of command auditory hallucinations. She hears voices pretty much continuously, but when she is not depressed, they do not talk of suicide. She has been divorced for many years and has trouble holding jobs due to her suspiciousness and odd responses to other people.

59. 35-year-old woman who wants her primary care physician to evaluate her for chronic fatigue syndrome. She does not have a history of viral or flu-like symptoms, just intense fatigue, hypersomnia (sleeping up to 11 hours per night), 10-lb weight gain, and generally low mood. She says she can feel better briefly when out with friends, but mostly she feels sad, discouraged to the point of hopelessness about becoming her normal self again, and worthless, because she is not the person she wants to be. While she says she would not intentionally hurt herself, she would be glad to "just disappear," if she could. She drinks socially, up to two beers every other weekend.

60. 50-year-old man who feels sad and confused since being laid off from his job 2 months ago. He can't seem to get himself to look aggressively for another one, saying he is too old and no one will hire him. He sleeps normally, except on the nights before job interviews, but he feels tired and dragged down many days. He drinks a beer with dinner every third night. Occasionally, he has bouts of restlessness and pacing, though he does not describe full panic attacks. He has some thoughts that life is not worth living, but none of hurting himself.

61. 64-year-old woman with 5-month history of depressed mood, markedly decreased sleep due to early morning awakening, 20-lb weight loss, crying spells and intensifying suicidal ideation. She says mornings are the hardest time, she feels so guilty about not getting up and doing all the things she should. After grieving the loss of her husband, who died 3 years ago, she became active in church groups and volunteer work. Now she just goes to work and comes home, since nothing feels worthwhile or enjoyable. She denies alcohol use and has no major medical problems except hypercholesterolemia managed with diet.

Item 62

62. The term schizoaffective disorder, most recent episode manic, connotes

  (A) someone who simultaneously meets criteria for a schizophrenic disorder and a manic episode
  (B) someone with mood incongruent psychotic features while manic
  (C) someone with a history of both manic episodes and of psychotic symptoms when they are not in either a manic or depressive episode
  (D) someone with schizophrenia who has a family history of bipolar disorder
  (E) someone with bipolar disorder who has a family history of schizophrenia

Items 63-65

Match the drugs below to the statements that follow; each term may be used once, more than once, or not at all

  (A) Fluoxetine, paroxetine, sertraline
  (B) Amitriptyline, imipramine
  (C) Nortriptyline, desipramine
  (D) Buproprion
  (E) Nefazodone
  (F) Trazodone
  (G) Tranylcypromine; phenelzine
  (H) Lithium, valproic acid, carbamazepine
  (I) Venlafaxine
  (J) Chlomipramine

63. Only dopaminergic antidepressant; does not affect serotonin or norepinephrine levels

64. Highly anticholinergic and antihistaminic antidepressants, often producing unacceptable side effects; lethal in overdose

65. Typically lowers blood pressure but may cause dangerous, even lethal hypertension in combination with foods containing tyramine; lethally interacts with meperidine or serotonergic drugs

Items 66-69

Match each pattern of toxicity to the neurotransmitters involved; each may be used once, more than once, or not at all.

  (A) Diarrhea, fever, myoclonus, delirium, hypertension, sweating
  (B) Constipation, dry mouth, blurred vision, urinary retention, dilated pupils, dry skin, increased temperature, delirium, heart block, arrhythymia, seizures
  (C) Severe hypertension, headache, stroke
  (D) Fever, elevated WBC, fluctuations in blood pressure, tachypnea, sweating, elevated creatinine phosphokinase (CPK)

66. Serotonin

67. Acetylcholine

68. Dopamine

69. Tyramine

Items 70-73

70. Which of the tracings in **Figure 9.2** below was recorded during REM sleep?

(A)
(B)
(C)
(D)
(E)
(F)

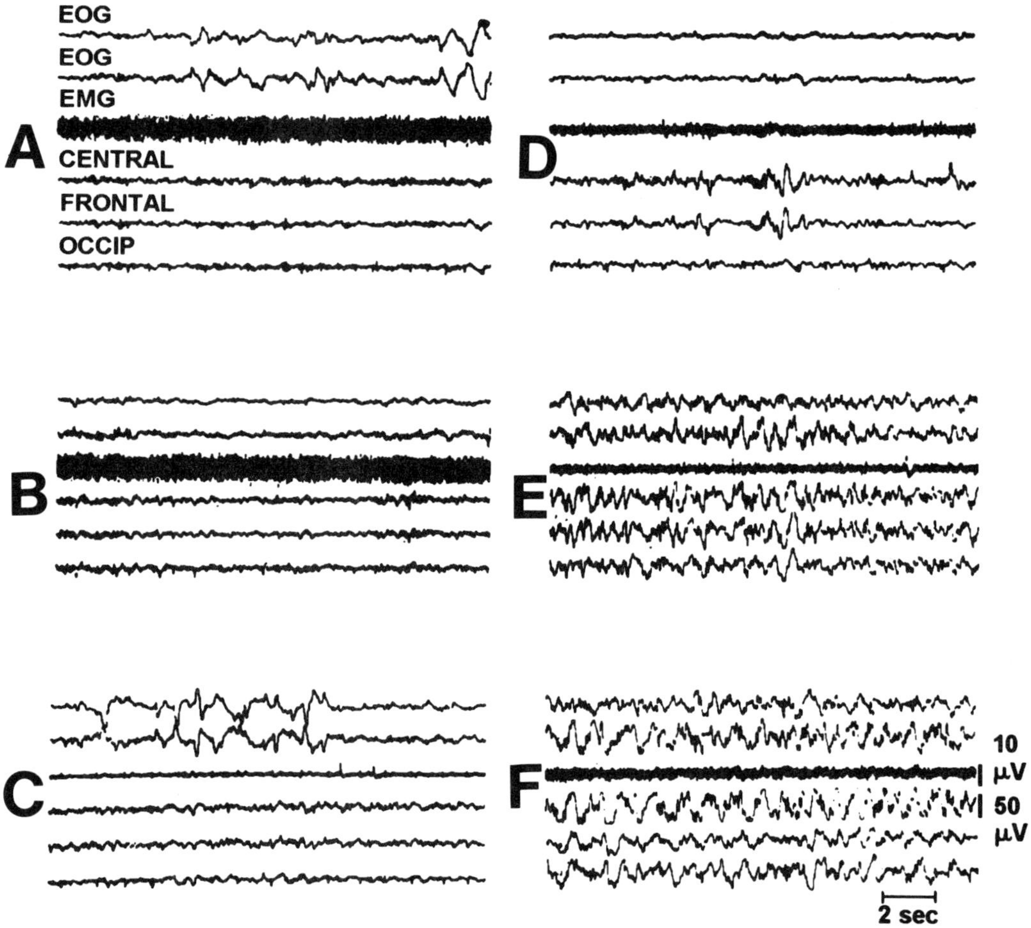

Figure 9.2

71. Which of the following EEG lead tracings in **Figure 9.3** below is charactertistic of stage 2 of sleep?

(A)
(B)
(C)
(D)
(E)
(F)

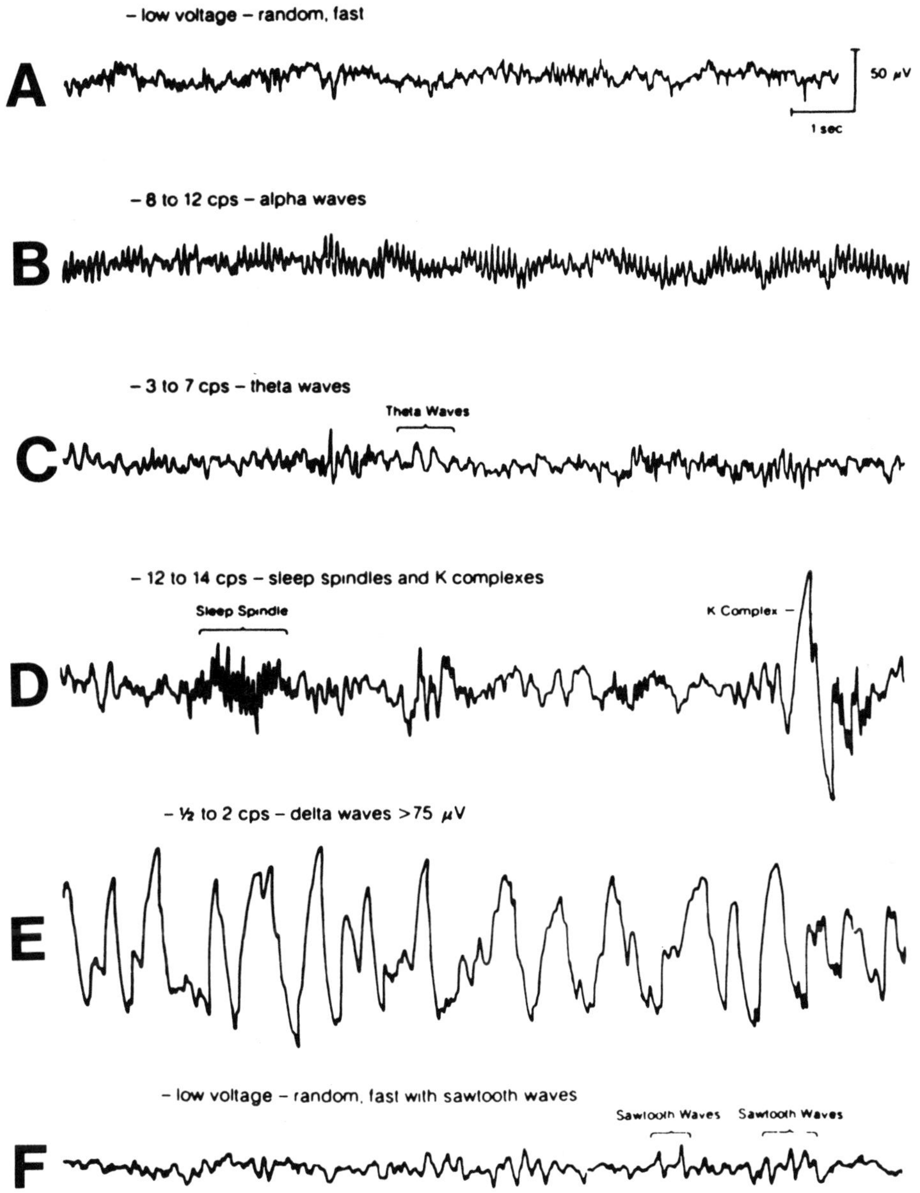

Figure 9.3

72. The regulation of REM sleep is principally

(A) noradrenergic
(B) cholinergic
(C) serotonergic
(D) dopaminergic
(E) None of the above

73. The regulation of nREM (nonREM) sleep is principally

(A) noradrenergic
(B) cholinergic
(C) serotonergic
(D) dopaminergic
(E) None of the above

Items 74-77

74. After a period of sleep deprivation, which phases will rebound (occur more intensely or more frequently) at the expense of other sleep stages?

(A) delta sleep only
(B) REM sleep only
(C) stages 1-2, REM
(D) delta and REM sleep
(E) none, total sleep will increase with roughly the same proportion of stages as sleep prior to the sleep deprivation

75. The most common auxiliary symptom in narcolepsy is

(A) hypnagogic hallucinations
(B) sleep paralysis
(C) cataplexy
(D) snoring
(E) enuresis

76. The difference between central and obstructive sleep apnea is that

(A) patients with obstructive apnea have increased thoracic over diaphragmatic respiratory effort during episodes
(B) patients with central apnea fail to show respiratory effort during apneic episodes
(C) patients with central apnea have longer and more frequent episodes
(D) patients with obstructive apnea more commonly awaken with headaches from muscle tension

77. A 25-year-old medical student complains that he cannot get to sleep before 4 AM then sleeps 7 hours, frequently missing morning classes. This case exemplifies

(A) advanced sleep phase syndrome
(D) REM sleep behavior disorder
(C) delayed sleep phase syndrome
(D) psychophysiologic insomnia
(E) adjustment sleep disorder

Items 78-80

Match the following vignettes with the appropriate treatment. Each may be used once, more than once, or not at all

(A) Bright light in the early part of the day
(B) Bright light in the later part of the day
(C) Improved sleep hygiene (avoid stimulants and alcohol, establish an effective bedtime routine, increase afternoon exercise, no nonsleep activities in bed); relaxation exercises
(D) Advise the patient to establish a fixed bedtime and stick to it
(E) Advise the patient to establish a fixed rising time and stick to it
(F) Advise the patient to stay awake 2 hours later each night until the onset of sleep advances to a normal bedtime, then stick to it
(G) Advise the patient to go to bed 1 hour earlier each night until reaching a normal bedtime, then stick to it
(F) Continuous positive airway pressure, possible surgery
(G) Occasional use of a sedative hypnotic
(H) Daily use of methylphenidate or another stimulant
(I) Prescription of nontricyclic antidepressant
(J) Prescription of any antidepressant
(K) Clonazepam, triazolam, carbidopa, baclofen, or gaba-pentin
(L) Referral to AA

78. Overweight 64-year-old man whose wife reports that he snores so loudly she has taken to sleeping in the spare room. He sweats profusely at night and complains of heartburn. Most mornings he wakens unrefreshed, with a headache. His blood pressure is typically 160/100. He takes several unrefreshing naps every day, even though this interferes with his work productivity.

79. 24-year-old graduate student who falls asleep during lectures, to the point when she must get other students' notes for most courses. She awakens from her naps feeling refreshed. Intense emotion causes her to abruptly lose muscle tone and collapse, without loss of consciousness. Some nights she experiences vivid hallucinations just as she is falling asleep.

80. 45-year-old woman with 4 month history of difficulty falling asleep and early morning awakening. She lies awake up to 2 hours at night and is up 1 hour before she needs to be, so that total sleep is diminished. She experiences daytime fatigue, low mood, crying spells, irregular eating, increased anxiety, and diminished self esteem. No active medical problems.

Item 81

81. Which of the following objective tests is abnormal during delirium from any cause?

(A) CT of the head
(B) EEG
(C) LP
(D) EKG
(E) serum glucose

STOP.

YOU HAVE COMPLETED THIS SECTION.

Notes

Behavioral Science

Answers and Tutorials

Answer and Tutorial on Item 1

The answer is: **1-C**. Because the **EEG** measures only the top few millimeters of brain electrical activity, epileptic foci deep in the limbic system are difficult to detect. When they fire without spreading to the rest of the brain, they may produce symptoms and behaviors that are easily mistaken for primary psychiatric disorders. Seizures confined to limbic structures are called partial complex seizures (formerly temporal lobe epilepsy). Recognized aspects of partial complex seizures include preseizure auras involving sensory distortions (olfactory and gustatory hallucinations, visual distortions; rarely, abdominal pain). During the ictal phase, patients may show stereotypic, elemental motor activity (standing and sitting, buttoning and unbuttoning), and disruptions of cognitive functioning (trance, depersonalization, repetitive thoughts). A partial seizure may also generalize to the rest of the brain, producing a **grand mal seizure**. Patients are typically amnestic for the ictal phase of either a grand mal or partial seizure and sometimes for events immediately beforehand (anterograde amnesia). Intense dysphoria, anxiety or rage may occur in conjunction with partial seizures and also in periods far removed from the actual seizure.

Organized, directed, **violent behavior** rarely if ever occurs during a seizure. However, violent behavior may occur interictally in patients with partial complex seizures or those with non epileptic EEG abnormalities in the temporal lobes. Interictal irritability is very common. Frequent *déjà vu* or *jamais vu* and feelings of depersonalization are other interictal clues that a patient may have partial complex seizures. Over many years, patients with partial complex seizures may develop personality changes, including passivity, unusual sexual behavior, loss of sexual interest, obsessiveness, religious preoccupations and even a chronic psychosis that closely resembles chronic schizophrenia. In patients with grand mal epilepsy, these changes are found more commonly in those with primary lesions in the **limbic system** than in those with other foci.

The diagnosis of partial complex seizures is sometimes hard to confirm. EEG abnormalities are most easily detected during the transition from waking to sleep, so it is best to study sleep deprived patients who fall asleep during the test. While partial complex seizures may be idiopathic, a clinical neurologic examination and brain imaging studies may detect structural lesions that account for the abnormal electrical activity. Projective psychological tests, though often helpful in studying personality and uncovering psychosis, suffer from lack of standardization and unacceptably low reliability. Thus, they have little place in standard neuropsychiatric evaluation.

Partial complex seizures respond best to **anticonvulsants**, with carbamazepine and valproic acid often more effective and less toxic than phenytoin, barbiturates or benzodiazepines. Lithium, which may reduce impulsiveness and violence, is analeptic (lowers the seizure threshhold), and not advisable as a single agent in patients with seizures. Behavior therapy is sometimes effective for compulsions, but not for those related to epilepsy. **Ergotamine** is used specifically for the treatment of **migraine headaches**.

Answers and Tutorial on Items 2-4

The answers are: **2-B; 3-A; 4-C**. Ablation or destruction of **limbic areas** highlights their role in the processing and storage of memory. Because of the protection afforded by the redundancy of having two hemispheres with overlapping functions, tumors, injuries or infarctions affecting limbic areas are often silent, unless they cause pressure effects or electrical excitation. Toxic or metabolic damage, which typically affects symmetrical areas, can, by contrast, have dramatic impact. The most common, clinically significant example is that of **thiamine deficiency**, which occurs in malnutrition, especially among **alcoholics**.

Acute thiamine deficiency produces **Wernicke's encephalopathy**. The cardinal features of this condition are delirium with ataxia, oculomotor dysfunction, especially 6th nerve palsy (intranuclear ophthalmoplegia) and sometimes anisocoria.

Administering glucose to someone on the verge of thiamine deficiency can precipitate acute encephalopathy, because thiamine is a cofactor for the cerebral metabolism of glucose. Wernicke's encephalopathy is prevented or rapidly reversed by the administration of thiamine.

Chronic thiamine deficiency causes alcohol-induced-chronic-amnestic disorder (**Korsakoff's syndrome**). The main sites of damage are paraventricular, symmetrical lesions in the mammillary bodies, the thalamus, and the hypothalamus. Lesions may also occur in the midbrain, pons, medulla, fornix and cerebellum. Cerebellar and ocular signs may not be present and diagnosis depends on a careful mental status exam. Patients with the alcohol amnestic syndrome have relatively preserved long-term memory, are socially appropriate, use language normally and can do simple calculations. Their profound recent memory loss seems so disproportionate to the rest of their mental status that observers may misdiagnose malingering—that is, willfully faking abnormality for some personal gain. Patients with the amnestic syndrome will occasionally try to conceal their deficits by confabulation, making up or agreeing to untrue scenarios given by the examiner. This is not the same thing as lying, but is often mistaken for it.

The presence of mild macrocytosis and elevated liver enzymes is a common incidental finding in chronic alcoholics and does not explain the behavioral changes described.

Answers and Tutorial on Items 5-6

The answers are: **5-D; 6-C**. Other clinically significant nutritional deficiencies and metabolic imbalances occur in **alcoholics**, affecting other parts of the nervous system and producing different mental status changes. Deficiencies of folate and vitamin B_{12}, which may co-occur, can cause macrocytic anemia, peripheral neuropathy, delerium or dementia. This patient has the classic loss of position and vibratory sense seen in peripheral neuropathy, macrocytic anemia (Item 6), and subtle mental status changes characteristic of early dementia.

The patient's normal reflexes are evidence against the deficiency of calcium or magnesium which can occur in alcoholics and lead to delirium, psychosis, hyperreflexia, tetany, seizures and death. Although this patient does not have symptoms consistent with ketoacidosis, it would be important to screen for this by measuring electrolytes, because alcoholics can develop ketoacidosis from alcohol, malnutrition, or from diabetes secondary to destruction of the pancreas.

Symptoms are often difficult to detect in intoxicated patients, and uncooperative behavior (even when the patient is sober) often leads medical professionals to perform cursory or inadequate medical evaluation. Physicians may be quick to apply pejorative psychiatric labels to alcoholic patients. While stocking and glove anesthesia or paresthesia are sometimes symptoms of hyperventilation or conversion disorder, burning sensations and a stocking distribution of the loss of position and vibratory sense are typical of peripheral neuropathy. Alcoholics suffer neuropathy both from alcohol itself and from associated vitamin deficiencies. Detection and differentiation of various alcohol-related neurological dysfunctions is crucial, since many have specific remedies. Left untreated, vitamin deficiency, electrolyte abnormalities, ketoacidosis or diabetes can lead to permanent, incapacitating neurological damage, even death.

Answers and Tutorial on Items 7-13

The answers are: **7-H; 8-B; 9-C; 10-E; 11-A; 12-H; 13-F**. **DSM- IV** assigns separate categories to anxiety disorders, personality disorders, somatoform disorders, and dissociative disorders. It is important to recognize that **anxiety**—as a symptom— appears in many psychiatric disorders in and outside of these categories. Thus, anxiety figures prominently in all forms of psychotic disorder, including brief psychotic disorder and schizophrenia, major depressions, avoidant, dependent, and borderline personality disorders, and stimulant intoxication or sedative withdrawal, among other common psychiatric problems.

All clinically significant forms of anxiety involve a mental state of dread or fear and somatic manifestations (eg, palpitations, churning stomach, diarrhea, urge to urinate, restlessness, sleep problems, muscle tension). In the anxiety disorders, these symptoms, by definition, lead to significant functional impairment.

Differentiating among the anxiety disorders requires classification of the patient's most prominent anxiety as persistent, as in generalized anxiety disorder, or brief and intense, as in panic disorder, social phobia, and simple phobia.

Bouts of acute, severe symptoms can occur superimposed on persistent, diffuse ones in **generalized anxiety disorder**. Between acute episodes, patients with mainly brief anxiety states may have persistent fear of their symptoms (anticipatory anxiety). Recognizing which aspect of the anxiety is most prominent and disabling requires clinical experience. At times, separation is not possible, and two or more anxiety disorders may be diagnosed concurrently.

The characteristic themes or triggers of patients' anxiety also help distinguish one anxiety disorder from another. In generalized anxiety, patients have fears concerning many aspects of their personal security, typically—money, health, the welfare of family members and so on. In **panic disorder**, patients fear the experience of panic itself; those who also avoid situations that they believe might trigger a panic attack, or where it would be dangerous or embarrassing to have a panic attack, are classified as having **panic disorder with agoraphobia**.

Patients with **social phobia** fear humiliation, scrutiny or rejection in interactions with others, sometimes only strangers, sometimes only in possible intimate relationships. These patients avoid the social situations they fear, for example, by limiting the kind of work they will do or being unable to form close attachments. Many will use alcohol to make threatening situations bearable. This pattern can progress to the development of frank alcohol abuse or dependence. Thus, the early identification and treatment of social phobia is an extremely important task.

Traumatic events, by definition, are events which evoke intense fear and horror in situations where the person feels helpless. People respond to such events in many ways. Those who use dissociation, a trance-like state that separates the events from the associated painful emotions, are most at risk to develop acute stress disorder. This disorder, by definition, subsides within a month. Symptoms that persist longer are classified as **posttraumatic stress disorder** (PTSD). Because dissociation is not complete, the cardinal feature of PTSD is intrusive reliving of the trauma in forced recollection, nightmares, or flashbacks. Intrusive symptoms typically erupt through a state of numbness, loss of interest, feelings of inability to relate normally to others, and a changed view of the future. The chief precipitant to anxiety in PTSD, then, is the welling up of unpleasant emotions related to a past traumatic event. Patients with PTSD also have symptoms of chronic hyperarousal, including sleep disruptions, irritability, low threshold for startle, hypervigilance, physical reactivity to reminders, and diminished concentration.

People with **borderline personality disorder** typically have problems soothing themselves and maintaining a consistent sense of their own identity either when alone or when involved in close relationships. Thus, the main precipitant to their often severe anxiety is disruption in relationships that sustain their shaky equilibrium—even minor separations, for example, can precipitate severe reactions. Classical psychoanalytic understanding of borderline personality "explains" this anxiety by analogizing it to the anxiety experienced by a 2- or 3-year-old child negotiating the stage of separation/individuation. This theory postulates that parental failure to encourage and support separation/individuation impairs the patient's sense of self and ability to regulate anxiety. More recent research suggests that borderline personality results from much more severe failures in parenting. Thus, 60-80% of patients with borderline personality disorder report experiencing abuse, especially sexual abuse, during childhood. Having been overstimulated or constantly vigilant against abuse in childhood, borderline patients develop high anxiety but cannot learn from trusted adults how to sooth and contain their feelings. Moreover, many pre-borderline children were abused at the stage when they were dependent on adults for basic survival. The threat of separation thus triggers not anxiety, but panic.

In addition to anxiety, borderline patients have symptoms similar to the numbing seen in those with PTSD, including a painful feeling of emptiness. Cutting, burning and other forms of self-mutilation, as well as suicidal gestures and attempts, are a cardinal feature of this disorder and are often explained by the patient as the only available means of coping with anxiety and emptiness.

Somatization disorder, though classified under somatoform disorders, overlaps with the anxiety disorders. In both, patients typically seek medical attention for cryptic physical symptoms. The symptoms of anxiety disorders are usually readily explainable as manifestations of autonomic arousal. Most anxious patients will, if asked, also be able to describe their fearful mental state. In somatization disorder, the symptoms are more varied and more difficult to explain. By definition, the patient complains of problems in at least four different organ systems—usually gastrointestinal, neurologic, urogenital, and cardiorespiratory. No clear physical basis for the complaints can be found. Often people with this disorder deny anxiety or psychic distress except for distress about their physical condition. The cause of somatization disorder is unknown. The disorder, which is most common in women, aggregates in families where there appears to be genetic risk for antisocial personality disorder in men. Somatization may also be another adult sequela of childhood traumatization or abuse.

Answers and Tutorial on Items 14-17

The answers are: **14-B; 15-E; 16-G; 17-C**. Systematic research has shown that the **MAOIs** and **imipramine/desipramine** are effective against various forms of anxiety, including panic. Increasing anecdotal evidence also supports the broad **anxiolytic properties** of the SSRIs. Because these antidepressants also induce anxiety and all require 3 - 4 weeks to bring about a therapeutic response (response latency), patients may not tolerate them, especially if used alone. The benzodiazepine receptor agonists alprazolam, clonazepam, and lorazepam are all effective against panic and have an immediate onset of action. Physicians initially often prescribe combinations of antidepressants and benzodiazepines and then wean the patient from the latter after a few weeks so as to minimize the potential for dependence and abuse.

While ineffective in the treatment of panic, **buspirone**, which is active at 5-HT_{1a}, 5-HT_2 and D_2 receptors, is useful in the treatment of generalized **anxiety**. It lacks the dependence/abuse problems of the benzodiazepine receptor agonists, partly because, like the antidepressants, it produces relief over a period of 3-6 weeks, but not immediately. Benzodiazepine receptor agonists also may relieve generalized anxiety symptoms. Since generalized anxiety disorder, by current definition, lasts at least 6 months, the likelihood that patients will become dependent because of persistent use is substantial. Nevertheless, maintenance on a benzodiazepine may be preferable to persistent, disabling generalized anxiety. When generalized anxiety exists in the context of a major depression, it often responds to antidepressant treatment. Thus, all three types of drugs are of use in the treatment of this symptom pattern.

Performance anxiety (stage fright or social phobia in performance situations) is the only type of anxiety that reliably responds to β–adrenergic receptor blockers. These drugs lack the potential for dependence, tolerance or abuse. In the low doses (20-80mg) required for relief of performance anxiety, they also produce minimal side effects. Why this type of anxiety responds so well to these drugs while other types do not is a mystery.

Clomipramine and SSRIs in high doses are the preferred treatment for **obsessive compulsive symptoms**. Other antianxiety and antidepressant drugs are much less effective for this problem.

Answer and Tutorial on Item 18

The answer is: **18-D**. The treatment of **anxiety disorders** usually requires a combination of specialized psychotherapy and psychotropic drugs. Drug therapy has improved a lot in recent decades, and effective drugs with limited side effects, minimal toxicity, and safety in overdose are currently available. While drug treatment often brings substantial symptomatic relief; however, drugs alone may not reverse the patient's functional disability, which usually involves avoidance of anxiety producing situations.

The availability of a wide variety of drugs to relieve anxiety is of great benefit to patients as shown by the statistic that 11% of the general population annually uses a benzodiazepine for purposes other than as a hypnotic.

Thioridazine, like all antipsychotic drugs (ie, phenothiazines/buterophenones—dopamine receptor antagonists) has marked anxiolytic properties, especially for the intense anxiety seen in the prodromal and active phases of psychosis. These drugs are generally safe in overdose. However, all dopamine receptor antagonists produce significant extrapyramidal or anticholinergic side effects. All except **clozepine** pose the long term risk of tardive dyskinesia, an irreversible and disfiguring neurologic condition. The availability of effective, safer alternatives makes the use of dopamine receptor antagonists unjustifiable, except in anxiety related to psychosis.

All classes of **antidepressants** (selective serotonin reuptake inhibitors [SSRIs], monamine oxidase inhibitors [MAOIs], cyclic antidepressants, trazodone, nefazodone, venlafaxine) relieve anxiety in depressed patients. SSRIs, cyclic antidepressants, and MAOIs also may be used in patients who are anxious but not depressed. Paradoxically, the antidepressants that most commonly given to relieve anxiety (fluoxetine, sertraline, phenelzine, desipramine) can also stimulate it. Treatment related increases in anxiety can occur early in treatment, when synaptic levels of neurotransmitters rise before compensatory changes occur in receptor sensitivities.

When side effects and therapeutic effects are balanced against each other, the best tolerated anxiolytic antidepressants appear to be the MAOIs and the SSRIs, especially for acute, intense anxiety, as seen in panic, social phobia, and posttraumatic stress disorder.

β-adrenergic receptor blockers (propranolol/atenolol and related drugs) may relieve some of the peripheral manifestations of a panic attack but do not affect the core experience of terror. Thus, β- blockers are generally not useful in panic disorder.

While it is an effective antidepressant, **clomipramine** has a very unfavorable anticholinergic/antihistaminic side effect profile. For this reason, it is used only for **obsessive compulsive disorder**. It is becoming the second choice drug, even for this condition, because the SSRIs are so much better tolerated (even if not quite as effective).

Answers and Tutorial on Items 19-21

The answers are: **19-B; 20-C; 21-D**. The patient displays all the elements of **panic disorder**. She describes intense but brief anxiety episodes with both bodily symptoms and exaggerated beliefs about the dangers of an attack. In addition, one can infer that she experiences fear of the attacks (anticipatory anxiety). She avoids situations that might be embarrassing in the face of panic, from which escape might be difficult, or help unavailable (agoraphobia).

Although patients with panic disorder or **somatization disorder** are both concerned about physical symptoms, by definition, somatization disorder includes symptoms in four different clusters: pain, gastrointestinal dysfunction, sexual dysfunction and pseudoneurological dysfunction. The occasional confusion between the two diagnoses may reflect the fact that both panic disorder and somatization disorder have shown a female predominance (2 or 3: 1 for panic disorder; 5:1 for somatization disorder) and tend to present in young adulthood. Panic disorder is more common than somatization disorder (1.5 to 3 % in the general population, rather than 0.5 %).

Paroxysmal atrial tachycardia is not necessarily accompanied by intense subjective anxiety and requires the characteristic doubling of the pulse rate and EKG evidence for diagnosis. Hypoglycemia rarely induces severe panic or anticipatory anxiety, except in the case of an insulin reaction. Patients are generally sweaty and hungry during an episode.

Specific phobias, by definition, involve reactions to discreet cues or situations, typically animals, aspects of the natural environment, blood/injection/injury, planes, elevators or enclosed places. The phobic stimulus may trigger a panic attack and avoidance, but only of the specific feared situation.

The medical evaluation of a person with panic disorder is influenced by the person's age and general health. Simple screening for physical factors that may present with symptoms of noradrenergic effects (arousal) generally focusses on conditions that have a significant likelihood of appearing in young people, especially young women. These factors include anemia, hyperthyroidism, and substance abuse (either stimulant use or alcohol/sedative withdrawal). These conditions are diagnosed by history, physical exam, bloodwork and urine toxicology. Any electrolyte deficiency, (especially hypocalcemia), may produce anxiety.

Much more extensive work-ups are only indicated if the patient has an unusual symptom or finding or does not respond to treatment. For example, if a click murmur is found, more extensive work-up for mitral valve prolapse, with echocardiogram and EKG, may be indicated. However, such studies are not routine. Indeed, the association between panic disorder and mitral valve prolapse may be not causal but coincidental. Both conditions are present in young women. In the absence of insulin use, hypoglycemia, even if present, is also often merely an incidental finding—that is, patients may show low glucose levels when they are not experiencing panic and may have normal glucose levels during a panic attack. Thus, a glucose tolerance test is not used in screening. The TRH stimulation test and dexamethasone suppression tests are of research interest in the evaluation of depression, especially with melancholic features, but are not relevant in panic disorder.

The prevailing psychotherapeutic approach to panic disorder with agoraphobia is **cognitive behavioral therapy**. Its core elements are psychoeducation, relaxation, changes in cognitive appraisal of the anxiety and the situations that provoke it, and gradual exposure to feared situations. Psychoeducation involves teaching people that anxiety, even panic, is an intrinsic physiological mechanism designed to protect the person in dangerous situations (the "fight or flight response") and not, in and of itself, dangerous. Relaxation exercises teach patients that they have the power to bring on a sense of relaxation, just as they have the power to bring on panic. Patients are encouraged to use relaxation and controlled breathing techniques as they expose themselves to the situations they fear. After prolonged exposure, with or without experiencing the anxiety, future vulnerability to panic in the same situation diminishes markedly. Changes in cognition—relinquishing the belief that panic symptoms are dangerous or will result in loss of control—follow from educational sessions, from specific techniques that challenge catastrophic beliefs, and from successful exposure. **Alprazolam** and **SSRIs**, but not buspirone or propranolol, are also common elements of the treatment of panic disorder.

Answers and Tutorial on Items 22-28

The answers are: **22-B; 23-D; 24-C; 25-A; 26-A; 27-E; 28-A.** The pattern of **subcortical clusters of cell bodies (nuclei)** that send axons to multiple areas of the neocortex and other subcortical areas is repeated many times in the organization of the central nervous system. Degeneration or other lesions of these focal brain centers provide unitary etiologies for otherwise confusing patterns of neurologic symptoms and behavior change. Loss of subcortical input causes widely dispersed brain areas to fail, producing behavioral, cognitive, emotional, and vegetative symptoms and signs. The cell bodies and axonal projections of the serotonin, norepinephrine, dopamine and acetylcholine subsystems of the brain have been mapped in recent decades. Recognition of these neurochemical subsystems has greatly furthered understanding of a variety of psychiatric illnesses, especially dementias and psychotic disorders.

A variety of peptide **neurotransmitters**, including substance P, neurotensin, cholecystokinin, somatostatin, vasopressin and oxytocin co-occur in monoamine transmitter systems. Less is currently known about the normal and pathological functioning of these substances, though they may eventually prove to equal monoamine transmitters in pathological significance.

Various psychopathological syndromes related to dysfunction of dopamine, acetylcholine and norepinephrine will be covered below, with reference to their activity in the normal brain. **Serotonergic neurons** in the midline raphe of the brainstem radiate to the cerebral cortex, hippocampus, hypothalamus, thalamus, septum, amygdala and spinal cord. Thus, 5-HT is a primary regulator of temperature, feeding, sleep, memory, aggression, and motivation. 5-HT also regulates the activity of other transmitter systems, specifically noradrenergic and dopaminergic. Secondary adrenergic effects partly account for the effect of serotonergic drugs in the treatment of depression and anxiety.

The monoamine transmitter **dopamine** (DA) affects many psychiatric disorders. The cell bodies of DA synthesizing neurons cluster in the **substantia nigra**, the ventral tegmental area (VTA), and the arcuate nucleus and periventricular area of the hypothalamus. The projections from the substantia nigra to the striatum (nigrostriatal tracts) regulate movement and, to some extent, mood. **Parkinson's disease** is characterized by loss of DA in the substantia nigra; blockade of DA receptors in the striatum accounts for the extra pyramidal (Parkinsonian) side effects of antipsychotic drugs. Dementia tends to occur late in the course of Parkinson's disease, indicating a role for dopamine in cognition as well.

Receptor (D_2) blockade in the **mesolimbic** and **mesocortical pathways** originating in the VTA contributes to the effect of antipsychotic (DA receptor blocking) drugs. This finding has, in circular fashion, contributed to the recognition that abnormalities in dopaminergic pathways are part of all psychotic illnesses, including **schizophrenia**.

Projections of the **mesolimbic pathway** to the nucleus accumbens subserve the sensation of **reward**. **Cocaine** and amphetamine exert their effects in part by increasing DA activity in this region. These drugs closely mimic the effect of spontaneously occuring mania, suggesting a possible role for DA in the pathogenesis of this condition.

The forth DA pathway, the **tuboinfundibular tract**, inhibits prolactin release from the anterior pituitary. The effect of DA blocking drugs on this pathway produces the side effect of galactorrhea.

Acetylcholine (ACh) neurons, originating in the **nucleus basalis of Meynert**, fan out through the neocortex. They radiate extensively to the hippocampus. Converging lines of research point to loss of ACh input as the primary biochemical lesion of **Alzheimer's disease** and senile dementia of the Alzheimer's type, (SDAT). Brain autopsies in SDAT have found degeneration of nucleus basalis neurons, as well as decreases in ACh and choline acetyltransferase (the enzyme that synthesizes acetylcholine). **Cholinergic drugs** (physostigmine and arecholine) improve cognitive function somewhat, while anticholinergic drugs impair it.

The characteristic lesions of SDAT (amyloid plaques), tangles, neurofibrillary degeneration, cell loss, granulovascular degeneration) seem to cluster in the cortical and hippocampal projection areas of subcortical ACh containing neurons.

Although these findings point to a central role for ACh in SDAT, other neurotransmitters, specifically norepinephrine and the peptides somatostatin and corticotropin, are also decreased. The presence of the **E4 gene** has also been found more frequently in patients with Alzheimer's disease, compared to controls.

The **dementia syndrome of depression**, formerly called "pseudodementia" because of its partial reversibility, connotes problems of concentration and memory during severe depressive episodes, especially in elderly people. Depression appears related to dysregulation of the **norepinephrine** (noradrenergic) (NE) **pathways** originating in the locus ceruleus. The dementia syndrome of depression, then, may reflect the loss of noradrenergic input to the cortex.

Answers and Tutorial on Items 29-33

The answers are: **29-H; 30-G; 31-A; 32-C; 33-D**. The **sick role** as defined by Talcott Parsons provides a useful way of understanding many of the problems that arise between physicians and patients. Rather than ascribe difficulties to faults or deficits in either person, social role theory, Item 29, would question how each individual might be deviating from the expectations of his/her role, and how the other party is attempting to re-establish role appropriate behavior.

Although it is desirable to educate patients about their conditions, this is not a necessary aspect of the sick role. Patients need only recognize they are in some way ill; the responsibility for understanding the illness belongs to the doctor role, though the doctor can (and should) share this understanding with the patient.

The sick role is necessary and useful in society, but undesirable or deviant. Patients are not fulfilling their normal obligations. They are expected to want to get well and relinquish the sick role as soon as possible. Indeed, the sick role is time-limited—patients who remain in it too long move into the more devalued, disabled role. People who are too eager to assume the sick role may be looked down upon as manipulative, malingering, or inadequate. Paradoxically, the sick role is given most readily to patients who are least eager to remain in it for any length of time.

Pseudo-parkinsonism is a term describing the extrapyramidal side effects of dopamine blocking drugs, a thoroughly real condition. Aberrant sick role behavior is a part of the other disorders on this list. **Factitious disorder** describes patients who make themselves ill in order to receive medical care, which gratifies deeply felt, though often disavowed, needs for acceptance, specialness, and legitimacy. People with **somatization disorder** express ambivalence and emotional distress though various bodily symptoms rather than language. In **conversion disorder**, patients express a more focal problem, often a response to a traumatic experience, through a single symptom or pattern of symptoms. Both somatization and conversion, by definition, cannot be confirmed as manifestations of illness by physicians, who then refuse to validate the patients in the sick role. **Malingering** describes patients who assume the sick role to avoid responsibilities or remain in it when it is no longer appropriate.

Each personality trait that people may exhibit is likely to influence the person's behavior in a given social role. **Histrionic personality style** implies that the person is flamboyant, dramatic, and often seductive or impulsive. Patients with this quality may describe their medical symptoms in dramatic terms, without being able to substantiate them on cross-questioning.

Paranoid patients mistrust physicians. They tend to scrutinize every bit of advice or information they are given, and will often be non compliant out of fear of unforeseen, negative consequences. Schizotypal patients tend to have idiosyncratic perceptions and odd reasoning that also can impair their ability to understand and follow medical advice.

Conversely, patients with deeply felt desires to be cared for by others will readily adopt the sick role when ill. The experience of receiving care may be so gratifying, however, that they have trouble appropriately relinquishing the sick role when they are better.

Narcissistic patients are, by definition, convinced of their own specialness and superior capabilities. Narcisisstic people have trouble allowing themselves to be dependent on others out of fear of appearing weak. Signs of illness threaten their sense of being above the normal constraints of life. Hoiwever, if they do acknowledge illness, they often become very demanding. They may insist that their illness is rare, severe, and special or they may become angry if treatment does not lead to perfect restoration of function.

Patients with **borderline personality traits** often manage distress by "splitting"—oscillating between one feeling and its opposite, without being aware of the incompatibility. They may express anger and resentment to one person and act helpless and deeply appreciative with another. This inconsistency has the tendency to divide treatment groups into those who respond to the borderline's angry, manipulative behavior and those who are privy to the person's underlying distress.

ANSWERS AND TUTORIAL ON ITEMS 34-35

The answers are: **34-F; 35-I**. The **Research Diagnostic Criteria (RDC)**, a detailed scheme for classifying the most serious and presumptively neurophysiologically based mental disorders for research purposes, provided a starting point for the modern DSMs. Reflecting this research heritage, disorders on the two primary axes are classified, whenever possible, in terms of symptoms that can be assessed reliably and behaviors that can be observed and quantified. However, the DSM is much broader and less rigorous than the RDC, being intended for clinical description, insurance reimbursement, many different kinds of research, and for communication between mental health disciplines or with legal authorities. Thus, the DSM strives to capture the whole range of conditions seen and treated by psychiatrists, many of which do not involve underlying brain dysfunction. It has appeared in three versions over ten years, with DSM-III published in 1980, DSM-IIIR a few years later, and **DSM-IV** in 1995.

The clinical comprehensiveness of the DSM accounts for its apparently arbitrary qualities, for example, the placing of both major psychiatric syndromes and various life problems on **Axis I**, because either may be a focus of clinical attention, grounds for research, or grounds for insurance reimbursement. Thus, Axis I provides detailed descriptive criteria for conditions ranging from severe disorders like schizophrenia, for which research is gradually elucidating genetic, physiological and psychosocial mechanisms; to life issues sanctified by custom as appropriate for psychiatric attention. The latter ("v codes") include bereavement, problems in intimate relationships, career problems, and the like.

Axis II provides a system for classifying personality, a subject that was always of greater interest to psychoanalysis than to biological psychiatry. Originally, Axis II included mental retardation because this was considered, like personality, to be an enduring quality of a person, rather than a discrete disease or disorder. In the years between DSM-III and DSM-IV, clinical use of the system blurred the definition of Axis II somewhat. It is now legitimate to use Axis II to describe habitual psychological defenses, even in the absence of a definable personality disorder.

Axis III in DSM-IV includes any medical condition, not just conditions relevant to the person's Axis I condition (the DSM-III standard).

Axis IV was originally a numerical rating of current psychosocial stressors, but this proved to be unreliable. In DSM-IV, meaningful psychosocial events are merely listed and may include remote events, eg trauma, that may be implicated in causing or exacerbating the patients' presenting problems.

Axis V has evolved from a 1-5 rating of current function to the use of the Global Assessment Scale, which combines occupational, relational and psychological functioning in numerical scores ranging from 1 to 100.

ANSWERS AND TUTORIAL ON ITEMS 36-39

The answers are: **36-A; 37-G; 38-E; 39-B**. Case I is a classic description of **mania** without clear evidence of psychosis. Thus, the patient is euphoric, pressured, and grandiose. Her disorganized appearance is consistent with her mild cognitive impairments (errors on serial sevens, slight disorientation, slightly reduced digit span) that are consistent with lack of attention/concentration or lack of motivation to respond accurately, but not of severe brain dysfunction. The difference between her judgment, as measured with a standardized question and as revealed in her history, is very typical in mania, where patients' behavior is often more disordered than their language and self presentation would lead one to expect.

Case II illustrates a **schizophreniform psychosis** in which cognitive functions are relatively intact, despite significant impairment in thought form, content, and mood.

Case III describes **depression**, in which mood is more disordered than thought.

Case IV is a realistic illustration of **Korsakoff's syndrome**, most typically a sequela of thiamine deficiency in chronic alcoholics. Although short-term memory loss is the most striking aspect of this disorder, patients typically have mild impairment in other cognitive functions (eg, disorientation in time, inability to remember a task long enough to complete it). Learned or rote material, which is tested by judgment questions, will be intact, but the ability to exercise good judgment requires being able to relate present circumstances to remembered ones. Patients who cannot remember the nature of their impairments cannot take them into account when making decisions.

Answers and Tutorial on Items 40-43

The answers are: **40-C; 41-D; 42-D; 43-B**. **Suicide**, the deliberate infliction of death on the self, was the first psychiatric problem to be studied epidemiologically and sociologically. This academic tradition has created a rich literature on variables associated with suicide attempts and completed suicide in large scale, retrospective, population based studies. These variables are called risk factors. Recognition of the presence of risk factors in individual patients is part of the evaluation of psychiatric patients. However, it should be noted that suicide is a rare event, even in very high risk populations. Counting up risk factors does not permit accurate prediction of suicide (or safety) in any particular case.

Despite the inherent unpredictability of suicide, all physicians should know that advancing age, male sex, substance abuse, depression, single status, recent losses, and poor physical health are the variables that account for the greatest percent of the variance in studies of suicide. Older, depressed, single, alcoholic men in poor health, then, should be assessed carefully, especially if they have sustained a recent loss. As a group, they tend to be non compliant and difficult to treat, so that physicians must make a conscious effort to push for active intervention when such patients describe suicidal thoughts, especially if they have made prior attempts.

In assessing the suicidal patient, mitigating factors are as important as exacerbating ones. The nature of a person's plans—choice of unavailable or nonviolent methods, the high probability of rescue, the presence of strongly held beliefs against suicide—as well as the absence of demographic risk factors, are to some degree protective. Being currently married with children lowers risk, though previously married people have higher rates than those who have never married. Regardless of protective factors, someone with suicidal plans is at greater risk that someone with passive ideation only.

Among psychiatric disorders, **depression**, which has a 15% mortality from suicide, confers the highest risk. However, suicide is a significant risk in many other disorders. Suicidal ideation is not a core criterion for schizophrenia, for example, yet the illness has a 10% mortality from suicide. Any psychotic patient should be queried about suicidal ideation and behavior, although suicide in this population tends to more impulsive (that is, less often preceded by expressed plans or intent) than it is in depression. Obsessive compulsive disorder, by itself, is not known to increase suicide risk. Patients with borderline personality disorder often make suicide attempts or are self-mutilating. Contrary to some popular myths, prior attempts are predictors of suicide, not signs that people do not intend really to kill themselves.

Suicide risk varies among physicians. In the US, male physicians do not have higher rates than males in the general population, perhaps because the rate among males in this country is so high. In Great Britain and Scandinavia, however, male physicians' risk is 2 - 3 times higher than that of the population. Women physicians in all countries are at higher risk than women in the general population, possibly because they also have a higher lifetime risk of mood disorders. While particular specialties, especially psychiatry, ophthalmology and anesthesiology, have higher suicide rates than others, the most important predictive variable among physicians remains the presence of a mood disorder or substance abuse. Other professional groups associated with increased risk include musicians, dentists, law enforcement personnel, lawyers, and insurance agents.

The finding of decreased 5-HIAA in the CSF of suicidal (and violent) patients has been repeated many times and points to a common dysregulation of serotonin activity that cuts across diagnostic categories associated with impulsivity and violence. This test is not used clinically. It is invasive, technically difficult, and the range of values overlaps between different subjects and controls, despite the significant difference in mean values.

Answers and Tutorial on Items 44-46

The answers are: **44-D; 45-E; 46-B**. Each of these cases requires clinical judgment. However, the case in Item 44 probably does not require hospitalization. Her suicide attempt was made with high probability of rescue, she was ambivalent at the time, she professes no ongoing suicidal intent, and there are people around to watch her. One of the immediate triggers of her suicidal behavior, alcohol, has presumably washed out of her system, and by history she should be able to follow instructions to avoid it. However, she has made a prior attempt, suggesting some long standing difficulties handling loss and separation. This is grounds for outpatient mental health treatment, which should be strongly urged.

The case of the widow illustrates the risk of impulsive, self destructive behavior in people with **organic brain disorders**. Depression is a common, undertreated sequela of stroke, especially strokes involving the left hemisphere. The lack of prior planning is not a protective factor in this case, since frontal lobe damage from the stroke or from multiple small infarcts related to hypertension may impair the capacity to plan. Mitigating against hospitalization, the patient seems to have no clear suicidal intent even after having hurt herself. Her method, though invasive, was of low lethality. Her antihypertensive medication is not particularly associated with depression, she avoids alcohol, and she seems likely to comply with outpatient treatment. Hospitalization would be indicated only if this patient could not be supervised at home. There is no reason to suspect that her social network would be unsupportive. Early follow up, with prescription of adequate doses of antidepressant medication, would probably be sufficient treatment. She might also be considered for partial hospitalization, again, supposing someone could be with her at night.

The man with the cocaine habit should be hospitalized. Although his drug abuse raises the possibility that he is manipulating to escape his current environment, intense depression is a physiological manifestation of cocaine abstinence. His recent high level of alcohol use, which is common in cocaine users, is enough to further depress him, and he has not had even a month of full abstinence, the time required for this effect to improve. His method is of high lethality, he faces a serious potential loss with the situation on his job, and his coping skills (increasing alcohol use) are highly dysfunctional. His social network, moreover, is thin and unreliable. The common crisis intervention technique of contracting for safety (promising to call or return if suicidality worsens) helps physicians decide in borderline cases whether to admit a patient to the hospital or not. Although refusal to make a contract may be a sign of manipulativeness, previously unknown patients should be taken at face value if they are unable to make such promises. The use of commitment or certification if the patient refuses voluntary treatment is controversial in a case where the person is cognitively intact. However, depression following cocaine withdrawal can be severe enough to impair competence and judgment by making patients hopeless about treatment. Commitment or certification, with early judicial review, would be defensible in this case.

Answers and Tutorial on Items 47-50

The answers are: **47-C; 48-D; 49-B; 50-A**. The 75-year-old widow's grief symptoms, though understandable, have persisted well beyond the usual 2 years of acute distress; she is now diagnosable as **depressed**. Interpersonal therapy for depression offers a protocol specifically for resolving depression after loss and is also compatible with antidepressant medication, which is indicated here. This patient might do as well in a support group for windows, if her depression is not so severe that it prevents her from attending. Reach for Recovery is a support program for women recovering from breast cancer surgery, not an appropriate resource in this phase of this patients's life. Her concern about cancer is a form of depressive somatic preoccupation and should not be the main focus of her current treatment.

The 35-year-old divorcé exhibits **alcohol abuse** proceeding to alcohol dependence. Individual psychotherapeutic approaches to this condition are generally ineffective. Alcoholics require at least 1 month of sobriety before they become candidates for antidepressant treatment. Many will find their depressive symptoms remit with abstinence alone. Thus, adjunctive antidepressant treatment is not indicated in this patient at the time of initial diagnosis, though it might be used later. Disulfiram, which precipitates a toxic reaction if patients drink alcohol, also cannot be used as an initial treatment, though it may help patients who achieve sobriety to maintain it. Professional assessment of the person's awareness of drinking as a problem is an important and necessary function.

Recommendations for self-help only succeed in patients who have some inkling that they need it. Efforts to educate patients about the damaging effects of alcohol in general and about the role played by alcohol in their particular case do contribute to the success of treatment.

The 25-year-old woman would likely benefit from **psychoanalytically oriented psychotherapy**. Her complaints are more about self-concept, maladaptive defenses, and patterns of relationships than symptoms. The patient is aware, but only partially, that her earlier experience plays a contributory role. The non directive stance of the psychoanalytic therapist would experientially encourage her to rely more on her own perceptions and judgment, by eliciting and relieving her discomfort in a situation where this is expected. While therapy might lead or encourage her to become more assertive, assertiveness training per se does not address the many levels of her difficulty. Simple encouragement to be more assertive might even endanger her if her partner were to react with overt abuse or battering. Family therapy with her parents would have been more appropriate before she left home—it is no longer the current behavior of the family, but her internalized reactions to past experience, that shape her problem.

Symptomatically, this patient's misleading facade, vagueness and blocking out of painful affect and memory suggest the use of dissociation as a prominent psychological defense. No available medical treatments improve dissociation per se, so none are indicated here. Dissociation in the course of partial complex seizure disorders may improve with valproic acid; methylphenidate improves focus in the context of attention deficit disorder; alprazolam can sometimes relieve the anxiety that leads to dissociative reactions, but at the cost of exposing patients to the risks of addiction. Recognizing and changing maladaptive defenses like dissociation is a core element of psychoanalytic psychotherapy, so this aspect of her case may resolve with therapy alone.

Answer and Tutorial on Item 51

The answer is: **51-B**. The most characteristic **mood congruent manic delusion** is belief that the person is special or has special powers (grandiose). Psychotic symptoms are not extremes of the continuum of normal experience in the way that pathological moods (anxiety, depression) seem exaggerations of normal experience. Psychotic symptoms include **hallucinations** (perceptions of stimuli that are not there), **delusions** (false beliefs not shared by members of a cultural group), and **thought disorder**. Although **schizophrenia** is the prototypical psychotic disorder, it is important to recognize that psychotic symptoms may occur in other psychiatric disorders, especially mania, severe depression, delirium and dementia. Although the neurological mechanisms that produce them are not well understood, psychotic symptoms indicate a degree of brain dysfunction and serious illness. Being able to recognize and correctly classify them is an important medical diagnostic skill.

Hallucinations, delusions, thought disorder and ideas of reference are typical **psychotic symptoms**. People with psychotic symptoms often lack insight into the unreality of their experience, that is, their symptoms are ego-syntonic. Ego-dystonic symptoms are those which patients recognize as irrational and abnormal, even if they cannot control them. Ego-dystonic obsessions are characteristic of obsessive-compulsive disorder; part of the anguish of patients with OCD derives from the awareness that their intrusive thoughts are senseless.

Schizoid personality disorder connotes a person who has little impulse towards involvement with others. Such people express little emotion, prefer solitary activities, are uninterested in sex, and seem cold and indifferent. The term schizoid was originally used to describe the premorbid personality of many schizophrenic patients, and these personality traits are often seen in that context. In DSM-IV, however, the criteria for schizoid personality disorder specifically exclude the psychotic manifestations of schizophrenia; people can be schizoid without inevitably developing psychosis.

Psychotic symptoms can occur as manifestations of a variety of metabolic disturbances. Physicians must avoid dismissing someone with hallucinations or delusions as "merely psychotic;" psychotic symptoms in medically ill people indicate acute brain failure and may presage death. Psychotic symptoms can be manifestations of life-threatening chemical deficits; **hypocalcemia** (also hypomagnesemia, hyponatremia) are among the most threatening. High cholesterol is usually asymptomatic, and hyperglycemia (along with other excess metabolic states like hypercalcemia or hypernatremia) more often produces depression or sedation than psychosis. Other metabolic causes of psychotic symptoms include **vitamin deficiencies** (especially B_{12} and folate), **endocrine imbalances** (especially thyroid or corticosteroids), hypoxia, **alcohol withdrawal** and various kinds of intoxication, including intoxication with prescribed drugs. In the past, CNS syphilis was a common cause of psychotic symptoms; in the age of AIDS, CNS infections are again important in the differential diagnosis of psychotic symptoms.

Delirium is a term which connotes a psychosis from serious bodily illness affecting the brain. By definition, it involves disruption of level of consciousness (indicating brain stem dysfunction). By contrast, simple problem solving ability, alertness and orientation are typically intact in schizophrenic psychoses. Being associated with severe illness, which rises with age, delirium is much more common in elderly patients; most psychiatric disorders with psychotic symptoms (except depression with psychotic features) typically arise before age forty. The exceptions to the rule that few organic causes of psychosis are relevant prior to age forty are drug intoxication/withdrawal states and the association of psychosis or delirium with HIV invasion of the central nervous system, or of CNS infections in AIDS. Delirium is typically of acute onset; schizophrenia, by definition, has a gradual onset.

The current definition of **schizophrenia** derives from the work of three European psychiatrists: Emil Kraepelin, Eugen Bleuler, and Kurt Schneider. Bleuler, who practiced in a sanitarium where he saw patients in the chronic and residual phases of illness, emphasized the social withdrawal (autism), ambivalence, and loss of emotional expressiveness (affective flattening) of chronic patients. The associational disturbances he recognized included thought disorder and the fragmentation of mental functions, from which the term schizophrenia derives. Schneider's contribution was to highlight the acute psychotic symptoms, including delusions he called ideas of reference (thought insertion, thought deletion, thought broadcasting, special personalized meanings from neutral stimuli, external control of perceptions or behavior). Kraepelin, who preceded both Bleuler and Schneider, noted the relationship between the psychotic manifestations of the illness and the long-term deterioration of personality and functioning that accompany it. The current criteria for the disease embody all three facets, namely, positive psychotic symptoms (Schneider), negative symptoms (Bleuler) and chronicity (Kraepelin).

In evaluating patients with psychotic symptoms, it is helpful to know the characteristic symptoms of different types of psychosis. **Visual hallucinations**, for example, are more common in **delirium** or **psychedelic intoxication** than in schizophrenia; **olfactory** and **gustatory hallucinations** are associated with **partial complex seizures**, and **tactile hallucinations** are seen especially in **delirium tremens**. Although auditory hallucinations are the most common type in schizophrenia, it is important to be aware that hallucinations in other sensory modalities do occur and that auditory hallucinations occur in nonschizophrenic psychotic states. The presence or absence of any one symptom or type of symptom does not determine any psychiatric diagnosis; most diagnoses depend on patterns of symptoms and a characteristic course.

Hallucinations are classified according to the sensory modality involved; **delusions** are classified by content. Although the content of a particular delusion does not, by itself, prove the presence of one diagnosis or rule out another, different psychiatric disorders do have characteristic delusions. Persecutory delusions are the most common form in both schizophrenia and in delusional disorder. When delusions occur in association with a pathologic mood state, they may be consistent with the reported or observed mood (mood congruent) or inconsistent with it (mood incongruent). Mood congruent delusions appear to be markers of the severity of the mood disturbance; mood incongruent ones are less easily explained, but are known to confer a worse prognosis.

The characteristic mood congruent delusions of depression are belief that the person is ill or deteriorating (somatic), poor (poverty), guilty of some terrible sin, or the belief that the world is coming to an end (nihilistic).

Answers and Tutorial on Items 52-56

The answers are: **52-C; 53-A; 54-J; 55-D; 56-G**. The two main diagnoses to be considered in the schizophreniform case are some form of **schizophrenia** or **schizophreniform disorder**. The patient has many schizophrenic symptoms, including disorganized behavior, decreased social and occupational functioning, auditory hallucinations and thought disorder. However, she does not meet the criterion for schizophrenia that symptoms, either psychotic, prodromal, or residual, be present for at least 6 months. This places her in the category of schizophreniform disorder.

The delusional patient fits the classic description, with nonbizarre delusions occurring in the absence of thought disorder, deterioration of social behavior, or extreme mood states. Being functionally intact and free of other psychotic symptoms distinguishes delusional disorder from schizophrenia; the absence of extreme moods rules out schizoaffective disorder.

The patient diagnosed with **schizoaffective disorder** has both manic symptoms (expansiveness, decreased need for sleep, impulsivity, especially related to spending, loss of judgment, disorganized behavior) and psychotic symptoms (auditory hallucinations). His lack of insight is characteristic of either disorder; the need to get history from a third party is typical. What distinguishes this from schizophrenia is that the patient appears to have a fully developed abnormal mood state; what distinguishes it from bipolar disorder, manic, with mood congruent psychotic features, is that the psychotic symptoms were present for a long time prior to the onset of the affective ones. The patient's relatively intact social adaptation—he is married and employed—are consistent with schizoaffective disorder and would be unusual in schizophrenia. His disorganized behavior and vegetative signs rule out delusional disorder.

The 30-year-old custodian meets the criteria for **schizophrenia, paranoid type**. He has had symptoms for more than 6 months, he has more than one psychotic symptom (hallucinations and delusions, especially bizarre delusions [impossibilities, such as implantation of electrical wires without a person's knowledge]), and he is socially impaired, isolated and holding a job below his level of education. He does not have prominent mood symptoms, ruling out schizoaffective disorder, and his use of substances is far too little to account for his symptoms, ruling out psychosis secondary to substance abuse. The paranoid subclassification refers to the nature of his delusions and to his stilted, quasimilitary social behavior. Although impaired, he is independent and able to function on a day-to-day basis—patients with paranoid type schizophrenia tend to be less impaired than those who are disorganized or catatonic. However, the different subtypes may not represent valid distinctions—the same patient may meet criteria for a different subtypes during different periods of exacerbation.

The high school student has all the features of **undifferentiated schizophrenia**, including insidious onset, prominent thought disorder, hallucinations, marked functional impairment, and peculiar affect. The premorbid social isolation is typical, and the early age of onset is a bad prognostic sign.

Answer and Tutorial on Item 57

The answer is: **57-B**. The **heterogeneity of schizophrenia** has presented a major challenge to medical research, resulting in a variety of explanatory hypotheses and controversies. Although European scientists in the late 19th and early 20th centuries postulated a cryptic organic etiology, mid-century psychiatrists developed the argument that schizophrenia arose most frequently from social or environmental causes in people with otherwise normal brains. In recent decades, converging lines of research, including genetic-epidemiologic studies, neuroimaging (**Figure 9.1**), functional neuroimaging, and pharmacologic treatment studies, have supported a return to the presumption that schizophrenia (though not necessarily a briefer psychotic condition) typically results from **organic brain dysfunction**. These studies suggest the partial localization of schizophrenic brain dysfunction to the **dopaminergic pathways** of the brain, especially those involving the prefrontal cortex. However, a variety of other neurophysiologic abnormalities may also be involved in the pathogenesis of schizophrenia; indeed, as currently defined, schizophrenia is probably not a single disease but a family of related diseases, with different underlying mechanisms. Social/environmental factors do affect the course of schizophrenia, and the possibility that social/environmental factors alone may produce some cases of the disease cannot be dismissed based on current evidence.

Schizophrenia can be realiably diagnosed cross-culturally using DSM or other standardized criteria. The general population **prevalence** of schizophrenia is approximately 1%. Patients may have neurological soft signs, indicating subtle or diffuse brain dysfunction, though these features are not always present. All of these facts support the likely link between organic dysfunction and schizophrenia. If the illness were induced by social/environmental factors, one would predict much higher rates in some cultures than in others, and the absence of the disease in cultures that lack the presumed causal factors. The presence of the same disease at roughly the same rate in different cultures thus supports causal biologic factors. Neurological soft signs include difficulty with spatial orientation, inability to simultaneously recognize multiple stimuli, poor coordination, pathological reflexes (frontal release signs), and incomplete lateralization. All are evidence of cortical or cerebellar brain dysfunction.

Studies that compare concordance for illness in mono- versus dizygotic twins are a standard methodology for demonstrating the contribution of genetic factors to a condition. In a genetic illness such as sickle cell disease, concordance will approach 100% in monozygotic twins, who share all their genes. The concordance rate in dizygotic twins will be the same as for siblings if no environmental factor related to twinship is involved in the pathogenesis of the disease. In schizophrenia, the concordance rate in monozygotic twins (around 46%) is higher than the concordance rate in dizygotic twins (14%). Statement B incorrectly overstates the concordance rates in both cases. The near 50% monozygotic twin concordance rate and the higher concordance between mono- and dizygotic twins are consistent with a **significant genetic contribution** to the illness. These findings also imply that full expression of the disease may require non genetic factors.

Family variables have been the most intensively studied non-genetic factor that might cause schizophrenia. Many families with a schizophrenic member are disrupted by irresolvable conflicts, emotional dyscontrol, detached or overclose relationships, and the like. Such difficulties may stem from both the abnormal social behavior of members with schizophrenia or those with high genetic loading for the illness, and from the difficulty normal family members have in dealing with the behavior of a psychotic person. Adoption studies have demonstrated that family environment does not, at least by itself, cause schizophrenia. Adoptions studies show both that children not biologically at risk for schizophrenia do not develop the illness when raised in dysfunctional adoptive families (including those with a schizophrenic member) while genetically at risk children develop schizophrenia even when raised in healthy families. However, family factors do play a role in the illness. Studies have repeatedly demonstrated increased rates of relapse and greater need for antipsychotic medication in patients who live in families where they are criticized and treated with hostility by an over-involved relative, usually a parent. Thus, family variables are exacerbating rather than causal factors in schizophrenia.

Answers and Tutorial on Items 58-61

The answers are: **58-E; 59-H; 60-J; 61-G**. **Depression** as a psychiatric symptom exists partly on a continuum with normal reactions to loss, disappointment, frustration, or rejection. It may differ from a normal mood only in being unduly persistent or severe, as when acute symptoms last for years following bereavement. Sometimes, depressed mood is qualitatively different from grief or sadness. People may describe themselves as empty or anguished rather than merely sad. Patients may also have psychotic symptoms—especially critical hallucinations and delusions—when they are depressed.

Because of the overlap with normal, the definition of depression as a disorder requires drawing an arbitrary line between illness and nonillness. By definition, a **major depressive episode** involves mood symptoms for at least 2 weeks, concurrent with neurovegetative changes in sleep, appetite, energy, capacity to experience pleasure, concentration, and motor behavior. In addition, depression involves characteristic beliefs or ideas, especially inappropriate guilt, thoughts of death or suicide, worthlessness, helplessness, loss of interest (apathy), and hopelessness. As defined in DSM-IV, a person needs five of the nine characteristic symptoms and one must be sadness or loss of interest or the capacity to experience pleasure (anhedonia). Disgust or revulsion, though clearly negative affects, are not among the criteria for depression.

As defined, the **syndrome of depression** is quite heterogeneous: people may sleep too little or too much, may gain or lose weight, may be retarded or agitated, have mostly ideational or mostly neurovegetative signs, and so on. Some of the different symptoms form characteristic patterns recognized as subtypes, to be covered below.

When **psychotic symptoms** occur in the context of a depressive episode, the distinction between mood congruent and mood incongruent delusions or hallucinations is a meaningful one. **Mood congruent delusions**, which include hypochondriacal beliefs, guilt, and nihilism in addition to delusions of poverty, are associated with a better prognosis than bizarre or incongruent ones. Depressed patients may also hear critical or derogatory voices.

Although mood congruent symptoms are less ominous than mood incongruent ones, any psychotic symptom in depression negatively affects outcome (and complicates treatment, see below). While the presence of psychotic symptoms does not require that a person be diagnosed with two disorders, at times that may be indicated. People with schizophrenia, for example, frequently experience depressive symptoms and sometimes have depressive episodes. In well established schizophrenia, subthreshhold levels of depressive symptoms are considered a part of the primary disorder. Depressive episodes in the course schizophrenia may prompt a diagnosis of schizoaffective disorder, which requires that the psychotic symptoms persist during some phase when the mood symptoms have abated. Younger depressed patients with psychotic symptoms may turn out to be bipolar; in older patients, the presence of psychotic symptoms should prompt evaluation for delerium or dementia. Schizophrenia, schizoaffective disorder, bipolar disorder, and delerium/dementia all confer a worse prognosis than depression alone.

The 50-year-old woman has **schizoaffective disorder**. She has a clear depressive syndrome, but by history she also has psychotic symptoms when not depressed. If she hallucinated only in close proximity to her depressive episodes, she would be classifiable as having major depressive episode with mood congruent psychotic features. Her poor social functioning is also more typical of a major psychotic disorder than of a mood disorder (though people with mood disorders often have social impairments that persist between episodes).

The 35-year-old woman has **major depression** with atypical features, specifically hypersomnia, weight gain, retardation, and preserved capacity for pleasure, despite a lack of initiative. Bipolar and Bipolar II patients often have atypical features when depressed. Atypical symptoms are also common in people who merit the qualifier "with seasonal pattern" (seasonal affective disorder, SAD in non technical terms). The patient in Item 59 is thus at greatest increased risk for a seasonal pattern or for manic episodes. It would be unusual for the two older patients to have first manic episodes so late in life (though they would be at risk if they had had previous ones).

The 50-year-old man has an **adjustment disorder** with depressed mood. There is an identifiable precipitant to his symptoms, he does not have a full blown depressive syndrome, and his symptoms have not lasted more than 6 months.

The 64-year-old woman has **major depressive episode** with melancholic features, specifically early morning awakening, anhedonia, diurnal variation with mornings worse, suicidal ideation, and guilt. Her mood differs from normal grief.

Middle-aged and older women are unduly prone to autoimmune disease, including **thyroiditis**. Hypothyroidism is high in the medical differential diagnosis of someone with either atypical or melancholic depression, especially if the person also has hypercholesterolemia. The high cholesterol does not cause the mood symptoms, but may be a marker for the thyroid dysfunction. LH/FSH are tests for documentation of menopause; they would undoubtedly be elevated in this 64-year-old patient, but of no diagnostic value. Whether recent menopause may precipitate depression in vulnerable women is a matter of some debate. The majority of perimenopausal women, however, experience only mild, transient mood symptoms; well-established menopause is not an adequate cause for a major depressive episode. Major depression with melancholia is associated with abnormal cortisol metabolism in roughly 50% of cases, but a single value would be uninterpretable—a dexamethasone suppression test would be required to uncover the abnormality.

The case of the 20-year-old man illustrates **dysthymic disorder**, a state of persistent mood symptoms more days than not, some vegetative symptoms but not a full depressive syndrome, and negative views of self and the future.

The case of the 60-year-old woman illustrates **major depression with mood congruent psychotic features** (accusatory hallucinations and delusions of poverty). The patient does not have a history of psychotic symptoms in the absence of depressed mood. Thus, she is not schizoaffective, depressed, the only other diagnosis on the list that might merit consideration.

Answer and Tutorial on Item 62

The answer is: **62-C**. Since antiquity, physicians have recognized that some patients experience both depressive episodes and episodes of excitement, increased energy, decreased need for sleep, and impulsivity. Kraepelin is credited with describing this pattern in modern terms and in noting that, in contrast to schizophrenia, patients with extreme mood swings do not typically follow a deteriorating course.

Up or **manic state**, by definition, includes both core mood symptoms—euphoria, irritability, or expansiveness—and neurovegetative changes: decreased need for sleep, increased energy, hypertalkativeness, changes in eating (weight loss or weight gain) and increased impulsivity, often leading to increased sexual activity or increased spending. Manic patients are typically distractible—intensification of concentration is, therefore, not a defining symptom.

Elevated moods are subclassified as manic, with or without psychotic features, and **hypomanic**. The presence of mood congruent psychotic features during a manic episode seems to be a marker of severity, and does not worsen the prognosis for recovery. Hypomanic states, which were only precisely defined in DSM-IV, are milder and briefer than mania. They are, by definition, non psychotic and do not impair function, although they must, again by definition, represent a clear, recognizable change from baseline.

DSM IV recognizes at least four different forms of alternating mood disorder: Bipolar or Bipolar I; Bipolar II; and cyclothymic disorder. Bipolar I differs from bipolar II in having full-blown manic, rather than hypomanic episodes. Cyclothymic disorder differs from both in that neither the depressed nor the elevated phases meet full criteria for manic or major depressive episode. The rapid cycling qualifier, connoting four or more discreet mood episodes in a year, represents another recognized subtype. Rapid cycling is more common in women than in men. It may be induced by antidepressant treatment and may be more refractory to treatment with lithium than other forms of bipolar disorder.

Genetics seem to play a greater role in bipolar than unipolar depressive disorders. Bipolar patients have increased rates of both unipolar and bipolar depression in their relatives; unipolar patients, by contrast, tend to have unipolar but not bipolar relatives. This finding partly reflects the fact that unipolar depression is 10 times more common than bipolar disorder and also more heterogeneous; any population of unipolar patients will include a much higher percentage of sporadic (nongenetic) cases, so that the number of patients with bipolar relatives will be small relative to the total. It is noteworthy that mood disorders tend to "breed true," that is, they are not associated with higher familial risk for other severe mental illnesses like schizophrenia.

Like depression, mania can be secondary to a systemic medical illness or condition. Stimulant intoxication, hyperthyroidism, and hypercortisolism are all recognized causes of manic syndromes. Almost any process affecting the CNS can cause mania, which has been reported from HIV and related infections, multiple sclerosis, uremia, and syphilis. However, depression or delerium are more common than mania as sequelae of severe medical illness.

Answers and Tutorial on Items 63-69

The answers are: **63-D; 64-B; 65-G; 66-A; 67-B; 68-D; 69-C.** Current **pharmacologic treatments for depression** include three distinct classes of antidepressant drugs and a handful of unique or novel agents. The three classes are the **cyclic antidepressants** (TCAs or CyADs), **monoamine oxidase inhibitors** (MAOIs), and **selective serotonin reuptake inhibitors** (SSRIs). CyADs are subdivided into the tertiary amine tricyclics (amitriptyline, imipramine, doxepin, chlomipramine, doxepin, trimipramine), secondary amine metabolites (nortriptyline, protriptyline, desipramine), and tetracyclics (amoxapine, maprotiline). MAOIs include phenelzine, tranylcypromine, and isocarboxazid. Fluoxetine, paroxetine, fluvoxamine, and sertraline comprise the SSRIs.

Drugs and drug classes vary mainly in pharmacokinetics, side-effects, and lethality in overdose. All increase synaptic levels of monamine neurotransmitters, by blocking reuptake (CyAD, SSRIs), inhibiting catabolism (MAOIs), or direct stimulation (trazodone, nefazodone). Flooding the synapse precipitates side effects, which may be immediate. Antidepressant effects correlate in time with the neuronal reaction to persistently increased levels of neurotransmitters, specifically down regulation of post-synaptic and feedback receptors, especially beta adrenergic receptors. β-adrenergic receptor downregulation occurs with all the currently available drugs, including the SSRIs. For this reason, although antidepressants differ meaningfully in terms of side effects and toxicity, all have roughly similar response latency (time to remission) and equal efficacy.

Information about pharmacokinetics, side effects, and toxicity can be organized according to class of drug—the novel agents must be learned separately. CyADs all have anticholinergic and antihistaminic side effects, especially sedation, orthostatic hypotension, dry mouth, constipation, urinary retention, sexual dysfunction, and weight gain. Abrupt discontinuation may produce cholinergic rebound effects—nausea, vomiting, diarrhea, and sleeplessness. Immediate increase in synaptic norepinephrine explains why these drugs (especially imipramine and desipramine) produce anxiety (which they may later relieve, due to down regulation).

Nortriptyline, desipramine, and protriptyline are all active, secondary amine metabolites of tricyclics with similar, but significantly milder, side effects. Chlomipramine is chlorinated imipramine (not a metabolite) with unique efficacy for obsessive compulsive symptoms but also very severe anticholinergic and antihistaminic side-effects. Amoxapine has

The mood stabilizers (**lithium** and the anticonvulsants carbamzepine and valproic acid) are included with this review of antidepressants because they often prevent and occasionally relieve depression in patients who are bipolar. ... n, has been used to augment the effects of ... and SSRIs, sometimes converting drug- ... to drug responders.

... some antidepressants have unique or ... interactions and toxicities as well as side ... erns of toxicity reflect syndromes related to ... ansmitters: anticholinergic delerium, the ... me, neuroleptic malignant syndrome (a ... icity relevant to antipsychotics), and the ... e acting as a false transmitter. As reviewed ... nolinergic toxicity (CyAD) includes delayed ... on, precipitation of acute glaucoma, and ... ated pupils, hot dry skin, constipation, and ... The "serotonin syndrome"—diarrhea, fe- ... onfusion, hypertension, and diaphoresis— ... en MAOIs are combined with serotonergic ... patients from SSRIs or MAOIs to the alternate ... olonged washout periods; combinations of ... ld never be given.

... tyramine, a pressor amine found in a variety ... ds including wine, most cheeses, and some ... AO is disabled, patients who ingest tyramine ... may experience severe, paroxysmal hyper- ... o stroke or death. A similar reaction may also ... nts' ingest sympathomimetic drugs, includ- ... over the counter cold preparations. (MAOIs ... ally with the narcotic meperidine by an ... nism.)

... olved in the pathophysiology of the neuro- ... syndrome (fever, delerium, rigidity, tachyp- ... CPK and WBCs) Amoxapine is the only ... ith dopamine blocking properties.

... use of antidepressants involves trying to ... ir side effects for therapeutic benefit, aware- ... and particular advantages or liabilities, and ... dling the problem of patients' non-response ... The first principle is "give enough for long ... idepressant effects are dose dependent and ... gs have significant response latency (market- ... contrary notwithstanding). While immediate improvement may occur, sustained improvement may be delayed for three to six weeks after starting treatment.

The most common prescribing error is underdosing or giving up too soon. Tricyclic effects have been correlated with blood levels, which can be measured clinically. With all other drugs, finding the appropriate or adequate dose requires trial and error. Patients' response to a three week trial of a standard "threshold" dose is determined first; nonresponsive patients then raise their dose to a maximum based on tolerance for side effects. Treatment must continue another three weeks before the physician can conclude that a given drug is ineffective.

Various patterns of symptoms appear somewhat more responsive to certain antidepressants than others. Patterns of side-effects help predict which drug may work best—patients with disrupted sleep do better with sedating drugs, patients who have lost weight will have greater tolerance for drugs that produce weight gain, and so on. More systematic studies have shown that patients with atypical features (hypersomnia, retardation, weight gain) respond better to MAOIs and possibly SSRIs than to tricyclics; melancholic features respond preferentially to tricyclics and possibly venlafaxine.

Because the guidelines for choosing antidepressants are so empirical, the best predictor of patients' response is their own past personal history with various classes of drugs. In a first episode, the history of family members' medication responses or nonresponses may help. The existence of concurrent medical problems also affects the choice of antidepressant—elderly patients, in particular, may have low tolerance for drugs with anticholinergic side effects and also for drugs commonly involved in drug-drug interactions.

When patients do not respond to a sustained trial of an antidepressant at an adequate dose, it is an error to conclude they are completely drug refractory and should be treated with psychotherapy alone. Augmentation of the primary drug with Lithium or L-triiodothyronine (T_3) may convert a nonresponder into a responder. Changing from one class of antidepressant to another may also be effective (changes from an MAOI to a TCA or SSRI require a 2-week washout to avoid severe toxic interactions). Finally, electroconvulsive therapy remains the most effective treatment for depression and may induce remission in patients who have failed to respond to trials of various drugs and combinations.

Answers and Tutorial on Items 70-73

The answers are: **70-D; 71-C; 72-A; 73-C**. An orderly progression of patterned brain activity occurs in cycles throughout **normal sleep** in human beings. This progression, called sleep architecture, goes from wakefulness (Stage 0) to drowsiness (Stage 1), sleep onset (Stage 2-appearance of sleep spindles and K complexes on EEG), deep or delta sleep (Stages 3 and 4—high voltage delta waves on EEG) and **rapid eye movement sleep** (REM). Brain activity during REM sleep closely resembles wakefulness (random fast activity or 8-12 cps, low voltage alpha waves with intermixed beta 13-35 cps waves) with eyes closed, with two differences: rapid conjugate eye movements and total muscular paralysis.

In **Figure 9.2**, **C**, which shows the eye movements on lines one and two and the lack of muscle movement on line 3, is a depiction of REM sleep. (A is stage 1, B is stage 2, C is stage 4).

Tracing **D** in **Figure 9.3** illustrates sleep spindles and K complexes, characteristic of stage 2.

Normal sleep architecture involves progression from stage 2-4 and back again, with periods of REM following stage 2 and occuring in place of stage 1 or 0. That is, people go into periods of deep (stage 3-4) sleep, approach wakefulness, enter REM, and then return to deep sleep. The REM periods lengthen in the latter third of the night and stage 3 and 4 gradually diminish. Both REM and deep sleep periods occupy 25% of total sleep time. The first sleep cycle of the night typically lasts 90 minutes and includes the longest period of deep or delta sleep. Neither REM nor brief awakening time typically occur during this phase of sleep.

The physiology of sleep is still obscure, but serotonin appears to regulate nREM sleep and norepinephrine seems the primary regulator of REM sleep. Acetylcholine is involved in maintaining the normal progression of sleep stages. These findings come from selective ablation studies, in which destruction or inhibition of serotonin containing raphe nuclei leads to total insomnia, destruction or inhibition of noradrenergic locus ceruleus neurons abolishes REM sleep, and loss of cholinergic function in dementia correlates with fragmentation of sleep. Dopamine is not implicated in the regulation of sleep in current physiologic models.

It is useful to contrast REM and deep sleep, the poles of the normal sleep cycle. Each occupies 25% of total sleep time. Deep sleep predominates in the first third of the night and may not occur at all in the last third. REM begins after the first 90 minutes of sleep and increases to its highest percentage as stage 3-4 disappears. People awakened during REM sleep typically report dreams; those awakened from stage three or four report no ideation. The arousal threshold rises from stage 1 to stage 4—patients in deep sleep are the most difficult to awaken. The arousal threshold during REM varies; patients in REM sleep are close to awakening by all physiological parameters except muscle tone. Deep sleep and REM both decrease in old age, though REM never disappears entirely. The absence of deep sleep in old age correlates with the complaints non-restful sleep and daytime drowsiness in elderly people.

Answers and Tutorial on Items 74-77

The answers are: **74-D; 75-D; 76-C; 77-B**. **Insomnia** is a common complaint, experienced by roughly 35% of people at some time in the past year in general population surveys. Half this number, 17%, have clinically significant sleep problems. Like most health problems, insomnia correlates with lower rather than higher socioeconomic status

While common, sleep problems are far from trivial. Insufficient sleep is a risk factor for traffic accidents and heart disease. It also diminishes cognitive efficiency, leading to decreased efficiency and productivity in the workplace.

After insufficient sleep, the body will try to make up for both missed sleep and REM sleep at the expense of the lighter stages of sleep. This phenomenon, called rebounding, suggests that both these stages have important physiological functions. REM rebound is often associated with intensification of dreaming or nightmares when people recoup sleep after a period of insomnia.

DSM-IV recognizes two categories of sleep disorders, the dyssomnias and the parasomnias. It also includes categories of sleep disorder due to other psychiatric conditions (eg, depression, psychosis, alcohol abuse or dependence) and sleep disorder from medical conditions other than alcohol. Dyssomnias are, by definition, disorders of initiating or maintaining sleep; parasomnias are abnormal sleep-related events (covered below). As an abnormal event occuring during sleep, somnambulism is a parasomnia.

The treatment of mild sleep disorders centers on adherence to a behavioral protocol that encourages sleep, called **sleep hygiene**. Good sleep hygiene includes eliminating barriers to restful sleep, including caffeine, tobacco and alcohol, over or undereating in the evening, exercising too late in the day, noise and extremes of temperature. All these measures reflect common sense. Behavioral research has contributed three other points of sleep hygiene: the importance of avoiding daytime naps, the helpfulness of a fixed rising time every morning (regardless of when the person goes to sleep), and advice not to stay in bed awake or involved in any non-sleep activity for any length of time.

The fixed rising time relates to the ease with which some people's sleep cycle creeps forward, because humans' biological clocks naturally run longer than 24 hours. Environmental regulators or *zeitgebers*, especially light, help keep circadian rhythms in sync with the normal day/night cycle. Fixed rising functions as a zeitgeber to prevent phase advance.

The avoidance of nonsleep activity exemplifies applied conditioning—people who read, work, watch TV, or merely fret about not sleeping while lying in bed condition themselves to wakefulness there. Using the bed for sleep and only sleep, by contrast, conditions the person to drowsiness in the appropriate place.

Narcolepsy is a dyssomnia in which a person experiences irresistible sleep attacks at inappropriate times. These may be harmless, as when a person falls asleep during a monotonous sedentary activity, or harmful. Narcoleptics may fall asleep in the middle of conversations or, most alarming, while behind the wheel. Decreased REM latency characterizes the sleep EEG in narcolepsy. Patients immediately enter REM sleep, without the normal 90 minutes between falling asleep and the first REM period. Genetics accounts for a remarkably high percentage of this disorder; 100% of narcoleptics have the HLA-DR2 histocompatibility antigen, compared with 20-35% of the general population. The proportion of afflicted first degree relatives in patients with narcolepsy is up to 50% in some studies.

In addition to the characteristic sleep attacks, narcoleptic patients have associated symptoms of cataplexy (sudden paralysis of motor activity while awake), hypnagogic hallucinations, and sleep paralysis (inability to move while falling asleep). All presumably represent the inappropriate occurrence of parts of REM sleep. Of the associated findings, cataplexy is the most common, occuring in up to 80% of cases.

Of all the sleep disorders, **sleep apnea** probably has the greatest medical significance. Sleep apnea connotes the presence of five or more periods per hour or 30 or more periods a night of cessation of respiration for 10 seconds or longer. In central sleep apnea, the person makes no respiratory effort during these times; in obstructive sleep apnea, abdominal and thoracic muscle activity increases, but the person cannot move air past nasal-pharyngeal obstruction. Pure central sleep apnea accounts for only 10% of cases; most sleep apnea is either obstructive or mixed. Each period of apnea terminates with momentary arousal, so that total sleep and sleep quality (decreased amounts of stage 3 and 4) both diminish.

During apnea, hypoxia, hypercarbia, and acidosis occur, predisposing the person to cardiac arrhythymias. Transient pulmonary and systemic hypertension (but not orthostatic hypotension) also occur and may become persistent in longstanding, severe cases. Behaviorally and symptomatically, apneic episodes are associated with snoring and snorting, sweating, sleepwalking, sleep talking, and gastroesophageal reflux. Patients may awaken with headaches, possibly related to the dilation of cerebral blood vessels during the night. Obesity, once thought to cause sleep apnea, may in fact be a sequela, due to decreased metabolism from recurrent hypoxia. Sexual dysfunction is another associated finding. Hypothyroidism, sinus or nasal obstruction, and acromegaly all predispose to sleep apnea. Untreated sleep apnea increases mortality.

Deficient total sleep and poor sleep quality in patients with sleep apnea lead to daytime sleepiness, often severe enough to impair work performance and safety behind the wheel. Personality changes (irritability and anxiety) also occur, along with mood disorders and significant psychosocial distress, especially marital and occupational problems. Compensatory abuse of alcohol (for anxiety) or stimulants (for sleepiness) can become problems in and of themselves.

Sleep apnea is more common in males than females (10:1), though the incidence in females rises after menopause. Incidence rises in both sexes with age; from 30-67% of elderly males are affected, leading to speculation that apnea contributes significantly to pulmonary and cardiovascular deaths in this group, especially during sleep.

The medical school student described above suffers from **delayed sleep phase disorder**. (Patients who fall asleep too early and waken too early have advanced sleep phase disorder.) Delayed sleep disorder may reflect the natural tendency of the human circadian cycle to run longer than 24 hours, effectively pushing the hour of sleep later and later in the absence of a daily structure that forces the person to awaken early. College and professional students are particularly prone to this pattern.

Nocturnal myoclonus (periodic limb movement disorder) and **restless legs syndrome** are two dyssomnias that may be easily confused with one another. Myoclonus refers to twitching or kicking of the lower extremities during sleep, leading to momentary arousals which patients typically do not recall. They do not experience any unusual sensations while awake; the diagnosis is typically made upon the history of a bed partner or by polysomnography. Restless legs (Ekbom's disease) is a sensory disorder; patients experience a creeping feeling and will move, stretch, or pace to relieve the symptom. This leads to difficulty falling asleep.

Both conditions are mainly idiopathic. Myoclonus may be associated with hepatic or renal failure, narcolepsy, and sleep apnea. Restless legs has been found in association with vitamin B_{12} or iron deficiency, pregnancy, temperature extremes, leukemia, rheumatoid arthritis and fibromyalgia. Sedative, alcohol, or other drug withdrawal, renal failure, and tricyclic antidepressants may contribute to either disorder. Restless legs may also occur in patients taking dopamine blocking drugs (antipsychotics). In this context it may represent the extrapyramidal side effect of akathesia. Either condition may interfere with the quality of sleep and with daytime functioning, though restless legs seems to have a greater association with mood disorders and psychosocial impairment.

Answers and Tutorial on Items 78-80

The answers are: **78-F; 79-H; 80-J**. The overweight 64-year-old man is a classic description of **sleep apnea**, which may sometimes be effectively treated with continuous positive airway pressure. Definitive treatment of obstructive sleep apnea may involve surgery to correct whatever nasopharyngeal problem produces the obstruction. Central sleep apnea, which is rarer and can be reliably differentiated from obstructive sleep apnea only by polysomnography, is harder to treat. Though it may respond to CPAP, this treatment can also make it worse. Various drug treatments have been tried; the treatment of last resort is either diaphragmatic pacing or mechanical ventilation. Patients should avoid all sedative hypnotics. Concurrent depression may require antidepressant treatment with less sedating (mainly nontricyclic agents) and concurrent anxiety will sometimes improve with buspirone.

The 24-year-old grad student has **narcolepsy**, manifested by sleep attacks from which she awakens refreshed, cataplexy and hypnagogic hallucinations. Efforts to ensure adequate nighttime sleep and prescribed naps may help, but stimulants like methylphenidate are specific remedies and the treatment of choice. Cataplexy responds to REM-suppressing agents like tricyclic antidepressants. Education and supportive psychotherapy may also be needed.

Restless leg syndrome is complicated by the inappropriate use of alcohol. Alcohol is a poor sedative because its short half life ensures patients will enter into withdrawal in the middle of the night; if they awaken, return to sleep may be quite difficult. Treatments for restless legs (and for nocturnal myoclonus) include the long acting benzodiazepine clonazepam or the short-acting triazolam (with drug holidays to minimize dependence), carbidopa, baclofen and, most recently, gabapentin. When an antidepressant is also indicated, nontricyclic agents are preferred.

Advanced sleep phase disorder is more common in elderly people. Use of extremely bright light in the early evening may be effective in pushing back the onset of sleep to a more socially appropriate hour.

Patients diagnosed with **delayed sleep phase disorder** may, when mild, respond to the advice to get out of bed at the same time each morning regardless of how long the patient has been asleep. Efforts to move the onset of sleep backwards in graduated steps always fail. Sleep phase advance, delaying the onset of sleep by 2 hours each day until reaching a normal bedtime, does work. This treatment requires strong motivation, because it forces the patient to miss 4 - 5 waking days and to stay up for several nights, disrupting social and occupational life to a severe degree. Once patients achieve a normal bedtime, they need to be very conscientious about sticking to it and to a fixed awakening time, or else their sleep will again naturally advance to its previous rhythm.

When a period of insomnia related to a particular stress leads to conditioned anxiety about not being able to sleep and anxiety about continued insomnia is classic psychophysiologic insomnia. Improved sleep hygiene, coupled with relaxation exercises (sometimes coupled with cognitive therapy to work on the patient's negative expectations about sleep), is often effective. Because the condition is chronic, the use of sedatives is likely to be ineffective due to the development of tolerance and/or dependence.

Answer and Tutorial on Item 81

The answer is: **81-B**. The **syndrome of delirium** occurs when global brain function is impaired from any cause. In all but rare instances, the impairment is acute and potentially reversible. The condition is often a medical emergency—acute brain failure is as ominous as acute heart failure and requires similarly aggressive treatment.

The cardinal features of delirium are acute or subacute onset, fluctuations between alertness and drowsiness, disorientation, perceptual distortions and hallucinations, decreased attention/concentration, and incoherence. Motor restlessness and sleep wake cycle changes are also common, with patients sleeping in the daytime and up all night, or napping and waking throughout the 24 hours. Agitation or paranoia are also common. Euphoria or any extreme mood may occur during a delirium, though anxiety or is more typical. In any case, prolonged mood elevation is not common. Mood, like other symptoms, fluctuates, so that delirious patients move from one mood state to another, just as their consciousness shifts from alertness to sleep.

The 40-50% 1-year mortality associated with delirium, the link to hospitalization for severe illness (ICU), and the preponderance of elderly patients all underline the severity of this condition. Because the symptoms of delirium are psychiatric, and the condition is associated with stigmatized patients (elderly, mildly demented patients and alcoholics), medical personnel often fail to make the diagnosis. Delirium is an urgent medical situation that requires urgent attention.

When delirium is suspected, the evaluation begins with a physical exam, including vital signs and fundoscopy. Elevated pulse, blood pressure and temperature are all common (especially in delirium secondary to infection or to sedative withdrawal). Frontal release signs, which may normalize with effective treatment, are common. Papilledema is rare, but when found indicates increased intracranial pressure as the cause of the abnormal mental status.

An EEG shows diffuse slowing in delirium from any cause. A more specific pattern (K complexes) occurs in delirium due to hepatic encephalopathy. All the other tests on the list are sometimes part of an evaluation for delirium, but relate to specific causes. The CT scan is probably the least useful, since delirium reflects metabolic more than structural pathology. An EKG will help diagnose delirium from severe arrhythymia leading to poor perfusion. Serum glucose is part of general metabolic screening, covered below, and an LP is needed in any patient with AIDS or a possible CNS infection. It is not a routine part of the workup in the absence of other factors suggesting infection.

Focal CNS lesions, usually infarcts or tumors, do not typically present with delirium, which represents pervasive brain dysfunction. All the other conditions on the list—sepsis, cation deficiency, drug related states and hypoxia—are high on the list of differential diagnosis of the causes of delirium.

Although reversing the underlying cause is the cornerstone of any treatment for delirium, mental status may not normalize immediately. Patients need to be managed carefully until they recover, to prevent self-injury. Manipulation of the environment by using light to encourage normal sleep wake cycles and reducing meaningless background ("white") noise may help the patient be less confused. High potency antipsychotic drugs are best for reducing agitation and sedating patients, except those withdrawing from alcohol or sedatives. These patients need benzodiazepines or other cross tolerant drugs to prevent DTs. Finally, reassuring contact with familiar people can be of great help, particularly if the person knows to keep communication simple and concrete and is willing to repeat things over and over to help the delirious person stay oriented.

Notes